# danielle walker's
# AGAINST all GRAIN

*for my precious Aila*

First Published in 2014 by Victory Belt Publishing Inc.

ISBN 13: 978-1-628600-42-1

Printed in the USA

RRD 0214


Lifestyle and cover photo team:

Photography—Jennifer Skog

Hair & Makeup—Lindsay Skog

Set Styling—PJ Rude of Milkglass Vintage Rentals

Accessories—Joy Dravecky Jewelry

# danielle walker's
# AGAINST all GRAIN

## meals made simple

gluten-free, dairy-free, and paleo recipes to make anytime

*written and photographed by*

# Danielle Walker

www.againstallgrain.com

*cover photography by* Jennifer Skog

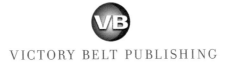

VICTORY BELT PUBLISHING

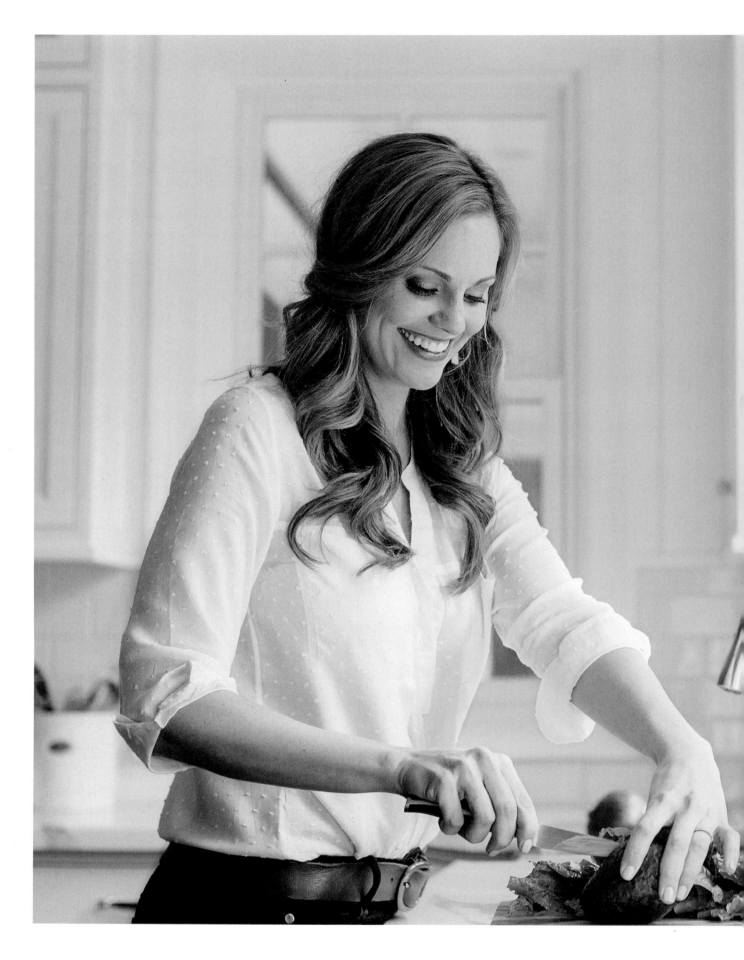

# contents

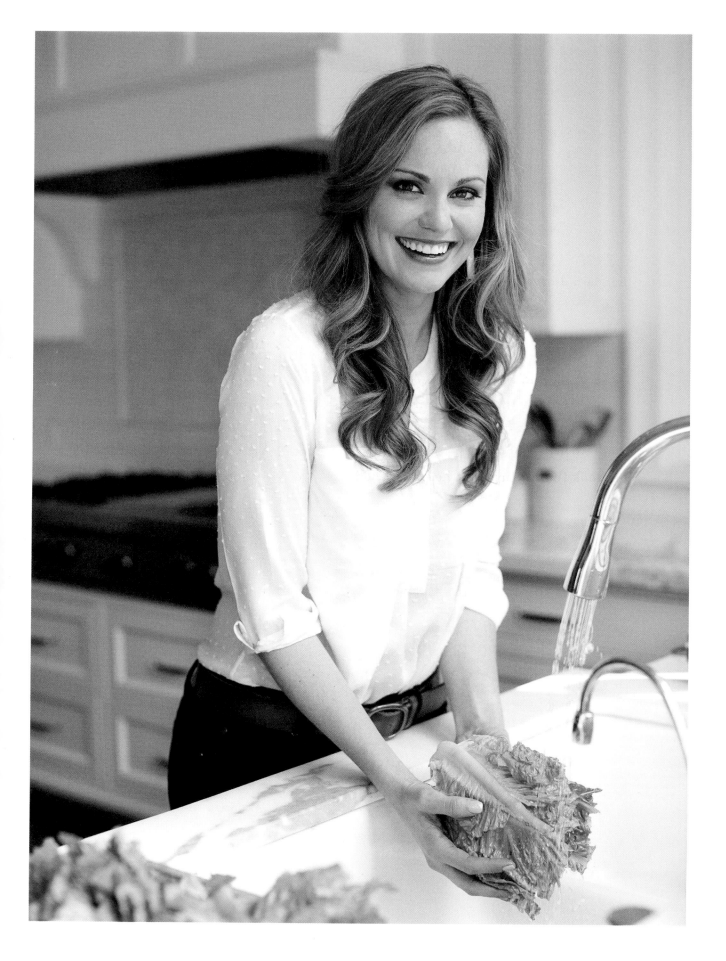

# *introduction*

In 2007, at the young age of twenty-two, and newly married, I was given
the grim diagnosis of an incurable autoimmune disease. The prospect of
living the rest of my life, through careers, motherhood, and grandchildren,
with an irreversible illness was an extremely disheartening prognosis and
left me feeling hopeless and alone. I had always dreamt of being a wife
and a mom, and those dreams seemed to be crashing down around me. I
remember lying in the hospital bed searching for answers from my doctor,
and the only question that I could mutter out amongst tears was, "Will I be
able to have children?" He assured me that I could live a normal life if I
just took the medications he prescribed.

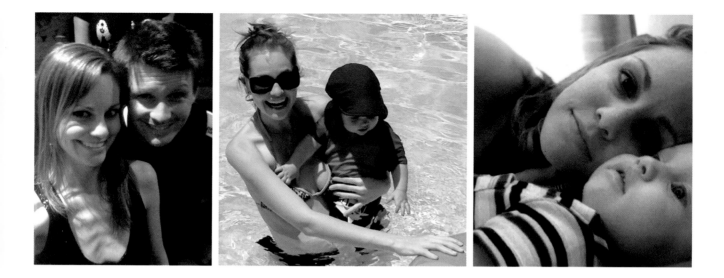

As we are taught to do by our mothers, I listened to my doctor and took the prescriptions. I was ushered out of the hospital with very little information as to what the disease was, how it was caused, the symptoms, or the forms of relief. I was not aware of the inexplicable episodes that were to come, which I now know as flare-ups. I also was not aware of the drastic side effects that the medications would begin to cause, or that the so-called normal life I was promised would be everything but.

For years, I suffered from the standard symptoms that accompany ulcerative colitis, as well as malabsorption, drastic weight loss, joint pain, and malnutrition. After countless doctor visits and trips to the emergency room and an expansive array of medications and high-dose prednisone steroids, I found myself hospitalized numerous times each year, admitted repeatedly for multiple blood transfusions due to morbidly low hemoglobin levels.

Left with a choice between major surgery and lifelong frequent IV treatments with harsh side effects, I began my own research to explore other options. After reading through community support boards and meeting a friend who had tried the Specific Carbohydrate Diet (SCD), I reluctantly gave it a try, eating only grain-free, sugar-free, starch-free, lactose-free, and unprocessed foods. Although no doctor would suggest, or even support, dietary change as a part of my treatment, I realized that I had take things into my own hands to achieve real results.

I noticed significant improvement within a matter of months, but committing to a new, drastically different diet was not easy, and I frequently fell off the regimen. I was able to conceive after quite some time of trying and, after experiencing a heartbreaking and rare loss with a first pregnancy, my son, Asher, was born in October 2010. When he was just nine months old, I had an extreme setback that caused me to be hospitalized for fourteen days, required multiple blood transfusions, and debilitated me for nearly four months. It was the darkest point of my life thus far and still conjures a flood of emotion when I recall it.

My son was not allowed to visit me in the hospital, and there were many times when I was at home in bed that I had to turn him away because I was too sick or exhausted to entertain him. My family and friends rallied during that time and became his surrogate mother, which was both comforting and tragic for me. Looking back on it now, I push away the feelings of guilt, knowing that he was young enough that he will never remember those months and will only remember me as his healthy mom who was present during his upbringing and attended each and every baseball game. He will never remember me uttering the words "Mommy is sick" or "Mommy cannot come downstairs today."

We all have a revelatory moment in our lives right before committing to an extreme lifestyle alteration. That was my moment, the point in my life when I realized that being incapacitated for months at a time was not an option now that I had a helpless life relying on me to care for him. It was no longer just my life, or even my ever-supportive husband Ryan's life, that was in jeopardy. There was a tiny human being who needed his mother, and during that final hospital stay I made the commitment to always be there for him.

As soon as I was released and gained enough strength to venture out, I began eliminating even more food groups, including all dairy and legumes, following a plan that closely mimicked the Paleo diet. After seeing dramatic progress after just forty-eight hours, I committed to the diet wholeheartedly and dedicated my free time to creating delicious comfort foods that could be enjoyed on a restricted diet. I started to become aware of the many different diseases and ailments that this style of diet can alleviate and decided to share my story and recipes on my blog, *Against All Grain*, in an attempt to ensure that no one else would have to feel as alone or lost as I did.

I began to gain a following of people suffering from a vast array of autoimmune diseases, autism spectrum disorders, diabetes, and so much more. Emails flooded in from people searching for hope and quality recipes that could make this diet sustainable long-term, which further fueled my desire to be a spokesperson for the movement. I never would have imagined, while lying in countless hospital beds, that everything I went through could be used to help bring hope to hundreds of thousands of people. As unbearable as it was, Ryan and I both agree now that we would not change any of it for the world. To be useful in such an impactful way, and out of such misfortune, is one of the most rewarding experiences I will ever have.

For an in-depth account of my health journey and the different stages I went through to find Paleo, see my first book, *Against All Grain*, and www.againstallgrain.com/my-journey

danielle walker | 9

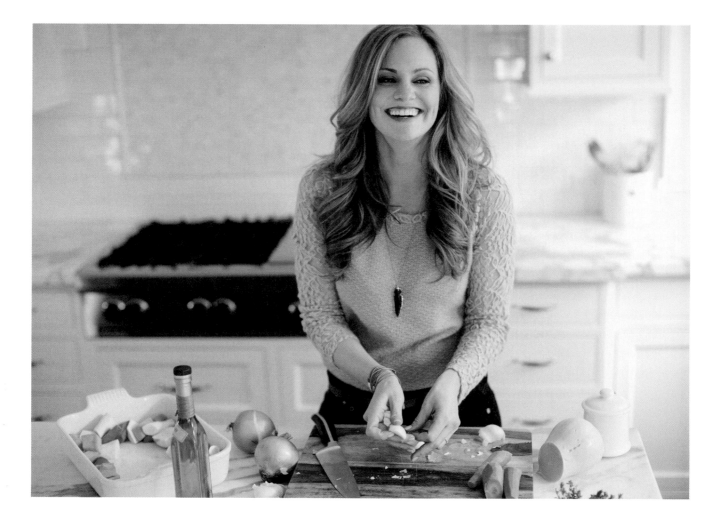

THE NUMBER-ONE CONCERN I HEAR from people attempting to transition to a Paleo lifestyle is about the amount of time and preparation involved. Undeniably, a real-foods, grain-free diet takes more of an effort and is not as convenient as purchasing ready-made food items, canned goods, or frozen meals at the grocery store.

This book was born out of a desire to alleviate those concerns and the pressure that so many families feel when they are cooking for a new diet. Learning which foods are acceptable and unacceptable is enough to consume someone completely in the beginning. Locating those foods, planning meals, cooking, and cleaning up is enough to send you running in the opposite direction. This is especially true if you are ill or are caring for someone who is, which is often why people find themselves turning to a grain-free or Paleo diet.

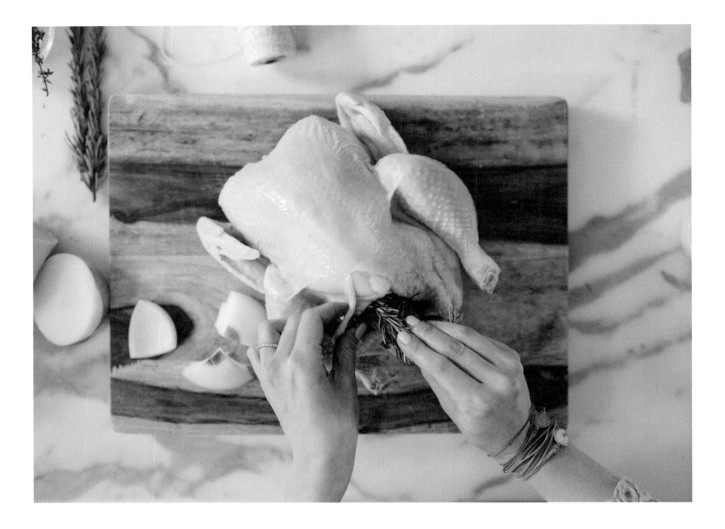

In 2013, I had the immense blessing of staying with a family close to us who was suffering greatly from autoimmune diseases. Both parents have been struggling with severe autoimmune diseases for many, many years and were so overwhelmed with their health struggles that cooking for a Paleo diet seemed out of their grasp. Their courageous and incredible nineteen-year-old daughter shouldered a lot of the burden of grocery shopping and preparing meals for the family and, quite honestly, did not know where to start. While she was a great cook and had helped care for her family for a long time, cooking from scratch and planning meals for the week was overwhelming.

The time I spent with them made me realize just how many people are in the same position. Whether there's an illness involved or not, people are busy. There are long workdays, school, after-school activities, and a plethora of other things that keep us busy day to day, leaving little time to think about meals. No matter how much time we dedicate to cooking during the week, dinner still seems to creep up on us without warning, and we're left frantically trying to throw something together. Well, except for the handful of people who are incredibly organized!

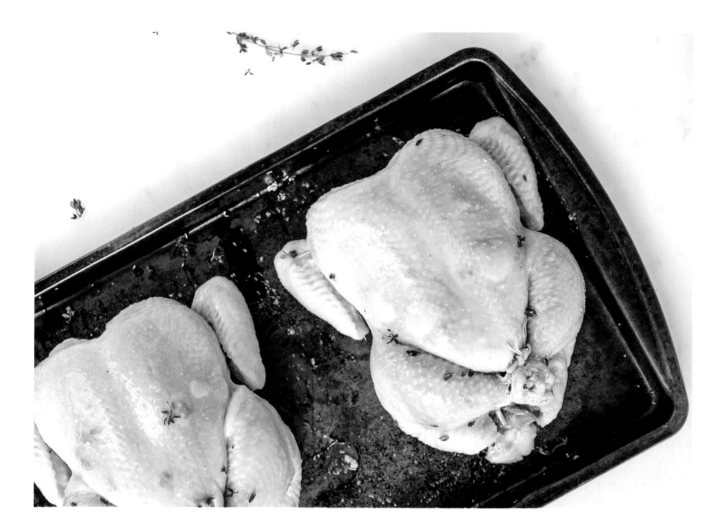

In a few days' time, my goal was not only to cook for them and stock their freezer, but also to break meal planning down to a level that felt accessible and less daunting. In those few days, I taught them how to utilize all the parts of a chicken and make several meals from one: We roasted two birds, served one for dinner, saved the other for quick lunches throughout the week, and used the bones to make a nutrient-rich and healing stock in the slow cooker (see page 242). Making homemade stock seemed intimidating to them at first, but they soon learned that it is as easy as throwing everything together and turning on the power.

We prepared a handful of slow cooker meals and put them in the freezer raw so that they could be pulled out when needed and thrown into the pot to cook throughout the day—providing a meal that is healthy and ready to eat when everyone returns home from their busy days. We doubled recipes and froze portions so that there would be leftovers to pull out at the last second when dinner is an afterthought, which it so often is for many of us.

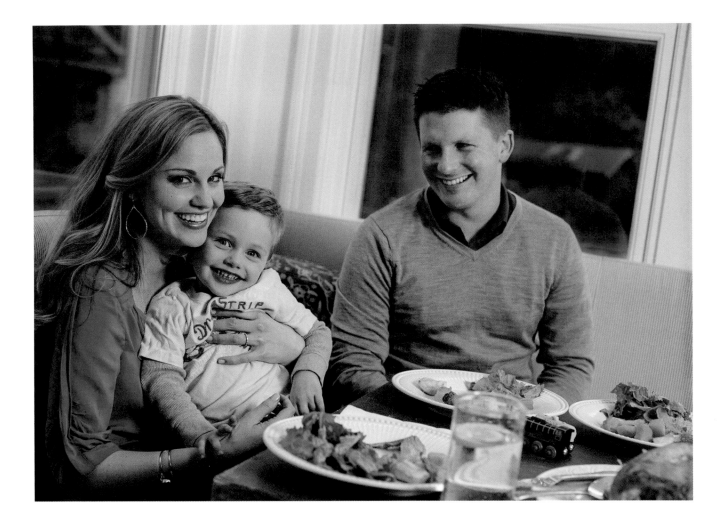

This way of cooking takes a bit of extra prep work but is, in the end, a lifesaver, and is just the thing that makes eating a healthy, grain-free diet sustainable. We are most susceptible to falling into old habits when cooking and eating in a new way feels uncomfortable, hopeless, or too difficult. I am also a strong proponent of keeping meals fresh and exciting. As an avid food lover, one of my biggest concerns prior to making the shift to Paleo was that I was embarking on a lifetime of grilled chicken and steamed broccoli, eliminating all the textures and flavors of foods that I loved.

I committed to changing my way of eating over a dozen times before it finally stuck. I often tell people during speaking engagements and book signings that if I have one regret, it is not diving in headfirst and staying committed. I waxed and waned for so long that I ended up causing more harm and spending more time being ill than was necessary, but we all learn and succeed at our own pace, and that was my journey. With this book, I hope to prevent that slippage for as many people as I possibly can.

*Danielle*

*danielle walker* | 13

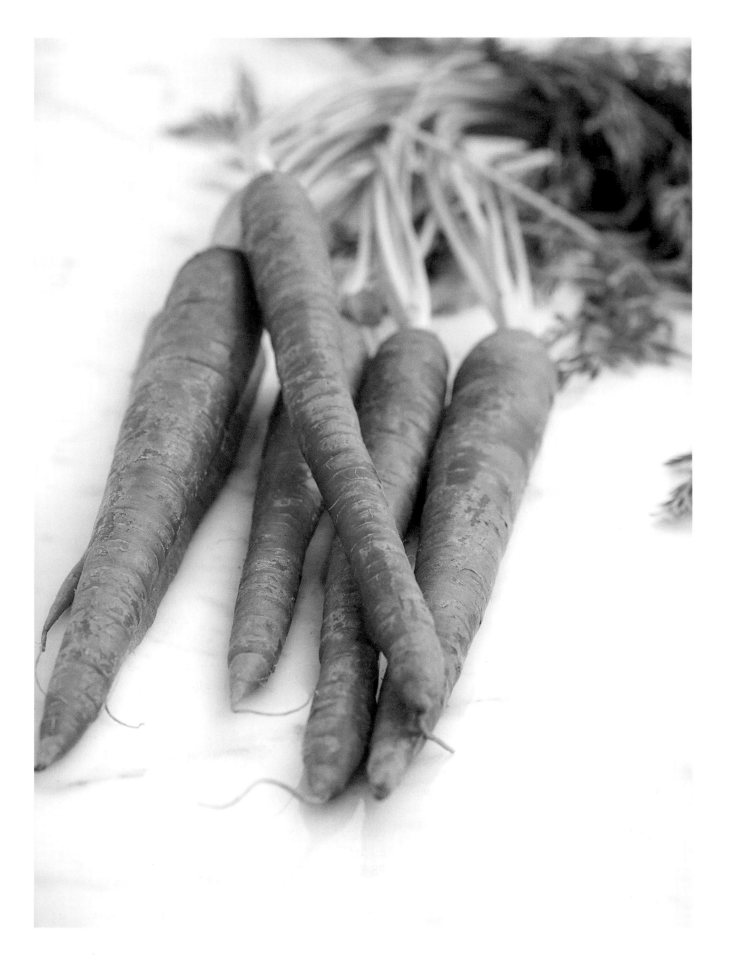

# how to use this book

In *Meals Made Simple,* I've set out to create meals that are full of flavor and texture but are simple enough to be practical for most families. Aside from actually cooking the meals, most people find that planning and preparation are what give them the most grief: figuring out grocery lists, planning for the week, and shopping for and preparing all the ingredients in a fashion that creates the least waste. This book takes the guesswork out of the process and alleviates stress and unease at the same time.

To that end, you will find a plan for eight weeks of dinners that will keep mealtime fresh and exciting and leave you feeling accomplished and satisfied rather than anxious (see page 44). The accompanying grocery shopping lists, broken down by week, will ensure that you are fully prepared at the beginning of each week and that you utilize the food you buy throughout that week. If Monday night's dinner calls for parsley or half a can of coconut milk, you will use that ingredient again in Wednesday night's dinner so that there is less waste and more money is saved. A handful of recipes in the book make large enough portions that you can set aside half and use it in a completely different meal during the week, saving you preparation time and keeping variety in your meals. Storage tips and time-saving make-ahead tips are included with each recipe to make everything as seamless as possible.

The following simple icons, found at the tops of the recipes, will help you navigate the recipe pages. At a glance, you will know whether a recipe fits within your dietary restrictions, or if it is an easy slow cooker meal or can be on the table in less than thirty minutes. (Complete lists of the recipes in these categories can be found at the back of the book beginning on page 296 for easier browsing.)

 These recipes are free of eggs.

 These recipes are free of tree nuts.

 These recipes are free of nightshades, which are often problematic for autoimmune and other inflammatory disorders. Nightshades include tomatoes, tomatillos, eggplant, white potatoes, and sweet and hot peppers.

SCD  These recipes contain only ingredients that are allowed on the Specific Carbohydrate Diet. Very often they are acceptable for the GAPS diet as well, since many of the rules overlap.

 These recipes are made in only one pot.

 These recipes are made in a slow cooker.

30 minutes or less  These recipes take a total of thirty minutes or less to prepare.

*danielle walker*  15

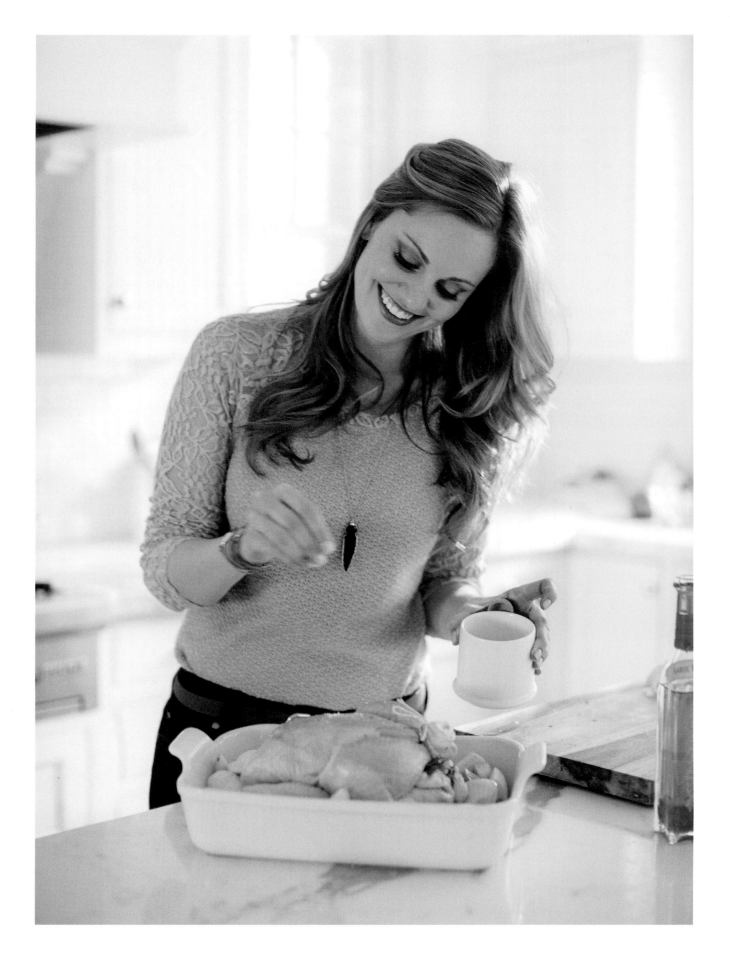

# my ingredients

A grain-free or Paleo pantry can look very foreign to someone who is new to the lifestyle, but once you stock your pantry with these staples, you will feel much more comfortable venturing into new recipes. Everything on this list can be found in health food stores, on Amazon, or through my website (againstallgrain.com/shop). For a list of my recommended products and brands, see the Shopping Resources on page 290.

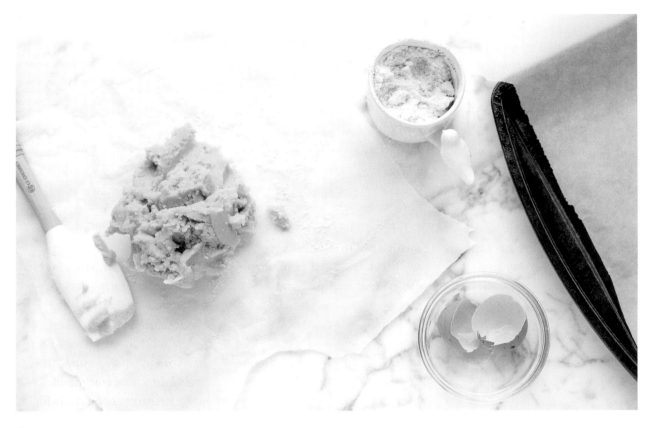

## flours

ALMOND FLOUR is high in protein, antioxidants, and heart-healthy fats and is a great substitute for gluten and grain flours. The best almond flour is made from blanched, skinless almonds that are finely ground into flour. The finer the grind, the better your baked goods will turn out. Coarsely ground brands such as Bob's Red Mill will result in overly moist products that sink in the center or have a grainy texture. I recommend purchasing your flour online from WellBee or Honeyville Farms.

CASHEW MEAL is similar to almond flour but is made from finely ground cashews. It can be found online or at Trader Joe's stores, or can be made at home by grinding raw cashews in a spice grinder or food processor. Cashew meal gives baked goods a more neutral flavor and can be substituted for almond flour if desired.

ARROWROOT POWDER is made from the starchy arrowroot plant and works as a substitute for cornstarch or potato starch. It is almost purely carbohydrate and has little nutritional value, so I try to use it in minimal amounts. It is, however, a wonderful gluten-free ingredient for baking or thickening when there are tree nut and coconut allergies. It is not to be confused with tapioca starch, which comes from the cassava plant and is less easily digested than arrowroot.

COCONUT FLOUR is made by drying and finely grinding the meat of a coconut. It is packed with dietary fiber and protein and is a naturally gluten-free flour alternative. The high fiber content also keeps the sugars from being absorbed into the bloodstream. It is a great alternative for those with nut or wheat allergies but can be somewhat tricky to bake with. Even an extra teaspoon can yield a different result.

# fats

COCONUT OIL is a healthy fat that is extracted from the meat of a coconut. It has many medicinal properties and is used in food as well as skincare products. It is heat stable, slow to oxidize, and resistant to rancidity, making it suitable for high-temperature cooking or frying. It is solid at room temperature (except when the room has no air-conditioning and it's summer!) and is wonderful to bake with. It is always best to use virgin coconut oil.

BACON FAT AND LARD sound a little out of the ordinary but can be wonderful fats to cook or even bake with. Cook a batch of pastured bacon, strain the leftover grease, and store it in the refrigerator to use as a flavorful ghee or butter substitute that holds up well to heat. Lard is made from rendered pork fat and is virtually flavorless and odorless, making it a great fat to bake with when dairy is not tolerated or the flavor of coconut oil would overwhelm a dish.

PALM SHORTENING is used as a butter substitute in many of my baked goods recipes. It has a firm texture and a high melting point, creating fluffy and cakelike delights. There is quite a bit of controversy surrounding the palm oil industry, so be sure to purchase this shortening from sustainable and eco-friendly sources, such as Tropical Traditions or Spectrum Organics. Grass-fed unsalted butter, ghee, or lard may be used as a substitute, but I do not recommend substituting coconut oil for texture and flavor purposes.

EXTRA-VIRGIN OLIVE OIL is superior to standard olive oil because it is cold pressed and not exposed to heat, making it lower in linoleic acid (omega-6). Be sure to purchase brands in dark bottles, and keep it in a cool place when not in use. Because extra-virgin olive oil can release free radicals when heated, there is a lot of concern in the Paleo community about using it in cooking; however, reaching its smoke point is fairly difficult unless it is used for frying. Though I opt to use ghee for higher-heat cooking, I do recommend extra-virgin olive oil as a dairy-free alternative for sautéing or baking and, of course, for salads and other cold dishes. Note, too, that if olive oil is used to sauté or roast vegetables that give off a lot of water, like zucchini, there is even less of a chance of it heating to its smoke point and oxidizing. It can also be mixed with another high-heat fat to further minimize the chances.

GHEE is my preferred fat to cook with, and I use it throughout this book. Ghee is clarified butter, which means that the milk solids have been almost entirely removed, leaving only the healthy butterfat behind. Very pure ghee is 99 percent pure butter oil but may have trace amounts of casein and lactose. Unless you are extremely sensitive, it normally does not cause problems, even if other dairy does. Because the recipes in this book are dairy-free, ghee is recommended but always has a substitute listed after it. If dairy is tolerated, grass-fed unsalted butter may be substituted throughout the book. Ghee can easily be prepared at home from grass-fed butter with a little time in the kitchen, and it can also be purchased online and in health food stores.

## milks

ALMOND MILK is easy to prepare (see page 240) and more delicious when homemade. If using store-bought, always buy the unsweetened original flavor and compare brands to find the one with the fewest ingredients and without carrageenan.

COCONUT MILK is made by puréeing the meat and water from a coconut. Avoid the boxed coconut milk "beverages" typically sold in the refrigerated sections of grocery stores, as they contain additives and stabilizers to retain a liquid consistency. Instead, look for canned coconut milk (in BPA-free cans) that contains only coconut and water and is preferably free of guar gum, which some people may be sensitive to.

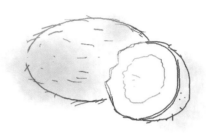

## sweeteners

HONEY is the most commonly used sweetener in this book. Raw, local, organic honey has incredible health benefits. It boosts both energy and the immune system, and locally produced honey can greatly help with seasonal allergies. Honey contains only monosaccharides (single sugars), making it easier for the body to absorb and process.

MAPLE SYRUP is a natural, unrefined liquid sweetener that I often use to enhance the flavors of baked goods or savory dishes. Use pure grade B maple syrup, or substitute honey if desired.

COCONUT CRYSTALS, also known as coconut sugar or coconut sap sugar, are produced from the sap of the flower buds of the coconut palm tree. They have been used as a sweetener for thousands of years and have a very low glycemic index.

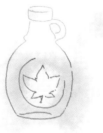

# condiments and seasonings

CHICKEN STOCK AND BROTH are similar and may be used interchangeably, but I recommend using stock, as it is made with bony parts and has a greater concentration of healthy gelatin from long-simmering the bones. Find my recipe for homemade stock on page 242. Because my stock is low in sodium, each recipe that uses it calls for the amount of salt needed based on the individual recipe. If you use store-bought stock or broth instead, be sure to buy a low-sodium product without sugars or additives and add salt to taste.

COCONUT AMINOS are made from naturally aged coconut sap and blended with sea salt. This soy- and gluten-free soy sauce substitute has a low glycemic index.

FISH SAUCE is a salty condiment used in Thai and other Asian cuisines. I also use it in recipes that would typically contain Worcestershire sauce, as it contributes a similar salty flavor. Look for bottles that contain only anchovies and salt, such as Red Boat brand.

SEA SALT brightens the flavor of any dish. I use a fine-grain Celtic or Himalayan pink sea salt, both of which are unbleached and unrefined and contain healthy trace minerals. If you are substituting table salt for the sea salt in my recipes, start with half the amount and adjust to taste.

TOMATO PRODUCTS sold in the United States often contain ingredients besides tomatoes, such as citric acid, calcium chloride, or other stabilizers. My preferred brands, Pomi and Bionaturae, are Italian, contain only tomato ingredients, and come in BPA-free containers. I often call for strained tomatoes, which are milled and strained of the seeds and skins to create a thick tomato puree.

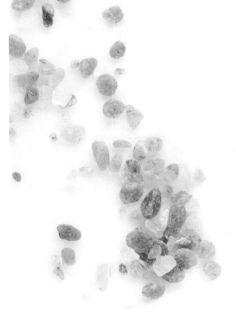

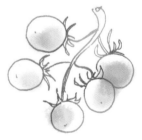

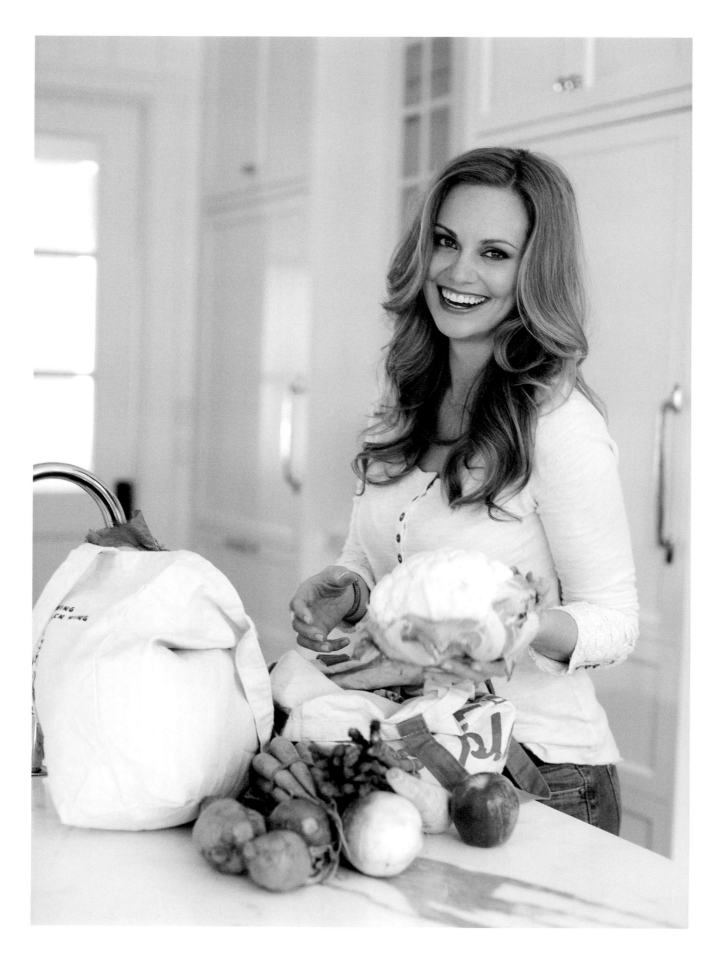

# shopping smart

When shopping in general, we all want the best quality possible for the lowest cost. This applies to food, too, though remember that when you're putting something in your body, quality is especially important. There are some tricks to buying good-quality food without blowing your budget, and the more experience you gain, the more you'll be able to fine-tune your shopping tactics to meet your needs.

# quality counts

I bought conventional meat for quite some time after going grain-free, not realizing the damage that it could be doing. I had not yet heard of organic or grass-fed meats and was unaware of the chemicals, additives, and poor diets that conventionally raised animals are subjected to, and in turn subjected my body to. Similarly, I continued to purchase conventional produce that was laden with pesticides and other chemicals. Once I became more familiar with what I could and could not eat, I focused on learning about quality ingredients and implementing a plan to purchase them, which helped take my health to another level.

## produce

Purchasing organic and local produce is essential in taking the right steps to eating a healthy diet. If you shop smartly, you'll notice an immediate improvement in your budget when you make the switch.

If buying all organic produce is not an option financially, opt for local fruits and vegetables from your farmer's market or take part in community-supported agriculture (CSA). To save here and there, you can choose to buy just the Dirty Dozen fruits and vegetables organic, as they are known to have the highest levels of pesticides, and save by purchasing local, conventional produce for the Clean Fifteen.

## meats

Switching to organic and 100-percent grass-fed meat was a difficult financial decision, but it was something that my family decided not to compromise on. Instead, we chose to cut down on eating out and buying coffees and spend the money where it was more worthwhile. Once we made the change, I noticed a significant difference in the way my body felt after consuming grass-fed beef versus conventionally raised beef that is fed a diet of grain, soy, and corn. I decided that if I wasn't going to be eating those foods, then the food I was eating should not have eaten them, either. However, if grass-fed meat, wild-caught seafood, and dairy products from grass-fed animals are not within your budget, you will still be making a big advancement in reducing inflammation simply by eliminating vegetable oils, grains, dairy, and processed foods from your diet.

1. apples
2. strawberries
3. grapes
4. celery
5. peaches
6. spinach
7. bell peppers
8. nectarines (imported)
9. cucumbers
10. cherry tomatoes
11. hot peppers
12. kale/collard greens

always
buy
organic

1. avocados
2. pineapple
3. cabbage
4. sweet peas
5. onions
6. asparagus
7. mangoes
8. papaya
9. kiwi
10. eggplant
11. grapefruit
12. cantaloupe
13. cauliflower
14. sweet potatoes
15. mushrooms

okay to buy
conventionally
grown
(low-pesticide foods)

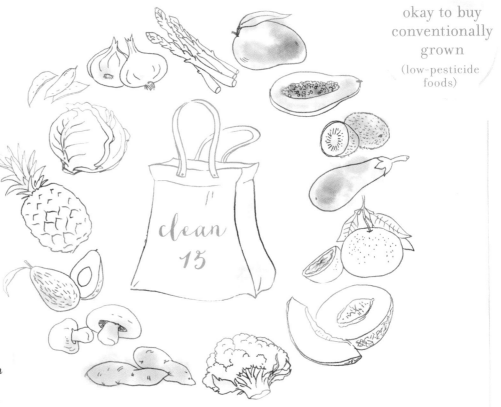

*The "Dirty Dozen" and "Clean Fifteen" lists are updated yearly. To check out the latest versions, visit www.ewg.org.*

# what do the labels mean?

Organic, grass-fed, natural, pasture-raised—what does it all mean? There are a lot of marketing tactics out there designed to make consumers think that they are purchasing the best items, but often the labels and jargon just leave people confused. Beef tends to be the most straightforward, but did you know that a package of meat can be labeled "grass-fed" even if the cows are given a grain-based supplemental diet?

To ensure that you're getting the best-quality ingredients, learn these terms before doing your shopping. They are listed in order of superiority, so start at the top and work your way down the list until you find one that fits within your means.

## 1. GRASS-FED

Cows are by nature grass-grazing animals. Yet, when they are fully grown, the diet of most cattle, organic and conventional, is switched from grass to grain in order to fatten them up and increase marbling. The grain can be genetically modified and often includes soy and corn. Beef from cattle that has been raised exclusively on grass has less saturated fat and more nutrients, such as omega-3 fatty acids, than grain-finished beef.

The U.S. Department of Agriculture (USDA) states that beef that is labeled "grass-fed" should have at least a partial grass diet and access to pasture year-round. The program is voluntary, however, without third-party verification. Labels that read "100% grass-fed" or "grass-finished" and are verified by a third party, such as the American Grass-fed Association, guarantee that the beef has been fed only grass and hay.

## 2. ORGANIC

Food labeled "organic" must be raised on a certified organic pasture and fed certified organic feed for its entire life. The USDA certification for organic meats prohibits the use of drugs, antibiotics, growth hormones, genetically modified feed, or animal by-products. The animals must have year-round outdoor access but are typically fed a diet of organic corn and other grains. However, this label does not address the treatment of the animals.

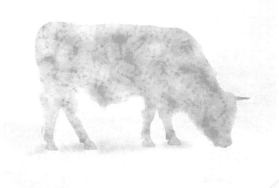

## 3. PASTURED

A label of "pastured" typically applies to poultry (including the eggs of laying hens) and pork, and is used to emphasize that the animals have been raised primarily outdoors on live pasture where they can dig or peck for insects, seeds, and whatever else they can catch. If possible, 100-percent pasture-raised animals are superior, as they are allowed to roam freely and forage on the ground as they were meant to, and are not given a feed of soy, corn, or other grains. The best source for this type of meat and eggs is local farmers.

## 4. NATURAL

The USDA defines "natural" and "all-natural" food products as those that are minimally processed and contain no artificial ingredients. These terms do not mean that a product is organic, free of GMOs, or even ethically raised.

## 5. FREE RANGE

Under USDA regulations, the "free range" designation means that the birds have been allowed access to the outdoors. However, there are no requirements for the amount of time the birds have access to the outside or the quality or size of the area. There are also no regulations on the supplemental feed that is given to the birds.

# protecting the budget

Who said eating healthy has to be expensive? When they evaluate the cost of mass-produced, packaged foods, a lot of families find that they end up spending less when they switch to a real-food diet. The amount of ingredients that need to be purchased, however, can be a shock—so here are some money-saving tips to help you eat healthy and not break the bank every time you go to the grocery store. Sticking to meats, fruits, and vegetables rather than Paleo baking ingredients such as nut flours and honey can also save money, so choose to purchase those items for special occasions.

**buy the whole bird or large cuts from larger animals**

Buying large segments of an entire animal directly from a rancher or farmer tends to be the cheapest avenue for purchasing meats, but that option can seen unapproachable for a lot of people, myself included! To make it more feasible, find a few friends who can go in on the purchase with you and divide it up evenly. Even with the possibility of sharing, however, freezer space or the required upfront payment can still be problematic. Following these grocery-shopping tips can help you shop for quality meats efficiently, but in a more attainable fashion.

Buy the whole chicken. At Trader Joe's, a whole organic chicken is around $5.99 a pound for an average four-pound bird. With two breasts, two thighs and legs, and other dark underside meat, you can roast it, eat the chicken, use the bones for stock, and use up leftovers in soups or on salads. A pound of boneless skinless breasts, or about two breasts, costs around $9.99, and you do not get to utilize any of the other parts. Whole organic chickens can even be found at wholesale clubs such as Costco for as low as $2.50 a pound.

Grass-fed ground beef is the cheapest form of beef and can be found for around $6 to $8 per pound, which in reality is double the price of conventional ground beef. Many families find that they can handle the cost of ground meat, but when they venture into buying large, tender cuts like roasts and steaks, the cost can be overwhelming. I suggest that you shop around for the cheapest price and find local vendors or online distributors, like US Wellness Meats.

The cost of a cut of meat usually correlates with how tender it is. Higher-priced cuts are better for quick cooking and grilling and will stay tender, but the lower-cost cuts are best cooked in a slow and low method, such as slow cooking or braising. Extra marinating time with an acidic ingredient such as pineapple or vinegar can also help tenderize less-expensive cuts of meat.

**buy whole vegetables**

While convenient, precut vegetables and fruit come with a premium price, so save your money and chop up your produce for the week's meals and snacks over the weekend and have them ready to throw into the pot when you are preparing your meal. Once they're cut up, store them in an airtight container in the refrigerator. If the fruit you are preparing is prone to browning, spritz it with a bit of fresh lemon juice to help preserve its color for a few days.

**buy in bulk**

Whether you are buying toilet paper or food, buying in bulk is and always has been the most cost-efficient way to shop, and this does not change when you follow a Paleo diet. When you see sales on meat, and if you have the freezer space, stock up on the cuts you like or plan to use in the future. If possible, shop at warehouse stores like Costco and Sam's Club and opt for organic meats. If you are feeding a smaller family, find a friend who may be interested in going in on a membership with you and purchase items that you can split between you.

Where you can find the best deals varies by city and region, so search for deals in stores or online and make a mental note once you find them.

If you have the storage space for excess dry goods, be it in the garage or in an additional closet, you will save money by shopping in bulk for Paleo foods and the new Paleo convenience snacks on the market. Things like almond flour, coconut milk, coconut flour, and nuts can be found at cheaper prices online and when sold in larger quantities. I always buy a five-pound bag of almond flour and store half in the fridge and half in the freezer. You can purchase a five-pound bag of almond flour for close to $0.41 per ounce online, but you will pay $0.90 per ounce when buying a small one-pound bag of lesser-quality flour from a health food store.

Most online vendors offer even deeper discounts for higher volumes and also frequently offer promotions like free shipping or buy-one-get-one-free sales. Keep an eye out for them, and stock up when you see special deals.

| | |
|---|---|
| buy online | Amazon and other online vendors, like Digestive Wellness and Barefoot Provisions, are great places to stock up on nonperishable items like nut flours, coconut aminos, and coconut milk. For a list of my favorite brands and websites, see page 290.<br><br>Amazon has two great promotions that we take full advantage of: |

1. *Get a Prime account and receive free two-day shipping in the United States all year long.*

2. *Use the Subscribe and Save option to save up to 15 percent on things like raw cacao, coconut milk, and other pantry items.*

| | |
|---|---|
| shop for seasonal produce | You can save a lot by shopping for fresh produce that is in season locally. Stores put a premium price on out-of-season produce because it is harder to find and usually in higher demand. Pick recipes that utilize what is in season, and do not be afraid to experiment with swapping produce for what you find in season and at a good cost. If possible, growing your own produce and herbs or joining a CSA will ensure you have high-quality seasonal produce and save you money at the same time.<br><br>Frozen vegetables can be a great alternative and are often less expensive than fresh vegetables that are out of season. Just make sure to thaw them properly before substituting them in a recipe. If you see fresh produce for a good price, you can also stock up and freeze it yourself. |
| plan ahead | Not only does being organized save time and make meal preparation simple, but it can save you money as well. Meal planning helps reduce waste by ensuring that you have a plan for everything you purchase. The result? No more finding spoiled food at the bottom of the refrigerator bins at the end of the week! By following the weekly meal plans on pages 44–47, you will use the more perishable items at the beginning the week and use up leftover ingredients in other recipes in the remainder of the week—so by week's end, everything will have been used up, and nothing will have gone to waste. |

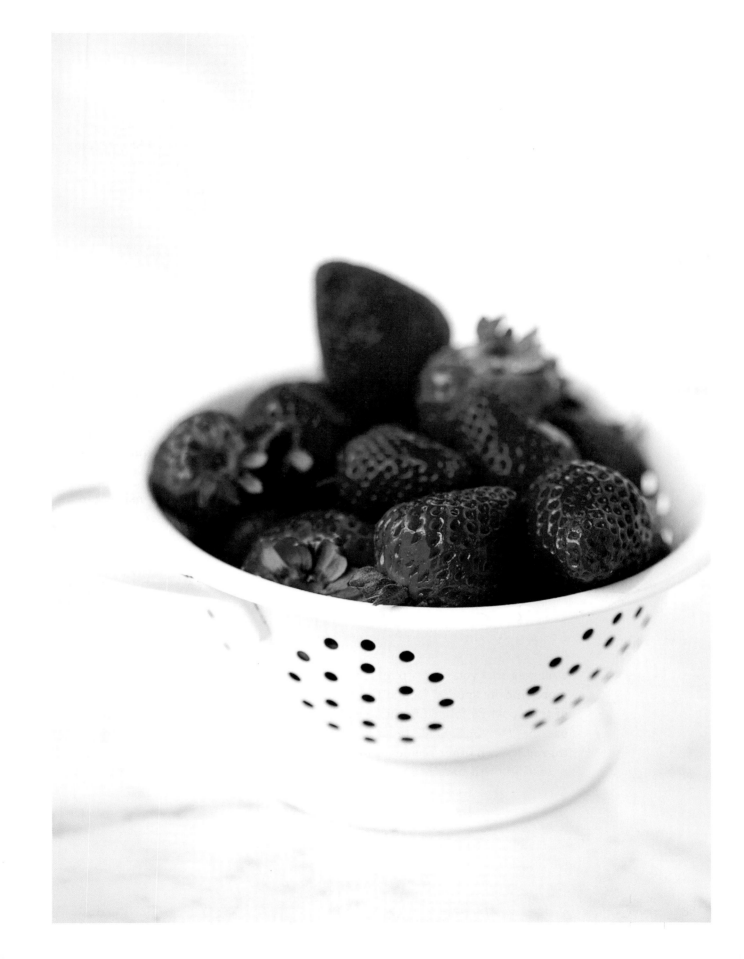

# grocery list for beginners

For those just starting out on a grain-free diet, the task of identifying hidden ingredients that are often snuck into food and deciphering marketing jargon can be slightly overwhelming. Use this basic grocery list to help guide you through the store when you are looking to buy basics and stock your fridge and pantry. For more specific grocery lists pertaining to the recipes in this book, see the meal plans on pages 44–47 and the meal plan grocery shopping lists on pages 300–307. (Note that this grocery list for beginners is also offered as a tear-out in the back of the book.)

## key words to look for

grass-fed

organic

pasture-raised

wild-caught

natural

local

sustainable

hormone-free

pesticide-free

GMO-free

## hidden ingredients and terms to avoid

agave nectar

cane sugar or juice

carrageenan

corn (*syrup, starch, dextrose, dextrin*)

xanthan & guar gum

hydrogenated oils

monosodium glutamate (MSG)

potato starch

sucrose, galactose, & maltose

## protein

*(100% grass-fed, organic, pasture-raised when possible)*

beef, bison, lamb, elk, etc.

poultry (*turkey, chicken, duck, etc.*)

pork

sausages, bacon, deli meat*

fish and shellfish (*wild-caught and fresh when possible*)

eggs

*\* Avoid added sugars, carrageenan, nitrates, sulfates, and MSG.*

## vegetables and fruits

Pick fruits and vegetables that are in season and local if possible. If you cannot afford to purchase all organic produce, consult the Dirty Dozen cheat sheet (page 25) for a guide on which to buy organic. Refer to the Paleo Cheat Sheet (page 35) for which vegetables are off-limits, such as white potatoes and corn.

| | | | |
|---|---|---|---|
| acorn squash | carrots | leeks | spaghetti squash |
| artichoke | cauliflower | lettuce | spinach |
| asparagus | celery | mushrooms | sweet potato |
| beets | cucumbers | parsley | Swiss chard |
| bell peppers | eggplant | parsnips | watercress |
| broccoli and broccoli rabe | fennel | pumpkin | yam |
| | herbs | radishes | yellow onion |
| Brussels sprouts | jicama | red onion | zucchini |
| butternut squash | kabocha squash | scallions | |
| cabbage | kale | shallots | |

apples
apricots
avocados
bananas
berries
cantaloupe
cherries
dates

figs
grapefruit
grapes
lemons
limes
mangoes
nectarines
oranges

papaya
peaches
pears
pineapple
plums
pomegranates
raspberries
strawberries

tangerines
tomatoes
watermelon
dried fruits (*without added sugar or preservatives*)

## fats
avocado oil

butter (*grass-fed and pastured*)

coconut oil (*virgin or expeller-pressed for mild flavor*)

duck fat

bacon fat

extra-virgin olive oil

ghee

lard (*pastured*)

macadamia oil

palm shortening (*sustainable and organic*)

sesame oil (*toasted or cold pressed*)

## baking
almond flour (*blanched*)

arrowroot flour

baking powder (*grain-free*)

baking soda

coconut crystals or palm sugar

coconut flour

cream of tartar

dark chocolate (*85% cacao*)

grade B maple syrup

honey

pure vanilla extract

raw cacao powder or cocoa powder

## nuts, seeds, and nut or seed butters (*purchase raw and organic when possible*)
almonds

cashews

flaxseeds

hazelnuts

macadamia nuts

pecans

pepitas (pumpkin seeds)

pine nuts

pistachios

sesame seeds

sunflower seeds

walnuts

almond butter

cashew butter

sunflower seed butter

tahini

## seasonings
fresh herbs

sea salt (*fine-grained*)

organic spices

## jarred and canned goods
organic tomato products (*no citric acid or sugars added*)
- *diced tomatoes in juices*
- *strained tomatoes or tomato puree*
- *tomato paste*

olives

curry paste

unsweetened applesauce

full-fat coconut milk

capers

pickles

vinegars (*apple cider, pure balsamic, champagne, red wine*)

fish sauce (*Red Boat brand*)

coconut aminos

# paleo—put simply

You may be coming to this book simply because you are grain-free, and you may be wondering, "What is Paleo?" Put simply, it is defined as "ancient or prehistoric." Following a Paleolithic-style diet means reverting to the foods that our bodies were intended to consume and process before the days of the agricultural revolution and processed foods.

# paleo cheat sheet

## eat

**FISH**
- *low-mercury*
- *wild-caught*

**GRASS-FED, PASTURE-RAISED MEATS**
- *beef*
- *bison*
- *lamb*
- *pork*

**POULTRY**
- *chicken*
- *duck*
- *turkey*
- *eggs*

**VEGETABLES,** including root vegetables

**FRUIT**

**FERMENTED FOODS**

**NUTS and SEEDS**

**HEALTHY OILS and FATS**
- *avocado oil*
- *bacon fat*
- *coconut oil*
- *ghee*
- *grass-fed butter*
- *olive oil*

## avoid

**GRAINS**
- *barley*
- *wheat*
- *rice*
- *corn*
- *rye*
- *cereals*
- *quinoa\**
- *breads*
- *oats*
- *pastas*

*\* While quinoa is not technically a grain, most people find that their bodies process it as such and are not able to tolerate it.*

**LEGUMES**
- *beans*
- *peanuts*
- *lentils*

**WHITE POTATOES**

**REFINED SUGAR**

**DAIRY**

**SOY**

**REFINED, HYDROGENATED VEGETABLE OILS**

**PROCESSED FOODS**

## key words to look for

grass-fed

organic

pasture-raised

wild-caught

natural

local

sustainable

hormone-free

pesticide-free

GMO-free

## words to avoid

agave nectar

cane sugar or juice

carrageenan

corn
*(syrup, starch, dextrose, dextrin)*

xanthan & guar gum

hydrogenated oils

monosodium glutamate (MSG)

potato starch

sucrose, galactose, & maltose

## swap this for that

| PASTA | RICE | WHITE POTATOES | MASHED POTATOES | MILK |
|---|---|---|---|---|
| spiral-sliced sweet potato or squash, spaghetti squash (pages 156, 166, & 204) | Cauliflower Rice (page 218) | white sweet potatoes, celeriac, parsnips | mashed parsnips (page 214) or cauliflower | coconut milk or Almond Milk (page 240) |

| SUGAR | CANOLA OIL | FLOURS | SOY SAUCE | TABLE SALT |
|---|---|---|---|---|
| raw honey, grade B maple syrup, coconut crystals | coconut oil, ghee | nut flours, coconut flour | coconut aminos | sea salt |

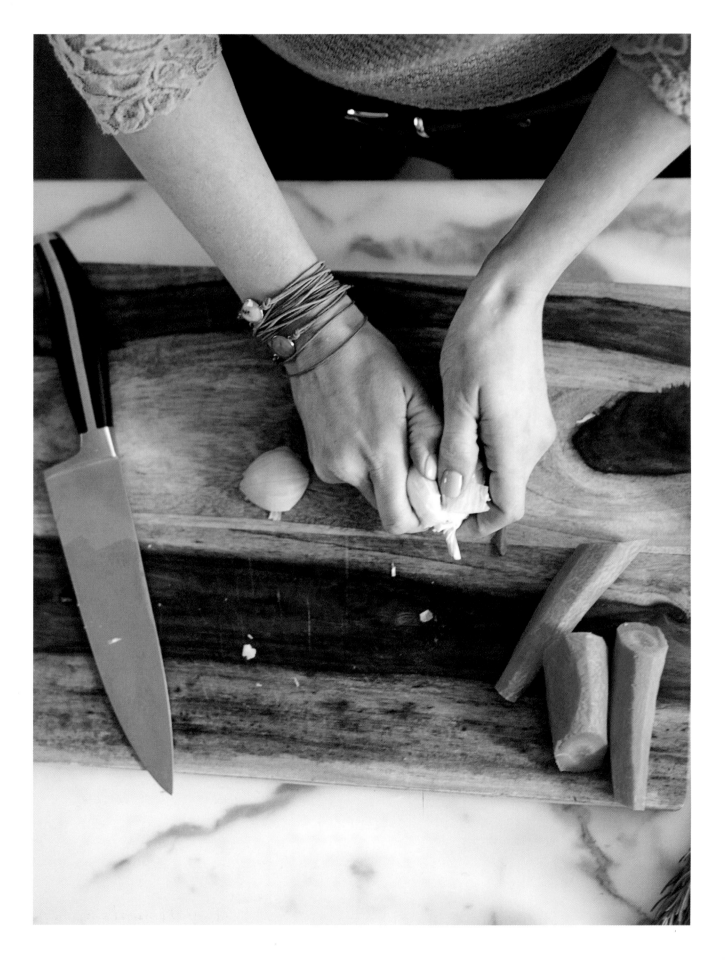

# my tools

Cooking for a whole-foods diet takes a little extra preparation time, but these tools will make you more efficient in the kitchen and help you achieve the best results.

blender

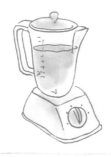

Grain-free and dairy-free cooking requires extra preparation, and a good blender can save you a lot of time. I use mine to create smooth doughs and batters, purée soups, and whip up smoothies. If you can afford one, a Blendtec is a fabulous machine that can pulverize virtually anything. Its twister jar is amazing for nut butters, salad dressings, mayonnaise, and single servings of smoothies.

food processor

This machine can chop or grate vegetables and fruit, grind whole nuts, and purée cooked vegetables. Most models have a greater capacity than blenders and therefore offer more versatility in food preparation.

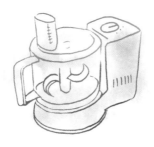

sharp knives

Eating a whole-foods diet entails quite a bit more preparation than a processed-foods diet, so a good set of sharp knives is a must. I had to save up and purchase my knives one at a time, but it was well worth it. I use the Japanese brand Shun, but Wüsthof and J.A. Henckels are also reputable brands. I recommend that every home cook have a paring knife, a 5½-inch Santoku or chef's knife, a carving knife, and a serrated knife in their arsenal. I also recommend that you have your knives professionally sharpened at least twice a year. You will be amazed at how much time a sharp knife can save in prep over battling with a dull one. My telltale sign that my knives need to be sharpened is that I am struggling to cut through ginger root!

parchment paper

Lining a roasting pan with parchment paper makes for easy cleanup, and covering the bottom of cake and loaf pans with a piece of parchment means that your breads and cakes won't stick. I always keep a large roll from Costco on hand.

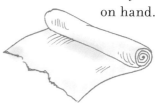

| pots and pans | My all-time favorite pots and pans are Le Creuset brand. They're made with nontoxic materials, heat quickly and evenly, and are a cinch to clean. Stainless-steel pots are also wonderful, and you can usually find whole sets discounted at stores like Costco and Home Goods. I recommend having at least a 2-quart saucepan, a 9-inch skillet, and a 3½-quart Dutch oven on hand. |

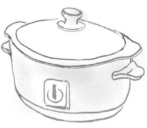

| slow cooker | A slow cooker, or Crock-Pot, is incredibly handy for a busy cook—and who isn't busy these days? There's nothing like coming home after a hectic day at the office or carpooling kids to a gazillion activities to a house full of delectable smells and a complete meal waiting for you. I use a 6½-quart slow cooker, and I recommend getting a model that is proportionately wide and shallow rather than narrow and deep. This size also works really well when you want to double a recipe. |

| spiral slicer | The winner in the creativity department, the spiral slicer (commonly known as the Spiralizer), is an inexpensive gizmo that can turn almost any vegetable into noodles, making meals more exciting for kids and adults alike. You can buy one for as little as $30, but a less-expensive julienne slicer will achieve somewhat similar results. |

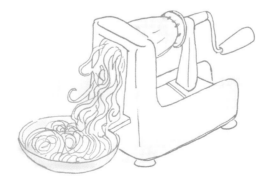

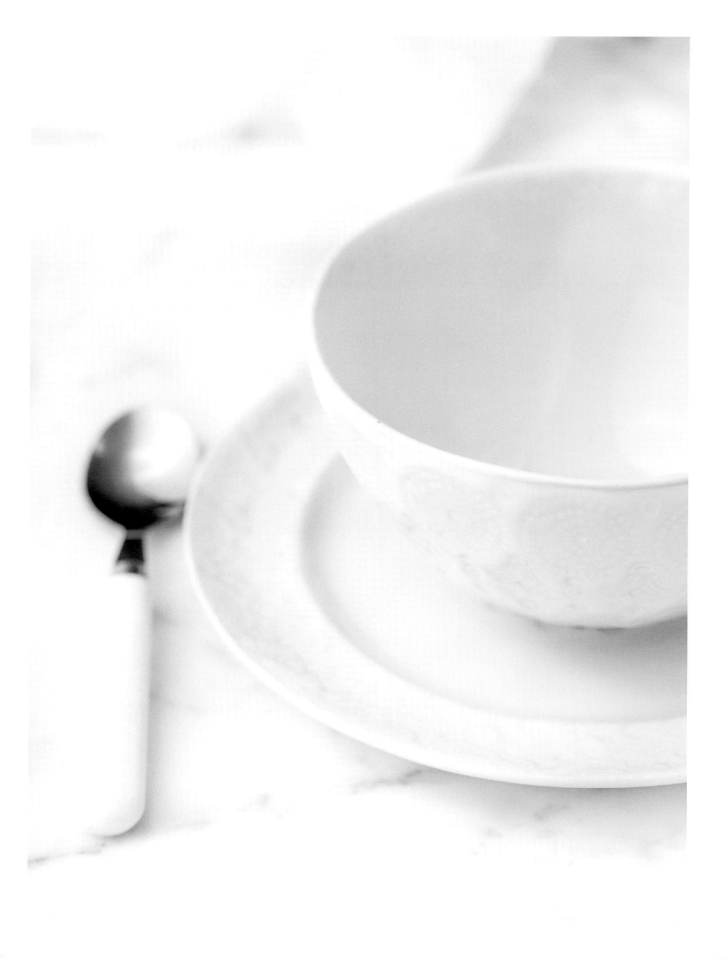

# making it simple

Aside from my personal tips, labeled "Tidbits," at the bottoms of the recipes, here are my top time-saving tips to help you get dinner on the table in the least stressful and least time-consuming manner. I have also included eight weeks of dinner ideas to get you started.

### 1.
plan ahead

Most people run into the most trouble when they get home from a long day and there is nothing to eat in the house. That is when take-out is awfully inviting, or when a trip to the grocery store goes awry and your cart ends up with many more indulgent items in it than necessary.

Sit down at the beginning of the week and use the grocery lists and meal plans (pages 44–47) to ensure that you are never in this predicament. Do your grocery shopping once a week to make your cooking more efficient and reduce the number of impulse food items you will likely buy during the week if you go in hungry and without a plan.

Take an hour on the weekend to prep the vegetables you will use for the week. Mince all your garlic for the week at once, chop all your onions, and use your food processor to shred or dice vegetables. Then pack them all up in resealable bags or containers and store them in the refrigerator for easy access and to shave time off of meal prep.

Take one day a week or month to make some of the refrigerator and pantry staples and store them so that they are ready to use at mealtime. Make a batch of my grain-free Wraps (page 262) and use them throughout the week for speedy lunches, and spend an afternoon making the sauces and salad dressings from the Basics section beginning on page 238 so that they're ready to go when you're in a pinch.

Also take time to strategize when following specific recipes. Read through the entire recipe and have all the tools and ingredients you need out and ready to go.

### 2.
double up

If you're going to go to the effort of cooking a nice meal and you know that you have a busy week ahead, double or triple the recipe. It may seem like a lot of work up front, but you will be thankful to have leftovers that you can pack for lunches or eat on the run. Many recipes can be frozen for later use as well. This will reduce your time and cleanup, plus it will alleviate the stress of cooking when it comes time to use the second meal.

### 3.
stretch it

Leftovers can get a little mundane. Instead of simply reheating them and eating them in exactly the same way, why not morph the initial meal into an entirely different one the next time around? The "stretch it" recipes on pages 52, 118, 134, 146, 152, 158, 160, 170, 176, 178, 180 and 184 were designed especially for this purpose. Once you get into the habit of morphing one meal into another, you'll see how easy it is to prepare an extra chicken breast, piece of meat, or fish fillet and use it in a new way—on salad, on pizza, or in a lettuce-wrapped sandwich.

**4.**
**stick to
one-pot and
slow cooker
meals**

Minimize cleanup and save time on the back end of a meal by sticking to the one-pot and slow cooker recipes in this book. Find a list of them on pages 298–299, or look for their icons. A slow cooker can be a lifesaver on a busy day, and the recipes typically double and freeze easily. Chop up all the ingredients the night before and throw them into the slow cooker in the morning before you leave the house. Or take one day at the beginning of the month and prep the ingredients for slow cooker meals that you can put in the freezer and pull out the day you need them—then the rest of the work is done in the slow cooker! I love to do this for my husband when I'm traveling, or when we have hectic weeks and I don't have time to plan meals. It's so convenient, and it beats going out to eat.

**5.**
**invest in a
food processor**

I discussed other time-saving tools in the My Tools section (page 37), but this tool deserves special mention here. Aside from my spiral slicer, which I use to make noodles, my food processor is one of the most-used tools in my kitchen. You don't have to spend a lot to get a good-quality machine; just make sure you find one that has grating and slicing attachments with it. A food processor with these attachments can save you hours in preparation time each week. Rather than standing over a cutting board with a knife, use it to slice, shred, and chop vegetables. You will be amazed at how quickly your meals come together.

**6.**
**when all else
fails, have a
backup plan**

Our backups are grass-fed, organic hot dogs with a salad, grilled burgers wrapped in lettuce, or a jar of organic spaghetti sauce to which I add some seasonings and ground beef and serve over spaghetti squash (see page 168 for my Shortcut Spaghetti with Meat Sauce). It's okay to serve something very simple now and then!

**7.**
**keep it fun**

Feeling stressed about getting something on the table for dinner, or taking packaged-food shortcuts that impair your health, is no fun. The meal plans and organization strategies in this book are meant to relieve meal prep anxiety, and I hope they make it more fun in the process. Another way to increase the fun factor and save time is to make it a social event. Take a full weekend day and cook a few different meals with a friend. One person can be chopping and prepping while the other cooks. Double or triple the recipes and divide up the bounty at the end of the day. It makes for great memories and keeps cooking fun!

# 8-week meal plans

I have designed eight weeks' worth of dinners to offer variety at mealtime and minimize waste. I left one day open each week to utilize leftovers or for special occasions and dining out.

Saturdays or Sundays should be used for shopping and prepping. The meals are designed to use the most perishable items first. Freeze fresh fish and poultry the day it is purchased and defrost it in the refrigerator the night before to avoid having to shop twice in a week. I've listed a few desserts if there are items to be used up, such as coconut milk, but of course you are welcome to enjoy dessert whenever you choose!

### day 1

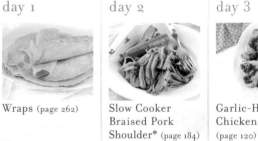

Wraps (page 262)

Slow Cooker Thai Beef Stew (page 160)

Coconut, Cilantro, & Lime Cauli-Rice (page 218)

### day 2

Slow Cooker Braised Pork Shoulder* (page 184)

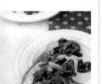

Catalan-Style Spinach (page 226)

*\* Reserve 1½ cups juices for Day 5*

### day 3

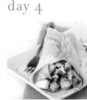

Garlic-Herb Chicken Thighs (page 120)

### day 4

California Chicken Wraps (page 128)

*Cook extra bacon and reserve leftover Herb Ranch Dressing for BLT Salad*

### day 5

Pork Ragu (page 186)

### day 6

BLT Salad (page 104)

*Use leftover Herb Ranch Dressing*

tidbits:
Take some time at the beginning of each week to prepare the basics you will use throughout the week. Stock your refrigerator with things like Mayonnaise (page 248), Chicken Stock (page 242), Wraps (page 262), and salad dressings (page 247) to make meal preparation quicker during the week.

Shopping list for Week 1 on page 300 and in the Tear-Out Guides

*week*
*1*

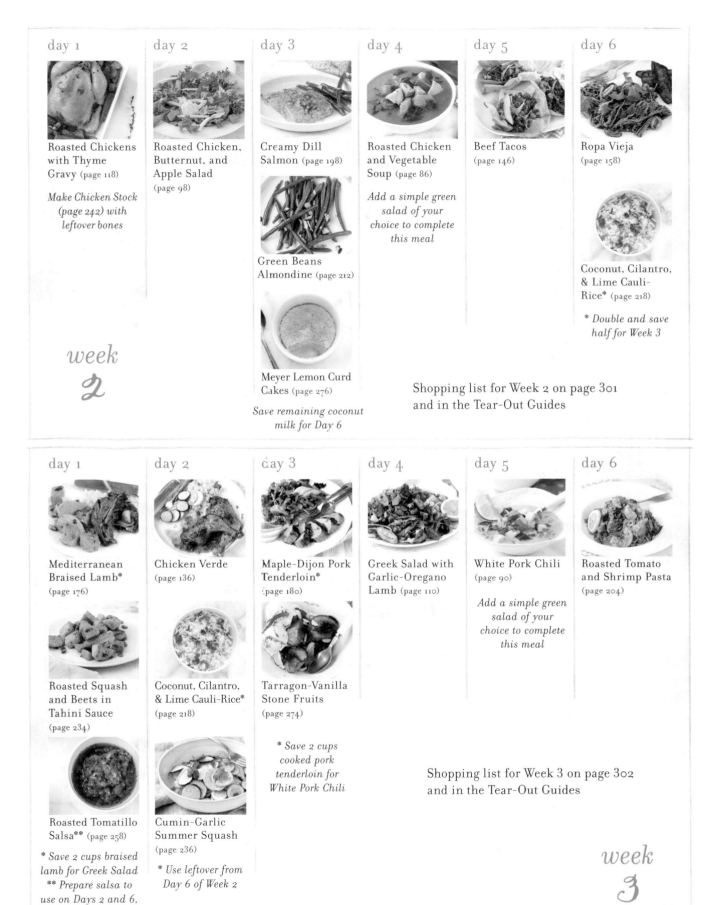

**day 1**

Roasted Chickens with Thyme Gravy (page 118)

*Make Chicken Stock (page 242) with leftover bones*

*week 2*

**day 2**

Roasted Chicken, Butternut, and Apple Salad (page 98)

**day 3**

Creamy Dill Salmon (page 198)

Green Beans Almondine (page 212)

Meyer Lemon Curd Cakes (page 276)

*Save remaining coconut milk for Day 6*

**day 4**

Roasted Chicken and Vegetable Soup (page 86)

*Add a simple green salad of your choice to complete this meal*

**day 5**

Beef Tacos (page 146)

**day 6**

Ropa Vieja (page 158)

Coconut, Cilantro, & Lime Cauli-Rice* (page 218)

*\* Double and save half for Week 3*

Shopping list for Week 2 on page 301 and in the Tear-Out Guides

---

**day 1**

Mediterranean Braised Lamb* (page 176)

Roasted Squash and Beets in Tahini Sauce (page 234)

Roasted Tomatillo Salsa** (page 258)

*\* Save 2 cups braised lamb for Greek Salad*
*\*\* Prepare salsa to use on Days 2 and 6, or buy store-bought*

**day 2**

Chicken Verde (page 136)

Coconut, Cilantro, & Lime Cauli-Rice* (page 218)

Cumin-Garlic Summer Squash (page 236)

*\* Use leftover from Day 6 of Week 2*

**day 3**

Maple-Dijon Pork Tenderloin* (page 180)

Tarragon-Vanilla Stone Fruits (page 274)

*\* Save 2 cups cooked pork tenderloin for White Pork Chili*

**day 4**

Greek Salad with Garlic-Oregano Lamb (page 110)

**day 5**

White Pork Chili (page 90)

*Add a simple green salad of your choice to complete this meal*

**day 6**

Roasted Tomato and Shrimp Pasta (page 204)

Shopping list for Week 3 on page 302 and in the Tear-Out Guides

*week 3*

45

## Week 4

| day 1 | day 2 | day 3 | day 4 | day 5 | day 6 |
|---|---|---|---|---|---|

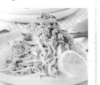

**Crab and Asparagus Linguine**
(page 200)

**Lemon-Oregano Chicken Kabobs**
(page 138)

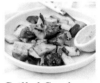

**Grilled Greek Summer Squash Salad** (page 106)

**Ginger Chicken and Broccoli**
(page 126)

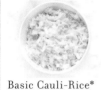

**Basic Cauli-Rice***
(page 218)

*\* Double and use leftover for Day 5*

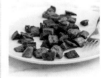

**Mexican Burgers**
(page 164)

**Smoky Roasted Sweet Potatoes**
(page 222)

**Chicken Curry**
(page 132)

**Basic Cauli-Rice***
(page 218)

*\* Use leftover from Day 3*

**Sausage and Peppers Arrabbiata**
(page 156)

*week* **4**

Shopping list for Week 4 on page 303 and in the Tear-Out Guides

---

## Week 5

| day 1 | day 2 | day 3 | day 4 | day 5 | day 6 |
|---|---|---|---|---|---|

**Barbecue Chicken**
(page 134)

**Jicama Apple Bacon Slaw**
(page 230)

**Barbecue Sauce**
(page 250)

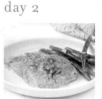

**Creamy Dill Salmon** (page 198)

**Green Beans Almondine**
(page 212)

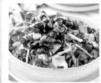

**Barbecue Chicken Chopped Salad**
(page 108)

**Slow Cooker Thai Beef Stew**
(page 160)

**Coconut, Cilantro, & Lime Cauli-Rice**
(page 218)

**Pesto Orange Roughy** (page 206)

**Roasted Basil Eggplant** (page 232)

**Garlic-Herb Chicken Thighs**
(page 120)

Shopping list for Week 5 on page 304 and in the Tear-Out Guides

*week* **5**

## Week 6

day 1

Pesto-Stuffed Prosciutto Chicken (page 122)

day 2

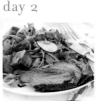

Beef Stroganoff (page 150)

day 3

Pineapple Beef Kabobs (page 162)

day 4

Poached Cod with Butternut Squash and Carrot Puree (page 202)

day 5

Meatloaf Meatballs (page 148)

Creamy Mashed Root Vegetables (page 214)

day 6

Chicken Tikka Masala (page 130)

Saffron Cauli-Rice (page 219)

*week 6*

Shopping list for Week 6 on page 305 and in the Tear-Out Guides

## Week 7

day 1

Roasted Chickens with Thyme Gravy (page 118)

*Make Chicken Stock (page 242) with leftover bones*

*Reserve 3 cups of shredded roasted chicken for Mexican Chicken Soup*

day 2

Rosemary-Lemon Pork Chops (page 174)

Lemon-Roasted Asparagus and Brussels Sprouts (page 224)

day 3

Greek Lamb Burgers (page 178)

Grilled Greek Summer Squash Salad (page 106)

day 4

Mexican Chicken Soup (page 88)

*Add a simple green salad of your choice to complete this meal*

day 5

Barbecue Salmon with Grilled Peach Salsa (page 208)

day 6

Beef Tacos (page 146)

*week 7*

Shopping list for Week 7 on page 306 and in the Tear-Out Guides

## Week 8

day 1

Maple-Dijon Pork Tenderloin (page 180)

*Save 2½ cups cooked pork tenderloin for Pork Stir-Fry on Day 4*

day 2

Barbecue Tri-Tip with Grilled Watermelon Salad (page 170)

*Save ¾ cups cooked Tri-Tip for Balsamic Steak Pizza on Day 5*

day 3

Peruvian-Style Chicken (page 116)

day 4

Pork Stir-Fry (page 182)

day 5

Balsamic Steak Pizza (page 172)

day 6

Hawaiian Chicken Burgers (page 124)

Grilled Sesame Asparagus and Scallions (page 220)

*week 8*

Shopping list for Week 8 on page 307 and in the Tear-Out Guides

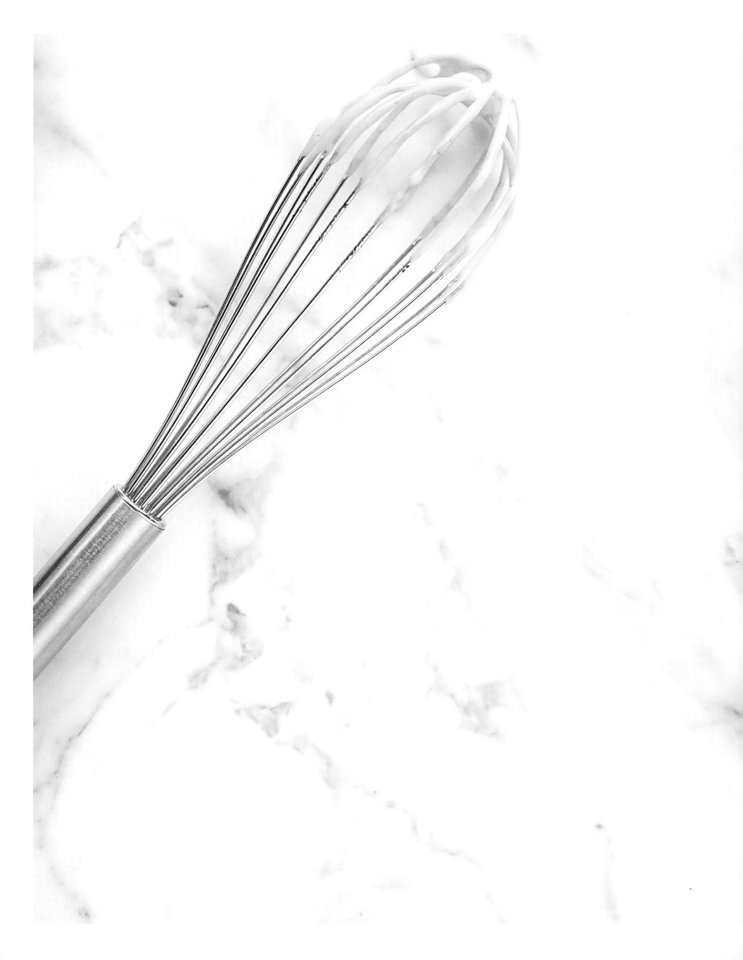

# breakfast

SCD

serves: 4 to 6
prep time: 15 minutes
cook time: 22 minutes

Frittatas are a fabulous way to use up leftovers, especially vegetables. Feel free to have fun with it—swap out the proteins and vegetables to make it your own and utilize what is in your fridge.

# southwestern frittata

## ingredients

- ½ pound ground beef
- ½ cup diced sweet potato, peeled*
- 2 tablespoons diced red onion
- 2½ teaspoons Taco Seasoning (page 244)
- ¼ teaspoon sea salt
- 2 cups baby spinach
- ½ cup diced zucchini
- 10 large eggs, beaten
- salsa, chopped fresh cilantro, or sliced avocado, for serving

\* *Substitute butternut squash for SCD.*

## method

1. Preheat the oven to 350°F.

2. In an ovenproof 10-inch skillet over medium heat, sauté the ground beef, sweet potato, onion, Taco Seasoning, and salt for 6 minutes, until the meat is mostly cooked through.

3. Add the spinach and zucchini and cook for 4 more minutes.

4. Pour the eggs into the pan and bake in the oven for 12 minutes, until the eggs have puffed up and are cooked through. Serve with salsa, cilantro, or avocado.

make-ahead tip:
Save time in the morning by chopping all the vegetables the night before!

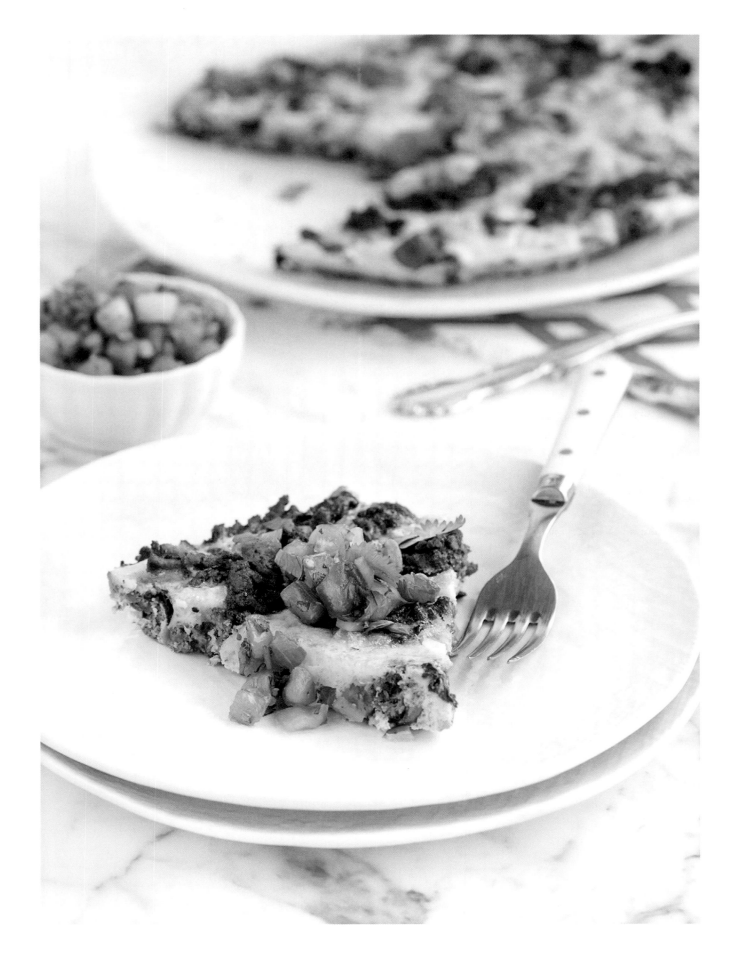

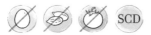 

serves: 6
prep time: 20 minutes
cook time: 20 to 22 minutes

Despite its name, this breakfast hash can be enjoyed year-round, with a couple of substitutions for the vegetables depending on what is in season. Eggs are optional, but the silky yolks really complete the flavor!

# autumn breakfast skillet

## ingredients

### SAUSAGE

- 1 tablespoon ghee or bacon fat
- 1½ pounds ground pork
- 2 tablespoons chopped fresh sage
- 1½ teaspoons sea salt
- 1 teaspoon fennel seeds*
- ½ teaspoon ground cloves
- ½ teaspoon cracked black pepper
- ¼ teaspoon ground nutmeg

### HASH

- 1 tablespoon ghee or bacon fat
- 1 small yellow onion, diced
- 2 cups diced butternut squash
- 1 cup diced apple
- 3 cups stemmed and coarsely chopped kale
- ½ teaspoon sea salt
- 6 fried eggs (optional)

*Fennel seeds are SCD legal if you have been symptom free.*

## method

1. Make the sausage: Heat 1 tablespoon of ghee in a large skillet over medium-high heat. Add the ground pork and other sausage ingredients and brown the meat until cooked through, about 8 minutes. Drain and set aside.

2. Make the hash: Return the pan to the heat and add 1 tablespoon of ghee.

3. Sauté the onion for 3 minutes, until fragrant.

4. Add the squash, apple, kale, and salt and continue cooking for 8 to 10 minutes, until the squash is tender.

5. Return the sausage to the pan, stir, and cook for another minute to heat through. Serve with fried eggs, if desired.

make-ahead tip:
Brown the sausage with the spices the night before. It can be stored in the refrigerator for up to 5 days.

stretch it:
Double the sausage mixture and use it in scrambles throughout the week, or form the meat into patties to serve between Biscuits (page 56).

tidbits:
You can save time by purchasing organic sausage. Just make sure to buy one without additives or sugar.

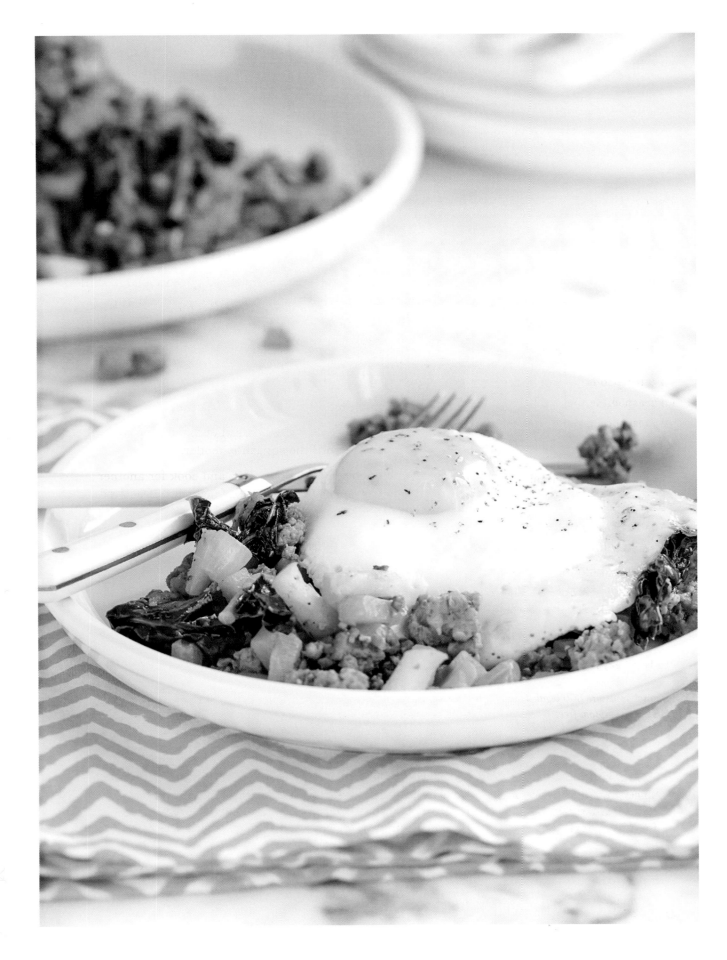

yield: 12 (8-inch) burritos

prep time: 15 minutes if using frozen Wraps

cook time: 15 to 25 minutes

Breakfast burritos are a great way to use up leftovers in the fridge, so don't feel like you have to use the exact ingredients listed below. Have fun and swap out the vegetables for what you have on hand, or add some greens to the mix, too. If you don't have leftover taco meat, cooked chorizo or breakfast sausage will work just as well. Because these burritos take a little extra prep time, I make a big batch and freeze them to provide quick, on-the-go breakfasts throughout the month.

# breakfast burritos

## ingredients

- 1 batch Wraps (page 262), at room temperature
- 2 tablespoons ghee or bacon fat, divided
- ½ cup diced red onion
- 1 small red bell pepper, seeded and diced
- 1 small yellow bell pepper, seeded and diced
- 1 small sweet potato, peeled and diced
- 1 teaspoon sea salt
- ½ teaspoon cracked black pepper
- 12 large eggs, beaten
- 2 cups leftover Beef Tacos filling (page 146)
- Roasted Tomatillo Salsa (page 258) or store-bought salsa
- 1 batch Guacamole (page 258)

## method

1. If making the Wraps fresh, begin to make them first. Save time by cooking the burrito filling in a separate skillet while the Wraps cook in batches.

2. To make the burrito filling, heat 1 tablespoon of the ghee in a deep skillet over medium-high heat.

3. Add the onion, bell peppers, sweet potato, salt, and pepper. Sauté for 10 minutes, until the vegetables have softened.

4. Stir in the remaining 1 tablespoon of ghee.

5. Pour in the eggs and let them sit for 30 seconds before stirring.

6. Gently move the eggs around the pan until they are almost cooked through.

7. Stir in the taco meat and continue cooking for 5 minutes, until the meat is warmed through.

8. To form the burritos, spoon about ¼ cup of filling into the center of each Wrap. Add salsa and Guacamole if serving immediately.

9. Gently fold the ends of the Wrap toward the center, then tightly roll the burrito. Place the burritos seam side down.

to freeze individual burritos:

Slightly undercook the eggs so they do not dry out when reheated. Let the burrito filling and Wraps come to room temperature before rolling the burritos, then wrap each one in plastic wrap or foil and store them together in an airtight container for up to 1 month. Reheat the burritos in a covered dish or wrapped in foil in a 350°F oven for 15 minutes. To microwave, wrap the burrito in a paper towel and heat for about 2 minutes. Add salsa and Guacamole after the burrito has been reheated.

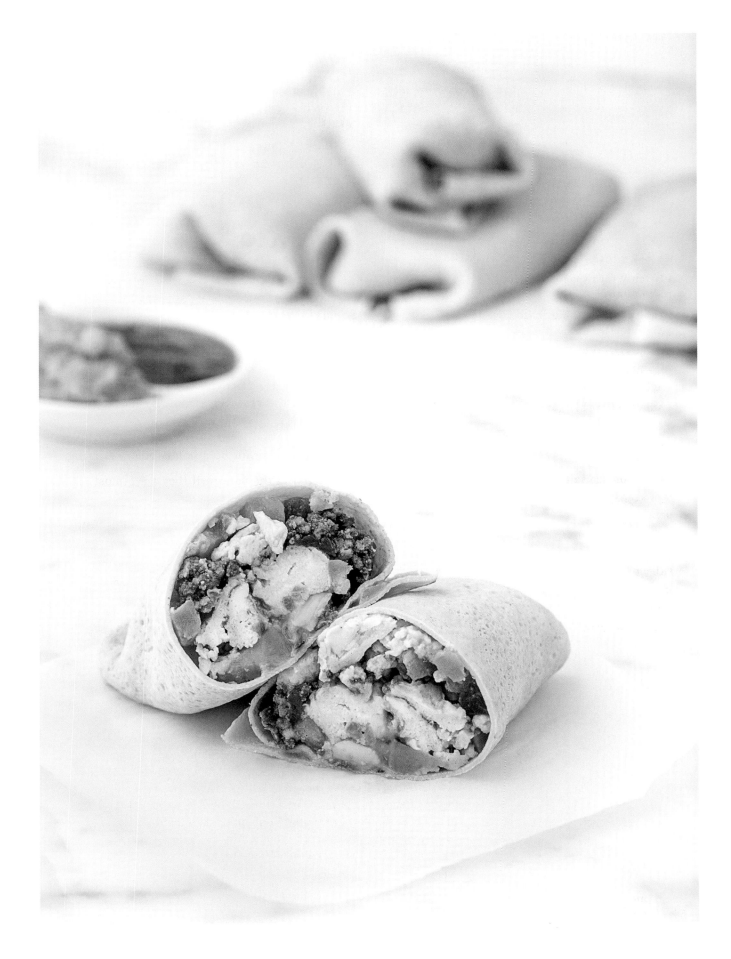

SCD

yield: 8 biscuits
prep time: 20 minutes
cook time: 18 to 20 minutes

These honey biscuits are wonderful served warm with jam for breakfast, or as a side for warm soups when the need for something breadlike arises. They are also used for Strawberry Shortcake (page 272) and can even be used for egg or sausage sandwiches.

# biscuits

## ingredients

- 3½ cups blanched almond flour, sifted
- ⅓ cup coconut flour, sifted, plus more for rolling out the dough
- 2 large eggs
- ¼ cup honey
- ¼ cup Almond Milk (page 240)
- 2 teaspoons apple cider vinegar
- 1 teaspoon baking soda
- ½ teaspoon sea salt
- ⅓ cup palm shortening or 5 tablespoons ghee

## method

1. Preheat the oven to 350°F. Line a baking sheet with parchment paper.

2. Place the flours, eggs, honey, Almond Milk, vinegar, baking soda, and salt in the bowl of a stand mixer and mix on medium until a loose dough forms.

3. Switch to a dough hook or use a pastry cutter to blend in the palm shortening, leaving pea-sized bits of the shortening visible in the dough.

4. Lightly sprinkle coconut flour on a sheet of parchment paper. Turn the dough out onto the floured surface. Gather it into a ball and form it into a 1-inch-thick circle, using your palms to flatten the top.

5. Use a round cutter to make biscuits, gathering the remaining dough into a ball and repeating the process until all of it has been used up. Alternatively, hand-shape 8 biscuits from the dough.

6. Place the biscuits on the prepared baking sheet.

7. Bake for 18 to 20 minutes, turning the sheet once midway through. Allow to cool slightly on a wire rack before serving.

make-ahead tip:
The texture of these biscuits is best when they are served fresh, but to have them on hand at all times, they can be stored in an airtight container in the refrigerator for 5 days or in the freezer for 6 months and rewarmed in a low oven. If frozen, thaw overnight in the refrigerator before warming.

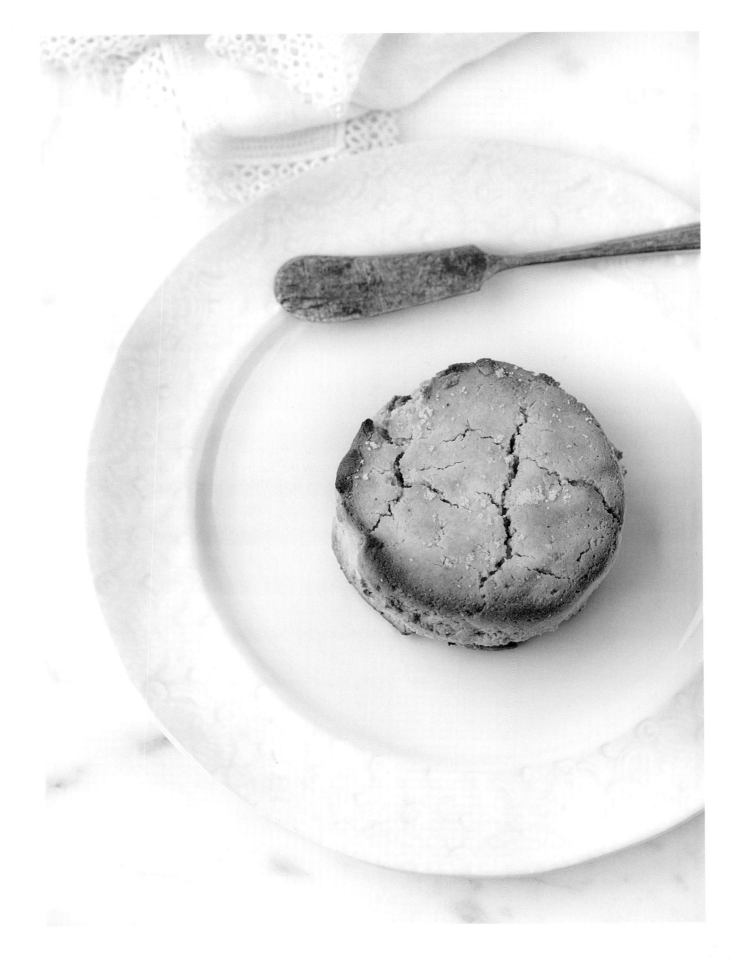

SCD

serves: 6
prep time: 20 minutes
cook time: 38 minutes

This crustless quiche is so packed with goodies that you will not even miss the time-consuming and overly filling pastry on the bottom. The Hollandaise Sauce is simple to make while the quiche bakes and adds an incredibly rich, velvety topping.

# quiche with bacon, zucchini, and chard

## ingredients

- ghee or coconut oil, for greasing the pan
- 6 ounces bacon, chopped
- 3 cups stemmed and chopped Swiss chard
- 1 medium zucchini, halved lengthwise and sliced
- ½ cup diced yellow onion
- 10 large eggs
- ¼ cup Almond Milk* (page 240)
- ¼ cup full-fat coconut milk
- ¾ teaspoon sea salt
- ¼ teaspoon cracked black pepper
- 1 batch Hollandaise Sauce (page 252), for serving

*For nut-free, use a total of ⅓ cup coconut milk and omit the Almond Milk.*

## method

1. Preheat the oven to 350°F. Lightly grease a 10-inch pie plate with ghee.

2. Cook the bacon, chard, zucchini, and onion in a skillet over medium heat for 8 minutes, until the bacon is cooked through and the vegetables have softened. Drain and transfer to the prepared pie plate.

3. In a bowl, beat the eggs with the milks, salt, and pepper. Pour over the bacon mixture.

4. Bake for 30 minutes, until the center is set but slightly soft.

5. Allow the quiche to cool for 15 minutes before serving with Hollandaise Sauce drizzled over the top.

make-ahead tip:
Make up to 4 days in advance and store in the refrigerator, tightly covered. Reheat in a low oven. Hollandaise Sauce is best fresh but can be gently reheated in a double boiler on low heat.

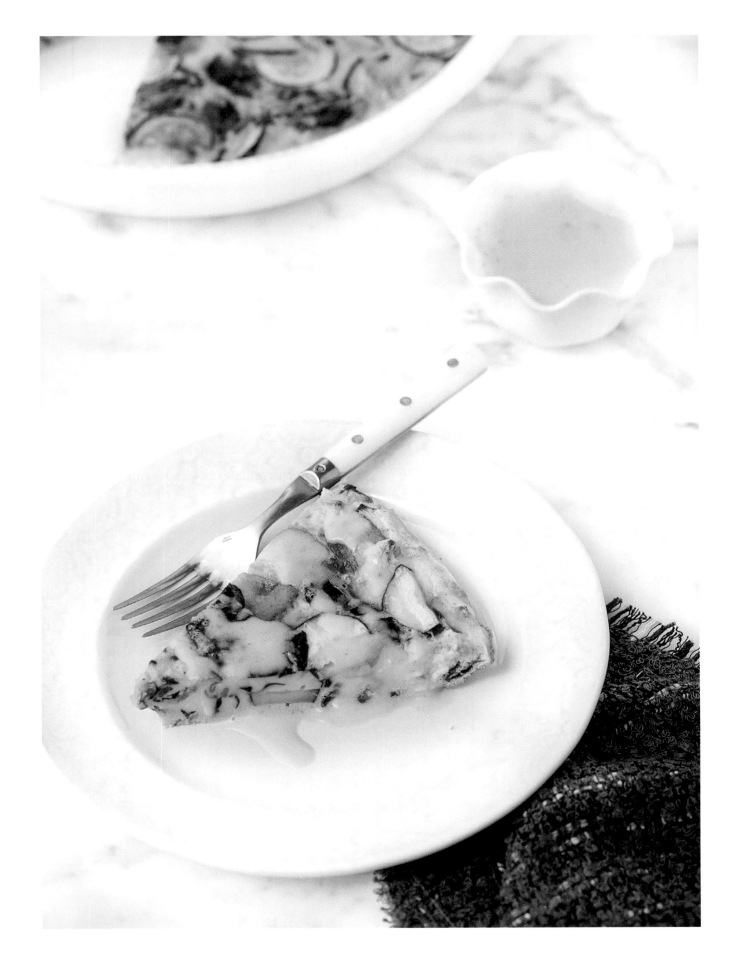

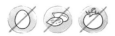

yield: 3 cups
prep time: 10 minutes
cook time: 21 to 23 minutes

There are so many people who cannot eat nuts, as well as schools that are nut-free, and I constantly get requests to change my ever-popular granola recipes into nut-free versions. This one uses a combination of seeds and coconut to provide the crunch, without grains or nuts.

# nut-free granola

## ingredients

- 2 tablespoons warm water
- 1 tablespoon chia seeds
- ½ cup honey
- 2 tablespoons coconut oil
- 2 tablespoons unsweetened sunflower seed butter
- ¾ cup raw pepitas
- ¾ cup raw sunflower seeds
- 2 tablespoons sesame seeds
- ½ teaspoon sea salt
- 2 teaspoons vanilla extract
- 2 teaspoons ground cinnamon
- 1 cup unsweetened coconut flakes
- ½ cup raisins

## method

1. Preheat the oven to 350°F. Line 2 rimmed baking sheets with parchment paper.

2. Mix the warm water and chia seeds in a small bowl and place in the refrigerator.

3. Melt the honey in a saucepan over medium-high heat. Simmer on medium-low for 5 to 7 minutes, until a candy thermometer reads 225°F. Stir in the coconut oil and sunflower seed butter and remove from the heat.

4. Meanwhile, combine the pepitas, sunflower seeds, sesame seeds, salt, vanilla, and cinnamon in a food processor. Pulse a few times, until everything is ground and resembles coarse sand.

5. Stir in the melted honey mixture, coconut flakes, and soaked chia seeds, then thinly spread the mixture on the prepared baking sheets.

6. Bake for 8 minutes, stir, then continue baking for another 8 minutes, until the granola is browned. Stir in the raisins, then allow the granola to cool completely before storing.

tidbits:

Unsalted raw seeds work best.

Pepitas may also be labeled pumpkin seeds.

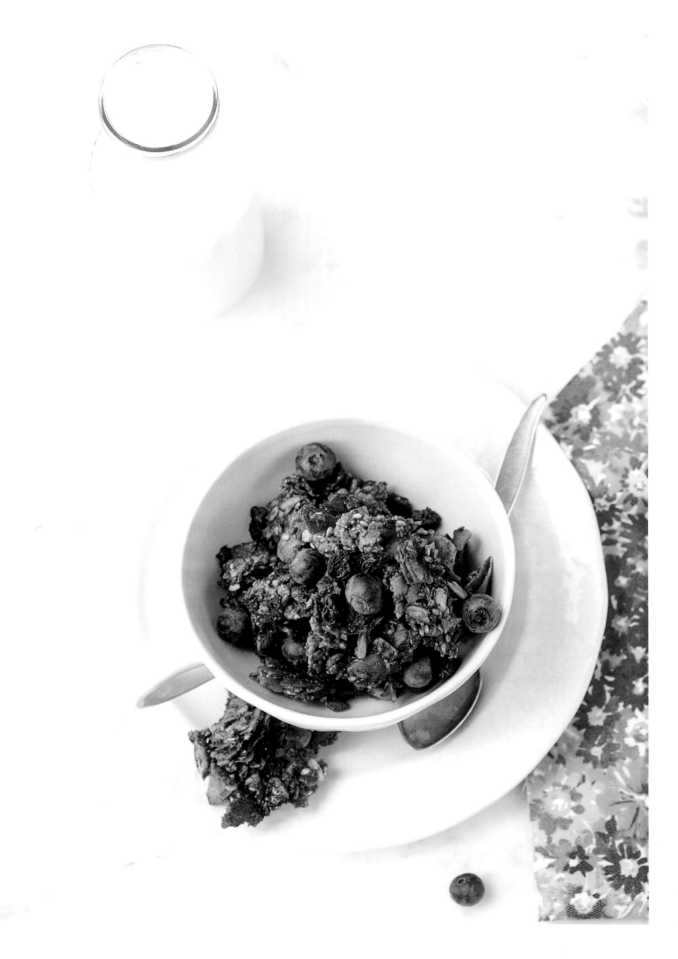

SCD

serves: 6 to 8
prep time: 20 minutes
cook time: 6 to 8 hours

Let breakfast cook while you sleep with this easy overnight casserole! There's nothing like waking up to the smell of bacon and sausage and having breakfast ready to go when you're drowsy and hungry.

# overnight breakfast casserole

## ingredients

- palm shortening or softened ghee, for greasing the slow cooker
- ½ pound bulk breakfast sausage, crumbled
- 6 ounces bacon, chopped
- ½ cup diced yellow onion
- 1 pound white sweet potatoes, peeled and shredded*
- 1 red bell pepper, seeded and diced
- 1 orange bell pepper, seeded and diced
- 16 large eggs, beaten
- ½ cup Almond Milk (page 240)**
- ¼ cup full-fat coconut milk
- 1 teaspoon sea salt
- ¾ teaspoon dry mustard
- ¼ teaspoon cracked black pepper

\* For SCD, substitute shredded celeriac.

\*\* For nut-free, use a total of ½ cup coconut milk and omit the Almond Milk.

## method

1. Grease a slow cooker insert well with palm shortening or softened ghee.

2. Cook the sausage, bacon, and onion in a skillet over medium-high heat for 10 to 12 minutes, until the sausage is browned and the onion is softened. Drain off the excess fat.

3. Place the shredded sweet potatoes in the slow cooker, packing them down slightly.

4. Add the meat and onion mixture and the bell peppers.

5. In a large bowl, whisk together the eggs, milks, salt, mustard, and pepper. Pour into the slow cooker.

6. Cover and cook on low for 6 to 8 hours.

tidbits:
Substitute or add in your favorite vegetables. Just be sure to choose vegetables that will stand up to the long cooking time and not get soggy. Mushrooms, asparagus, broccoli, or winter squash would all be great additions.

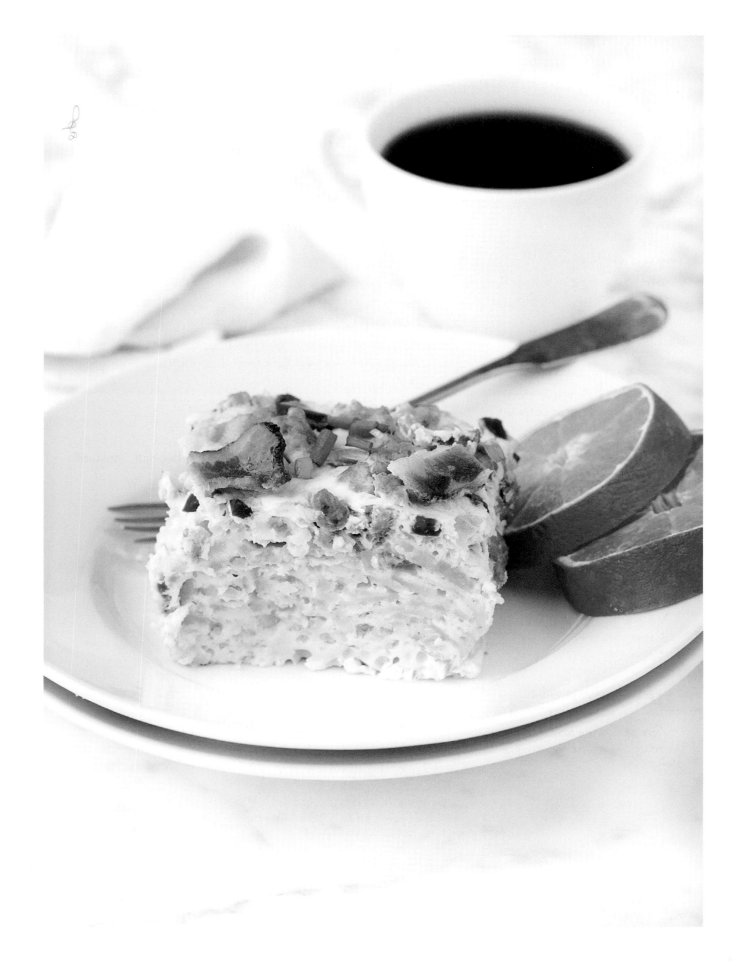

yield: 1 (8½-by-4½-inch) loaf
prep time: 10 minutes
cook time: 60 minutes

There's nothing better than a fluffy loaf of rich pumpkin bread with all the flavors of the fall and winter seasons! I worked diligently to create this loaf especially for those who are sensitive to nuts and coconut, and it has been a longtime favorite on my blog ever since. See my blog, againstallgrain.com, for an SCD-friendly version.

# pumpkin bread

## ingredients

- 2 large eggs
- ¾ cup unsweetened sunflower seed butter or tahini
- ½ cup grade B maple syrup or honey
- ½ cup pumpkin puree
- 3 tablespoons softened palm shortening, ghee, or coconut oil, plus more for greasing the pan
- 2 teaspoons fresh lemon juice
- 1 teaspoon vanilla extract
- ½ cup arrowroot powder
- 1½ tablespoons ground cinnamon
- 2 teaspoons ground nutmeg
- 2 teaspoons grain-free baking powder (see Tidbits)
- ½ teaspoon grated lemon zest
- ½ teaspoon ground ginger
- ¼ teaspoon sea salt

## method

1. Preheat the oven to 350°F. Lightly grease an 8½-by-4½-inch loaf pan, then place a piece of parchment paper on the bottom of the pan.

2. In a high-speed blender or food processor, combine the eggs, sunflower seed butter, maple syrup, pumpkin puree, palm shortening, lemon juice, and vanilla. Purée for 30 seconds, until smooth and creamy.

3. Add the arrowroot powder, cinnamon, nutmeg, baking powder, lemon zest, ginger, and salt. Blend for 30 seconds, until well combined.

4. Pour the batter into the prepared loaf pan. Bake for 60 minutes, until a toothpick comes out clean when inserted in the middle.

5. Remove the loaf from the oven and allow to cool in the pan for 15 minutes. Remove from the pan and allow to cool completely on a wire rack before eating.

tidbits:

Hain baking powder contains potato starch but is grain-free and does not use the standard cornstarch. To make a starch-free baking powder, mix 1 teaspoon baking soda with 2 teaspoons cream of tartar, then measure the 2 teaspoons called for. My purpose for using baking powder here is to prevent the loaf from turning green with the use of sunflower seed butter.

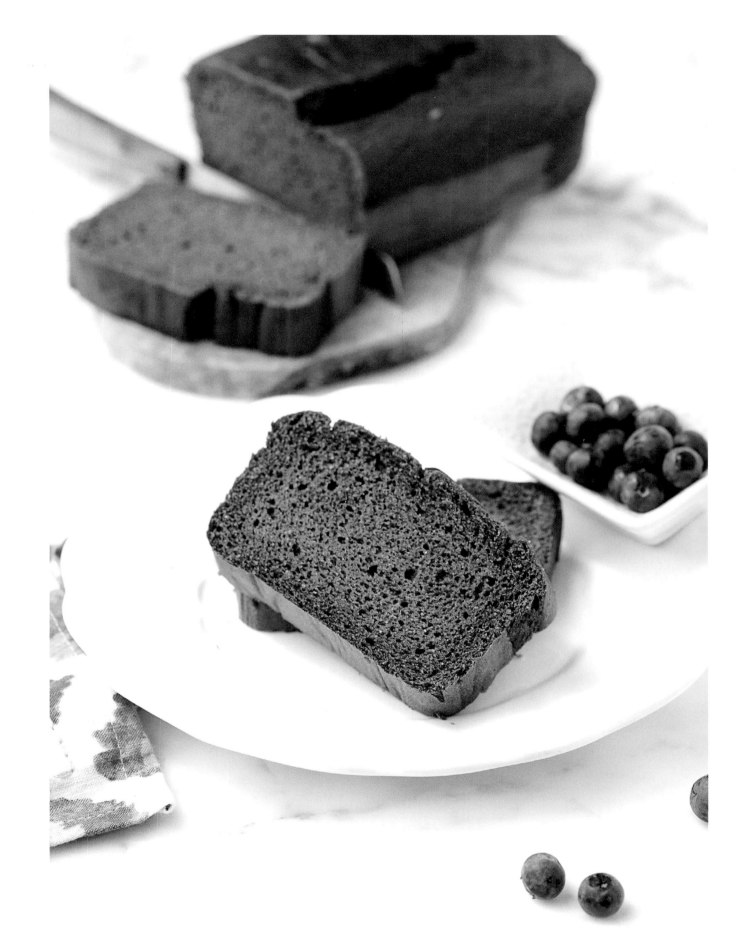

yield: 24 waffles

prep time: 5 minutes

cook time: 15 minutes

Whether you are serving these waffles immediately or making a large batch to freeze for quick and easy breakfasts on the run, they are simple to whip up and will become a family favorite.

# freezer waffles

## ingredients

- palm shortening or coconut oil, for greasing the waffle iron
- 6 large eggs
- 1 cup Almond Milk (page 240) or full-fat coconut milk
- 2 cups Pancake Mix (page 260)
- ¼ cup melted ghee or coconut oil
- ¼ cup coconut crystals or honey
- 1 teaspoon vanilla extract

## method

1. Preheat a waffle iron and lightly brush with palm shortening.

2. Place all of the ingredients in a blender or food processor, in the order listed.

3. Blend on high for 30 seconds. Scrape the sides of the blender container with a spatula and blend again until smooth.

4. Pour batter into the waffle iron in the amount recommended in the manufacturer's instructions, and close the lid. Cook until the indicator light goes off.

5. Repeat until all of the batter has been used.

make-ahead tip:
Allow the waffles to cool completely and then freeze them individually on a tray before placing together in a freezer-safe bag or container. Freeze for up to 6 months, and reheat in the toaster directly from the freezer.

tidbits:
I find that these freezer waffles stick the least and stay an even brown color when the waffle iron is greased with palm shortening; however, ghee or coconut oil will work as well.

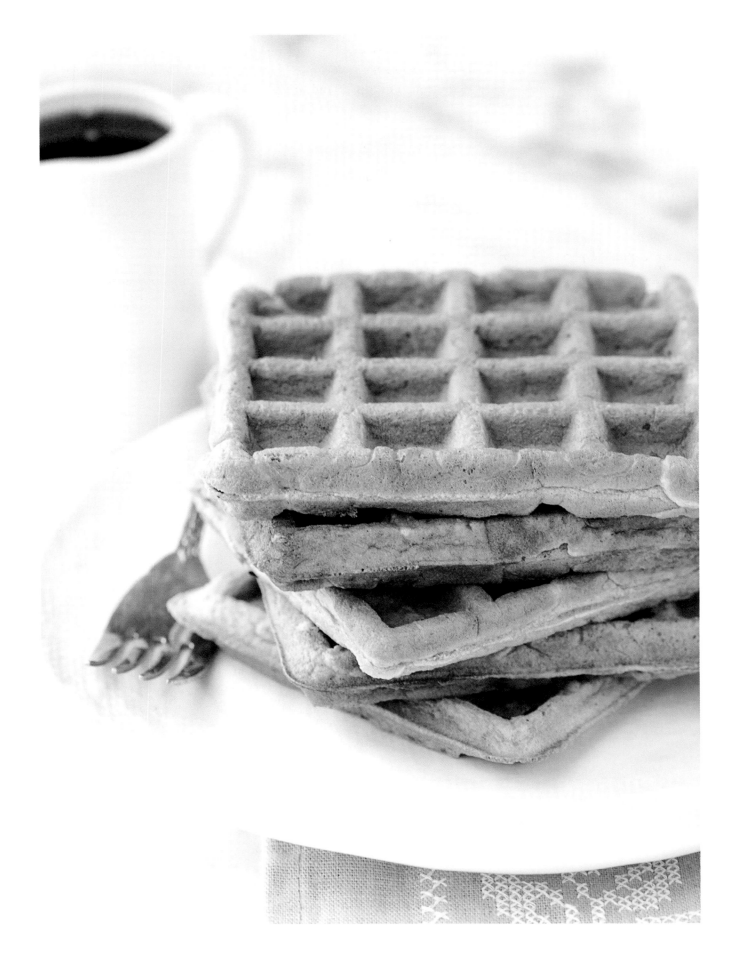

yield: 24 (4-inch) pancakes
prep time: 5 minutes
cook time: 15 minutes

This is the same batter recipe that was used for the waffles on the previous page, but these instructions are for tried-and-true pancake lovers or those who do not own a waffle iron. The same batter produces both fluffy pancakes and waffles, without alterations.

# fluffy pancakes

## ingredients

- palm shortening, for greasing the pan
- 6 large eggs
- 1 cup Almond Milk (page 240) or full-fat coconut milk
- 2 cups Pancake Mix (page 260)
- ¼ cup melted ghee or coconut oil
- ¼ cup coconut crystals or honey
- 1 teaspoon vanilla extract

## method

1. Heat a well-seasoned cast-iron skillet or griddle over medium heat. Add a teaspoon of palm shortening and swirl to coat the pan.

2. Place all of the ingredients in a blender or food processor, in the order listed.

3. Blend on high for 30 seconds, until smooth. Scrape the sides of the blender container with a spatula and blend again if necessary.

4. Pour about ¼ cup of the batter per pancake onto the pan and spread lightly into a 4-inch-wide circle. Cook for 2 to 3 minutes on the first side, until bubbles form on the surface and the sides lift easily. Flip and cook for 1 to 2 more minutes.

5. Repeat with the remaining batter, adding a little more oil to the pan if the pancakes begin to stick.

make-ahead tip:
Allow the pancakes to cool completely and then freeze them individually on a tray before placing together in a freezer-safe bag or container. Freeze for up to 6 months, and reheat in the toaster directly from the freezer.

tidbits:
I find that these pancakes flip the best and stay an even brown color when the pan is greased with palm shortening; however, ghee or coconut oil will work as well.

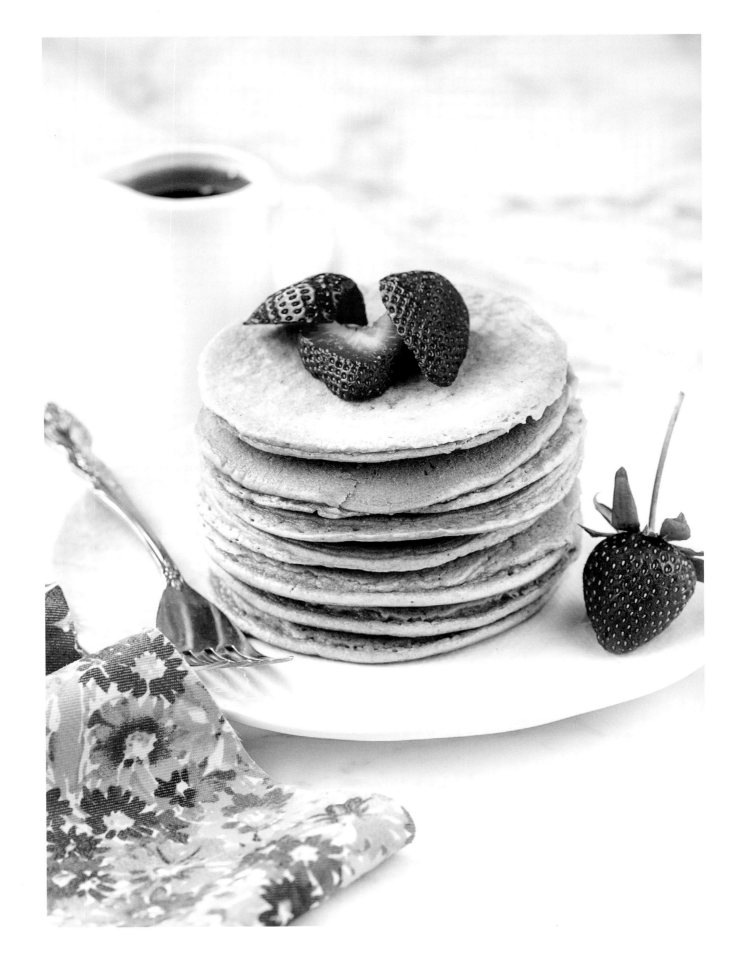

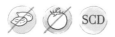

serves: 4

prep time: 5 minutes

cook time: 15 minutes

Shirred eggs are so easy to prepare and make an elegant breakfast. The eggs are nestled in a vessel of ham and baked with a hint of coconut milk for creaminess and some fresh herbs for brightness.

## shirred eggs with ham

### ingredients

- 1 tablespoon bacon fat or ghee
- 8 slices ham or prosciutto
- 8 large eggs
- 2 tablespoons full-fat coconut milk
- pinch of sea salt and cracked black pepper
- 2 teaspoons chopped fresh thyme, tarragon, or chives
- mixed greens, for serving (optional)

### method

1. Preheat the oven to 375°F.

2. Melt the bacon fat in a 10-inch cast-iron skillet over medium-high heat and swirl to coat the pan.

3. Overlap the ham pieces in the bottom and up the sides of the skillet and cook for 2 minutes.

4. Remove the pan from the heat and gently crack the eggs on top. Drizzle the coconut milk over the eggs and sprinkle with the salt, pepper, and herbs.

5. Place the pan in the oven and bake for 10 to 12 minutes, until the whites are set but the yolks are still soft. Check frequently to ensure that the eggs are not overcooking.

6. Serve directly from the skillet or over a bed of greens.

tidbits:

For even more decadence, add a drizzle of Hollandaise Sauce (page 252) over the top after the eggs have baked.

I frequently cut the recipe and make this dish just for myself using a 5-inch personal-sized skillet. The baking time will vary based on the pan size, so watch the eggs closely.

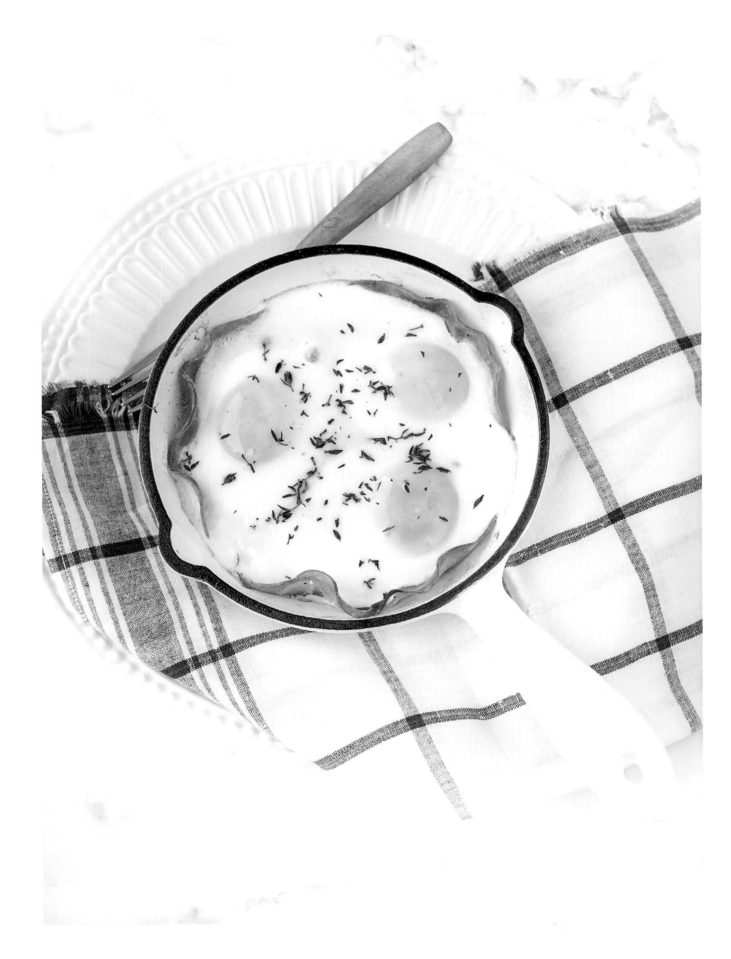

There's something about the aroma of blueberries baking in the oven with a sweet dough surrounding them. You can just smell the juices popping out of the skins and sweetening with the heat. I make a big batch of these muffins and keep them in the freezer for quick breakfasts on the run.

# blueberry muffins

## ingredients

### MUFFINS

- 2 large eggs, at room temperature
- 2 tablespoons fresh lemon juice
- 1/3 cup palm shortening or ghee, softened
- 1 teaspoon vanilla extract
- 1/3 cup honey
- 1/2 cup warm water
- 1¾ cups Pancake Mix (page 260)
- 1/2 teaspoon ground cinnamon
- 1/2 cup fresh blueberries

### TOPPING (OPTIONAL)

- 1/3 cup raw pecan halves
- 1 tablespoon unsweetened shredded coconut
- 1 tablespoon solid coconut oil
- 1 tablespoon blanched almond flour
- 1 tablespoon coconut crystals or honey
- ¾ teaspoon ground cinnamon
- 1 large date, pitted
- pinch of sea salt

## method

1. Preheat the oven to 350°F. Place a heatproof dish filled with 2 cups of water on the bottom rack. Position another rack in the center of the oven.

2. Place all of the muffin ingredients except the blueberries in a high-speed blender or food processor in the order listed and blend for 30 seconds. Scrape down the sides, then blend again until very smooth.

3. Stir in the blueberries by hand.

4. Grease 10 cups of a 12-cup muffin tin or line with paper cups. Spoon the batter into the cups, filling each cup two-thirds of the way full.

5. If making the streusel topping, place all of the topping ingredients in a food processor and pulse a few times, until the mixture resembles coarse sand. Sprinkle the topping over the batter.

6. Place the muffins in the oven on the center rack and bake for 20 to 25 minutes, until a toothpick inserted into the center of a muffin comes out clean. Remove to a wire rack and let cool. Store any leftovers in the refrigerator for up to 1 week or in the freezer for up to 6 months. Thaw to room temperature or in a warm oven.

make-ahead tip:
Double this recipe and store half in the freezer. Defrost in a toaster oven or oven when ready to consume, or at room temperature for 2 hours.

tidbits:
The steam bath increases the rise and keeps the almond flour from browning while baking, resulting in moist and fluffy muffins.

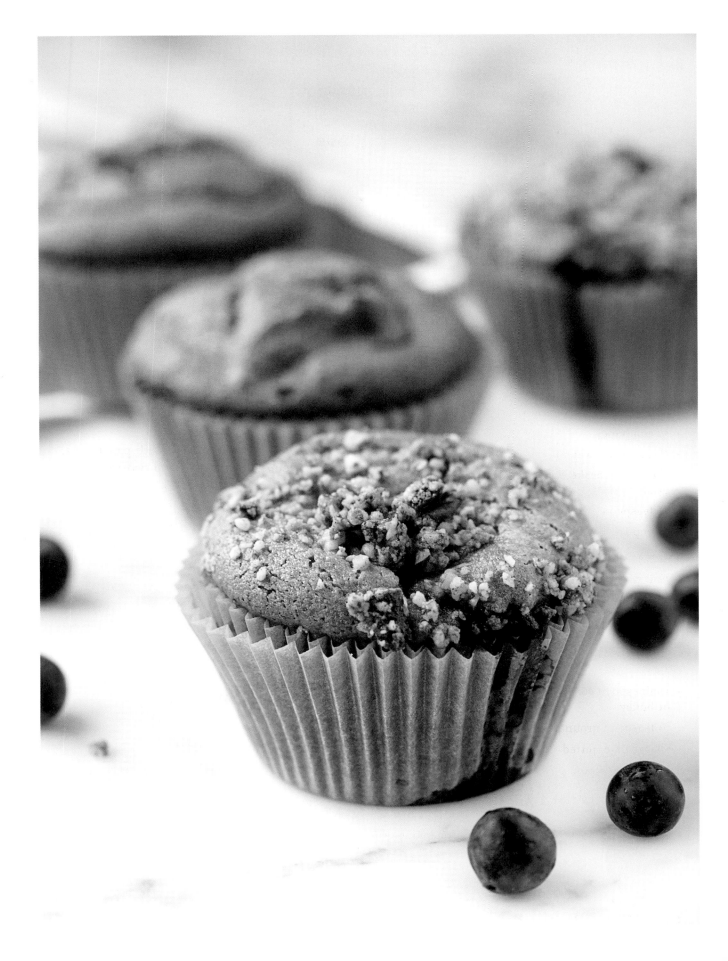

yield: 12 sandwiches
prep time: 40 minutes
cook time: 20 minutes

These sandwiches use two other recipes—my Biscuits (page 56) and homemade breakfast sausage (page 52)—to create a breakfast that can be frozen and defrosted when you are on the run and need something quick! Once the base sandwich is made, you can dress it up with any of the optional condiments.

# sausage breakfast sandwiches

## ingredients

- 1½ batches Biscuits (page 56)
- 1 batch sausage (page 52)
- 1 tablespoon ghee or bacon fat
- 12 large eggs
- 2 teaspoons Almond Milk (page 240) or water
- ¼ teaspoon sea salt
- ¼ teaspoon cracked black pepper
- optional condiments: Mayonnaise (page 248), Pesto Sauce (page 256), Guacamole (page 258)

## method

1. Prepare the Biscuits according to the method on page 56.

2. While the Biscuits bake, combine the sausage ingredients listed on page 52 in a bowl and form the mixture into 12 patties.

3. Heat the ghee in a large skillet over medium heat. Cook the sausage patties for 3 to 4 minutes on each side, until cooked through. Remove the sausage patties from the pan and set aside on paper towels.

4. In a bowl, whisk the eggs with the Almond Milk, salt, and pepper. Scramble the eggs in the skillet over medium-high heat for 8 to 10 minutes, until firm.

5. Cut the Biscuits in half and divide the sausage patties and eggs evenly among the sandwiches. Top with condiments, if desired.

make-ahead tip:
To freeze, let all of the ingredients cool to room temperature before assembling the sandwiches, and leave off any optional condiments. Wrap the sandwiches individually in foil or parchment paper and store together in a resealable bag or container in the freezer. To reheat, place a wrapped frozen sandwich in a 400°F oven for 25 minutes, until heated through, or wrap in a paper towel and heat in the microwave for 2 minutes.

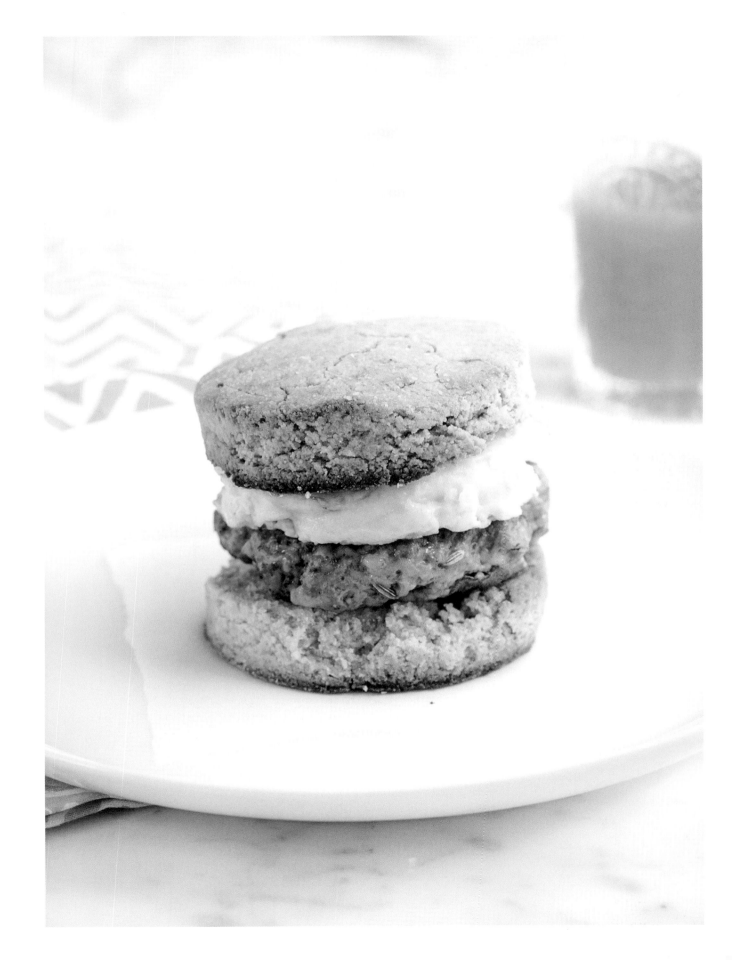

Whip up one of these smoothies on a busy morning and add your favorite supplements for an extra boost. We often add Great Lakes gelatin or L-glutamine to ours for gut health!

serves: 2

prep time: 5 to 10 minutes

## quick smoothies

### banana choco-malt

#### ingredients

- 1½ cups Almond Milk (page 240) or ¾ cup coconut milk and ¾ cup water
- 1 medium banana, frozen or fresh
- ½ cup crushed ice
- 2 or 3 dates (Medjool or Deglet Noor), pitted
- 2 tablespoons unsweetened almond butter
- 2 tablespoons cacao powder
- 1 teaspoon golden flaxseeds
- 1 cup baby spinach

### asher's "green" smoothie

#### ingredients

- 1½ cups cold water or unsweetened apple juice
- 1 small banana, frozen or fresh
- 1 cup frozen mixed berries
- ½ small avocado
- 1 cup chopped fresh kale

### cucumber melon mint cooler

#### ingredients

- 1 cup cold water or unsweetened apple juice
- 1 cup peeled, seeded, and diced cucumber
- 1 cup peeled, seeded, and diced green apple
- ½ cup diced honeydew melon
- ¼ cup chopped fresh mint
- 1 teaspoon honey
- 1 teaspoon fresh lime juice
- ½ cup ice cubes

### island breeze

#### ingredients

- 1½ cups coconut water
- ½ cup frozen strawberries
- ½ cup frozen mango chunks
- 1 medium banana, frozen or fresh

#### method

Place all of the ingredients in a blender in the order listed. Blend on high until smooth.

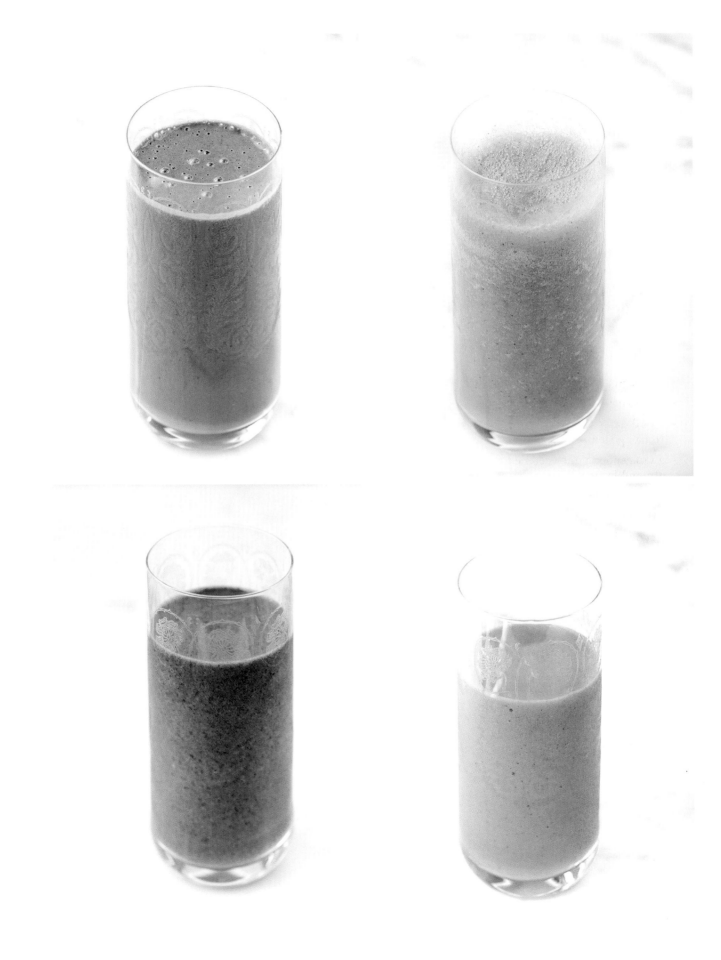

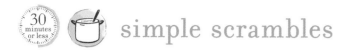 

## chorizo veggie scramble

serves: 2
prep time: 10 minutes
cook time: 6 minutes

### ingredients

- 1 tablespoon ghee
- ½ cup chopped Swiss chard
- ¼ cup diced zucchini
- ¼ cup sliced chorizo sausage
- ¼ cup halved cherry tomatoes
- 6 large eggs, beaten
- pinch of sea salt and cracked black pepper
- 1 avocado, sliced, for serving

### method

1. Melt the ghee in a large skillet over medium heat.

2. Sauté the chard, zucchini, chorizo, and tomatoes for 2 minutes, until the vegetables are mostly cooked.

3. Add the eggs and scramble until cooked through, about 3 to 4 more minutes.

4. Season with salt and pepper and top with avocado slices before serving.

tidbits:
Check the chorizo ingredients carefully. Look for sausage that has a natural pork casing and does not contain any additives or sugar.

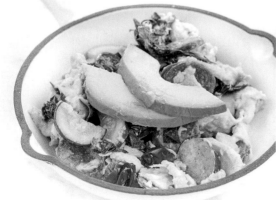

## smoked salmon and sweet potato scramble

serves: 2
prep time: 12 minutes
cook time: 12 minutes

### ingredients

- 3 tablespoons ghee, divided
- ¾ cup peeled and shredded sweet potatoes
- 1 tablespoon sliced leek
- 6 large eggs, beaten
- 1 teaspoon chopped fresh dill
- 2 ounces smoked salmon, thinly sliced
- pinch of sea salt and cracked black pepper

### method

1. Melt 2½ tablespoons of the ghee in a large skillet over medium heat.

2. Sauté the sweet potatoes and leek until browned and crispy, about 8 minutes. Remove from the pan and set aside.

3. Return the pan to the heat with the remaining ½ tablespoon of ghee. Add the eggs and dill and scramble until cooked through, 3 to 4 more minutes. Remove from the heat and stir in the crispy potato mixture and the salmon.

4. Season with salt and pepper.

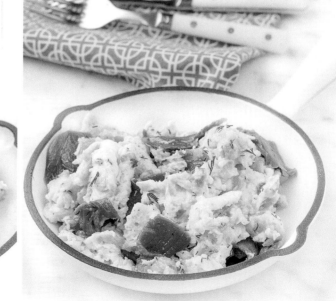

# green veggie scramble

serves: 2
prep time: 8 minutes
cook time: 6 minutes

## ingredients

- 1 tablespoon ghee
- 1 cup baby spinach
- ¼ cup chopped asparagus
- 6 large eggs, beaten
- ½ avocado, diced
- pinch of sea salt and cracked black pepper

## method

1. Melt the ghee in a large skillet over medium heat.

2. Sauté the spinach and asparagus for 2 minutes, until the spinach is wilted and the asparagus is crisp-tender.

3. Add the eggs and scramble until cooked through, about 3 to 4 more minutes. Remove the pan from the heat.

4. Stir in the avocado and season with salt and pepper.

# bacon mushroom scramble

serves: 2
prep time: 10 minutes
cook time: 13 minutes

## ingredients

- 4 slices bacon, diced
- ½ cup sliced mushrooms
- 6 large eggs, beaten
- pinch of sea salt and cracked black pepper

## method

1. Cook the bacon in a large skillet over medium heat, about 5 minutes. Drain half of the grease and return the bacon to the heat.

2. Add the mushrooms and sauté for 3 to 4 minutes, until softened.

3. Add the eggs and scramble until cooked through, 3 to 4 more minutes. Season with salt and pepper.

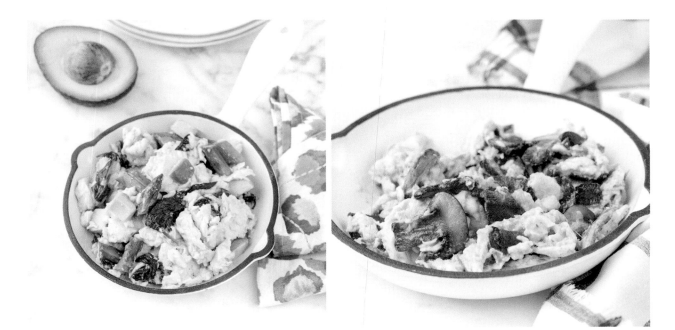

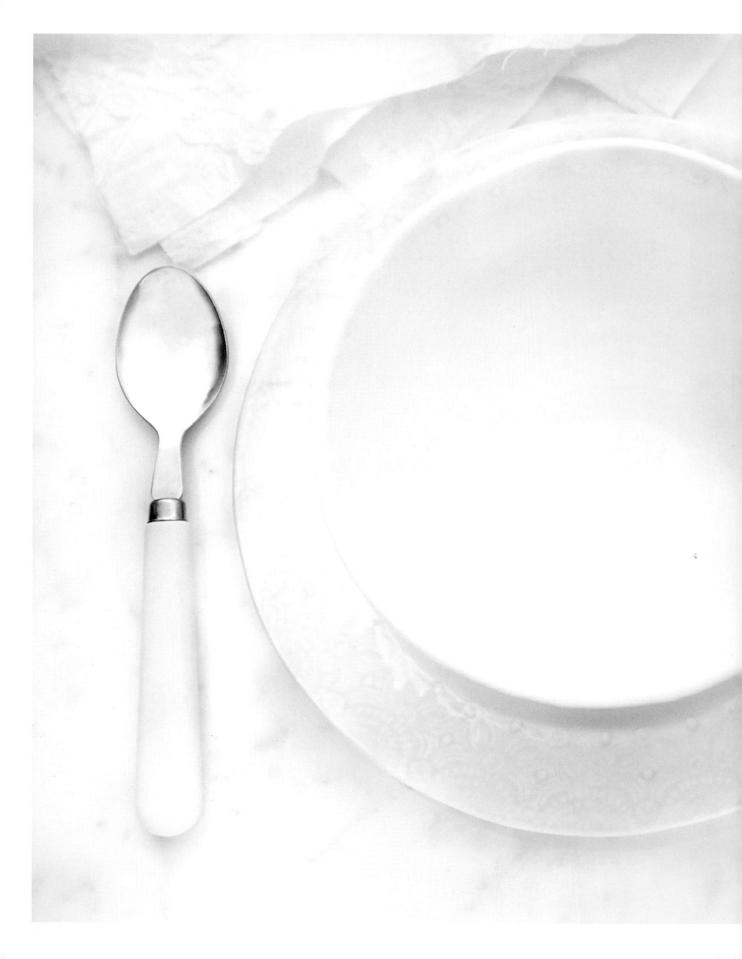

# soups and hearty salads

italian wedding soup / 82

minestrone soup / 84

roasted chicken and vegetable soup / 86

mexican chicken soup / 88

white pork chili / 90

roasted beet and bacon salad / 92

spa salad / 94

buffalo chicken salad / 96

roasted chicken, butternut, and apple salad / 98

chicken waldorf salad / 100

warm taco salad with creamy avocado-cilantro vinaigrette / 102

BLT salad / 104

grilled greek summer squash salad / 106

barbecue chicken chopped salad / 108

greek salad with garlic-oregano lamb / 110

tuna salad / 112

SCD

serves: 8
prep time: 20 minutes
cook time: 18 minutes

This colorful dish marries seasoned meatballs and greens to make a hearty and comforting soup.

# italian wedding soup

## ingredients

### MEATBALLS

- ½ medium yellow onion
- ⅓ cup chopped fresh parsley
- 1 large egg
- 1 clove garlic, minced
- 1 tablespoon almond meal or 2 teaspoons coconut flour
- 2½ teaspoons nutritional yeast
- 1 teaspoon sea salt
- ¼ teaspoon cracked black pepper
- 1 pound ground beef
- ½ pound lean pork

### SOUP

- 1 tablespoon extra-virgin olive oil, ghee, or bacon fat
- 2 cups peeled and diced carrots
- 1 cup diced celery
- 10 cups Chicken Stock (page 242)
- 2 to 3 teaspoons sea salt, divided
- ¼ teaspoon cracked black pepper
- 3 cups baby spinach

## method

1. Make the meatballs: Run the onion through the grating attachment of a food processor or grate with a box grater. Combine it with the remaining meatball ingredients.

2. Form the meat into bite-sized meatballs and place on a rimmed baking sheet. Cover and refrigerate until ready to use.

3. Make the soup: Heat the olive oil in a large stockpot over medium-high heat. Sauté the carrots and celery for 5 minutes.

4. Pour in the Chicken Stock, 2 teaspoons of the salt, and pepper and bring to a boil.

5. Reduce the heat to medium and add the meatballs. Cover and cook for 8 minutes, until the meatballs are cooked through and begin floating to the top.

6. Stir in the spinach and cook for an additional 5 minutes, until wilted.

7. Season to taste, adding up to an additional teaspoon of salt.

> **make-ahead tip:**
> Uncooked meatballs will keep for 2 days in the refrigerator or 3 months in the freezer.
>
> To freeze, place the uncooked meatballs on a rimmed baking sheet lined with parchment paper. Once frozen, transfer the meatballs to a freezer-safe bag or container. Pull the meatballs out the night before and thaw in the refrigerator, or place the entire sealed bag in the sink and run warm water over it until thawed.
>
> **tidbits:**
> Nutritional yeast is used in place of the traditional Parmesan cheese. Substitute ¼ cup grated Parmesan cheese if dairy is tolerated.

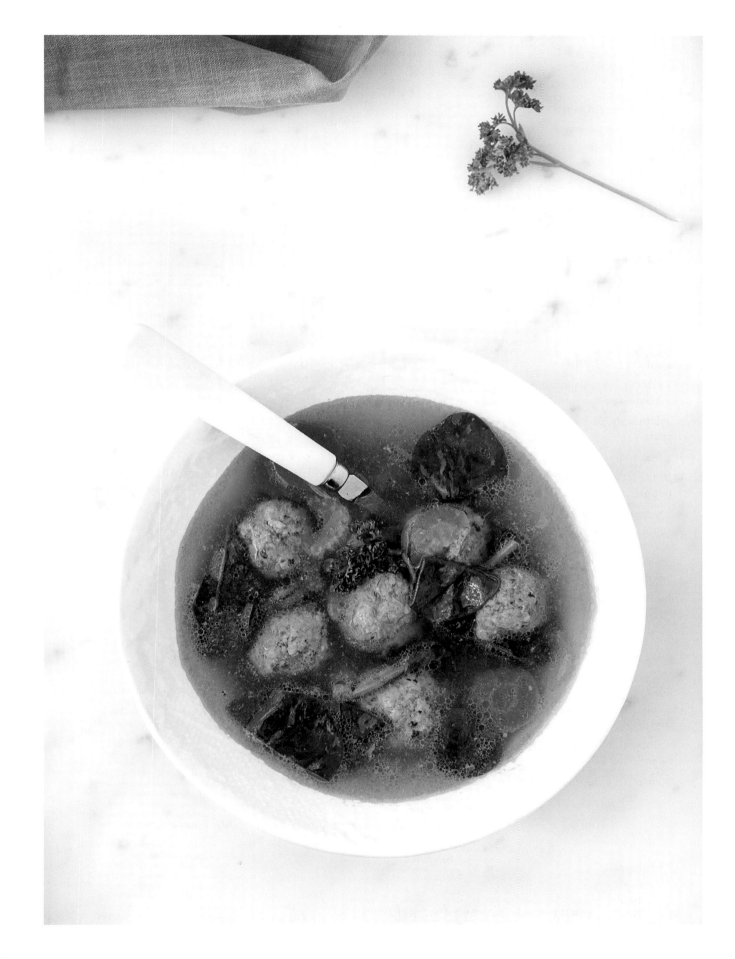

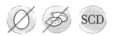

serves: 8 to 10

prep time: 20 minutes

cook time: 6 to 8 hours

Minestrone is a classic, hearty Italian soup that is usually full of vegetables and sometimes meat. While it is known for including beans or pasta, this version omits the legumes and grains and makes up the difference in flavor with added veggies!

# minestrone soup

## ingredients

- 2½ pounds ground beef, turkey, or chicken
- 1 medium yellow onion, chopped
- 4 cloves garlic, minced
- 3 stalks celery, thinly sliced
- 3 cups shredded carrots
- 2 cups peeled and diced celeriac
- 9 cups Chicken Stock (page 242) or low-sodium beef stock
- 24 ounces strained tomatoes
- 1 (18-ounce) jar diced tomatoes
- 3 tablespoons white vinegar
- 2 tablespoons Italian seasoning
- 1½ tablespoons sea salt
- 1 tablespoon dried parsley
- 1 tablespoon ground cumin
- ¾ teaspoon cayenne pepper
- ½ teaspoon cracked black pepper
- ½ pound yellow squash, halved lengthwise and thinly sliced into half-moons
- ½ cup chopped fresh basil, plus more for garnish

## method

1. Brown the ground meat in a large skillet over medium-high heat, until cooked through. Use a slotted spoon to transfer the meat to a slow cooker insert, leaving the fat in the pan.

2. Add the onion, garlic, celery, carrots, and celeriac to the pan and sauté over medium heat for 8 minutes, until the vegetables are slightly tender. Drain and add the vegetables to the slow cooker.

3. Add the remaining ingredients, except the squash and basil. Cover and cook on high for 6 hours or on low for 8 hours.

4. Add the squash and basil during the last 30 minutes if cooking on high or 1 hour if cooking on low.

5. Adjust the seasoning if necessary, and serve with a garnish of fresh basil.

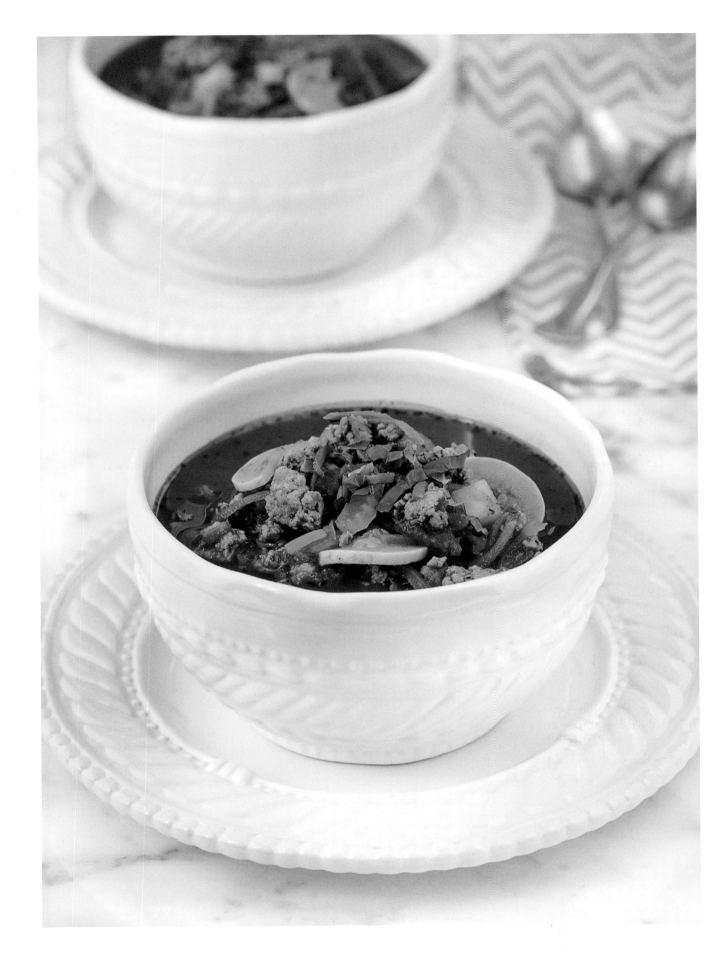

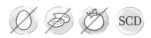

serves: 8 to 10
prep time: 15 minutes
cook time: 30 minutes

Roasted vegetables give this soup the most sensational flavor and a smooth, creamy texture. It is a fabulous way to use up leftover Roasted Chicken (page 118) or rotisserie chicken that you picked up from the market.

# roasted chicken and vegetable soup

## ingredients

ROASTED VEGETABLES

- 6 cloves garlic, peeled
- 1 small sweet potato, peeled and cubed*
- 4 cups peeled and cubed carrots
- 4 cups peeled and cubed butternut squash
- 2 yellow onions, quartered
- ¼ cup melted ghee or coconut oil
- pinch of sea salt and cracked black pepper

SOUP

- 12 cups Chicken Stock (page 242)
- 4 cups cubed cooked chicken
- 2½ teaspoons dried parsley
- 1½ teaspoons dried thyme leaves
- 1½ teaspoons dried rosemary
- 1 teaspoon dried oregano leaves
- 1 tablespoon sea salt
- ½ teaspoon cracked black pepper
- 1 cup water
- 5 cups baby spinach

* For SCD, eliminate the sweet potato and increase the butternut squash to 4½ cups.

## method

1. Preheat the oven to 425°F.

2. Roast the vegetables: Place the garlic and vegetables on a rimmed baking sheet. Drizzle on the ghee, sprinkle with the salt and pepper, and toss to combine. Roast for 20 minutes, until the vegetables are tender.

3. Meanwhile, bring the Chicken Stock to a simmer in a large stockpot. Add the chicken, herbs, salt, and pepper. Keep warm while the vegetables are roasting.

4. Pick out the onion quarters from the pan of roasted vegetables and place them in a blender. Add half of the remaining vegetables to the soup, and place the other half in the blender. Purée the vegetables with the 1 cup of water.

5. Add the vegetable puree and baby spinach to the soup. Simmer for 5 to 10 minutes, until the spinach is wilted and the soup is hot. Adjust the seasonings to taste.

make-ahead tip:
Roast the vegetables up to 3 days in advance and store in the refrigerator.

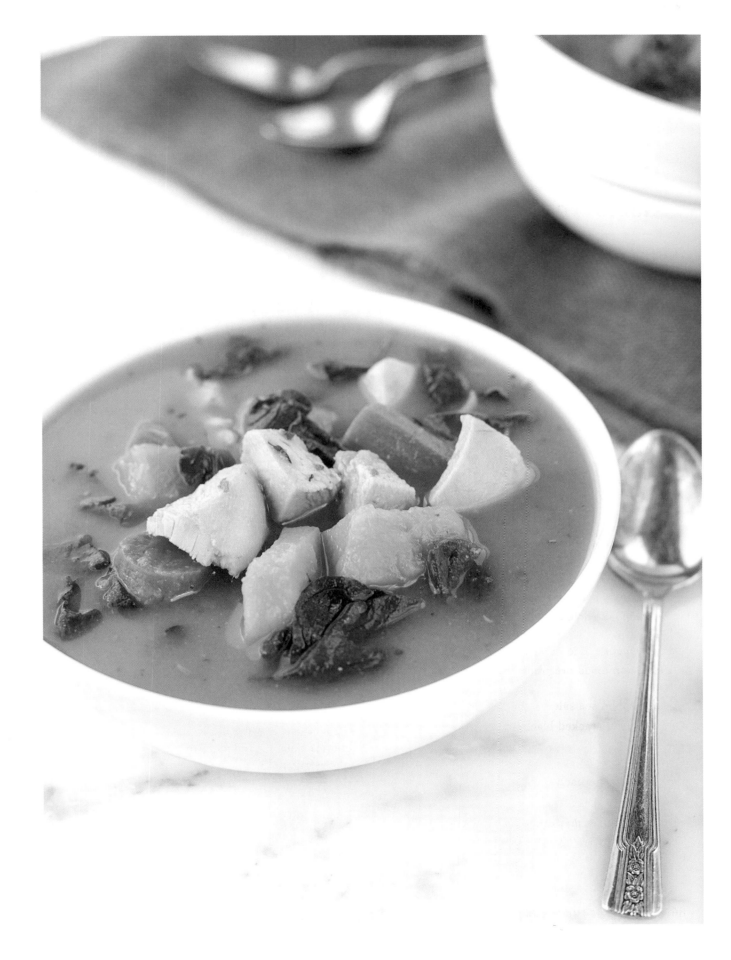

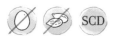

serves: 4 to 6
prep time: 20 minutes
cook time: 6 to 8 hours

Here's a soup that can be thrown together in a snap and is full of bold Mexican flavors. The best part is that it simmers in a slow cooker all day, so it's easy and no fuss! When seeded, the poblano peppers are fairly mild, giving the soup just a hint of chili heat and a distinctive smoky flavor.

# mexican chicken soup

## ingredients

- 9 cups Chicken Stock (page 242)
- 5 large carrots, peeled and cut into ¼-inch-thick discs
- 1 yellow onion, diced
- 2 small poblano peppers, seeded and chopped
- 6 cloves garlic, thinly sliced
- 4 Roma tomatoes, chopped
- 1½ cups tomato juice
- 3 tablespoons Taco Seasoning (page 244)
- 1 tablespoon sea salt
- ½ teaspoon cracked black pepper
- 3 cups shredded leftover Roasted Chicken (page 118)
- juice of 2 limes
- ½ cup chopped fresh cilantro leaves
- 2 avocados, diced, for serving (optional)

## method

1. Place the first 10 ingredients in a slow cooker. Cover and cook for 8 hours on low or 6 hours on high.

2. During the last 30 minutes, add the chicken, lime juice, and cilantro to the slow cooker. Serve with avocado, if desired.

tidbits:
To use fresh chicken, place 1½ pounds of boneless, skinless chicken breasts or thighs in the slow cooker with the other ingredients in Step 1. Remove the chicken at the end, shred it, then return it to the pot before serving.

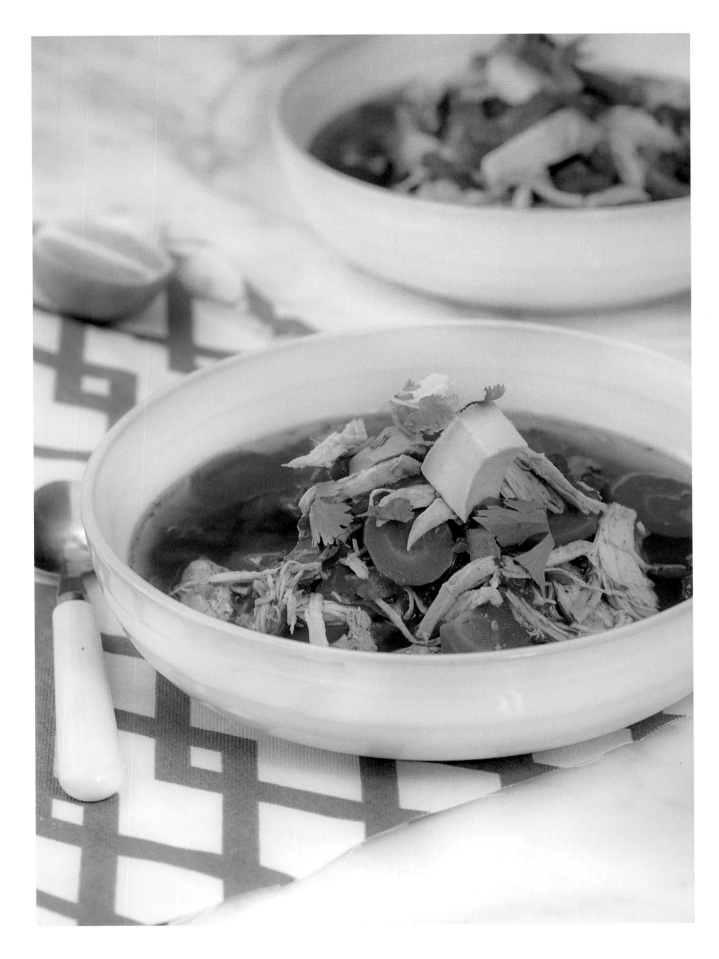

serves: 6 to 8

prep time: 12 minutes

cook time: 22 minutes

This creamy white chili comes together quickly because it uses leftover Maple-Dijon Pork Tenderloin (page 180). It has become an all-time favorite in our home. The mild spiciness paired with the creamy broth and vegetables is so comforting and satisfying!

# white pork chili

## ingredients

- 2 tablespoons ghee or bacon fat
- ½ medium yellow onion, chopped
- 3 cloves garlic, minced
- 2 poblano peppers, seeded and chopped
- 1½ cups diced white sweet potatoes
- 2 teaspoons ground cumin
- 2 teaspoons dried oregano leaves
- 1 teaspoon sea salt
- ¼ teaspoon cracked black pepper
- 1½ cups diced zucchini
- 1 cup hard cider (see Tidbits) or dry white wine
- 4 cups Chicken Stock (page 242)
- 2 cups diced leftover Maple-Dijon Pork Tenderloin (page 180) or other leftover pork
- 1 cup Roasted Tomatillo Salsa (page 258) or store-bought salsa (see Tidbit on page 136)
- ½ cup raw cashew butter
- 1 tablespoon fresh lime juice

## method

1. Heat the ghee in a large stockpot over medium-high heat. Sauté the onion and garlic for 2 minutes, until fragrant. Add the peppers, sweet potatoes, cumin, oregano, salt, and pepper and sauté for 5 minutes more, until the vegetables begin to soften.

2. Add the zucchini and cider and bring to a boil. Reduce the heat and simmer for 5 minutes. Add the remaining ingredients, cover, and cook for 10 minutes longer, until the vegetables are soft and the pork is warmed through.

make-ahead tip:
Chop all the vegetables the night before and make or purchase the salsa beforehand to speed up prep work and get this soup on the table in 30 minutes.

tidbits:
Hard cider is a fermented alcoholic beverage made from apples and typically is naturally gluten-free, but double-check the bottle before you purchase it.

Leftover Roasted Chicken (page 118) works equally well in this recipe!

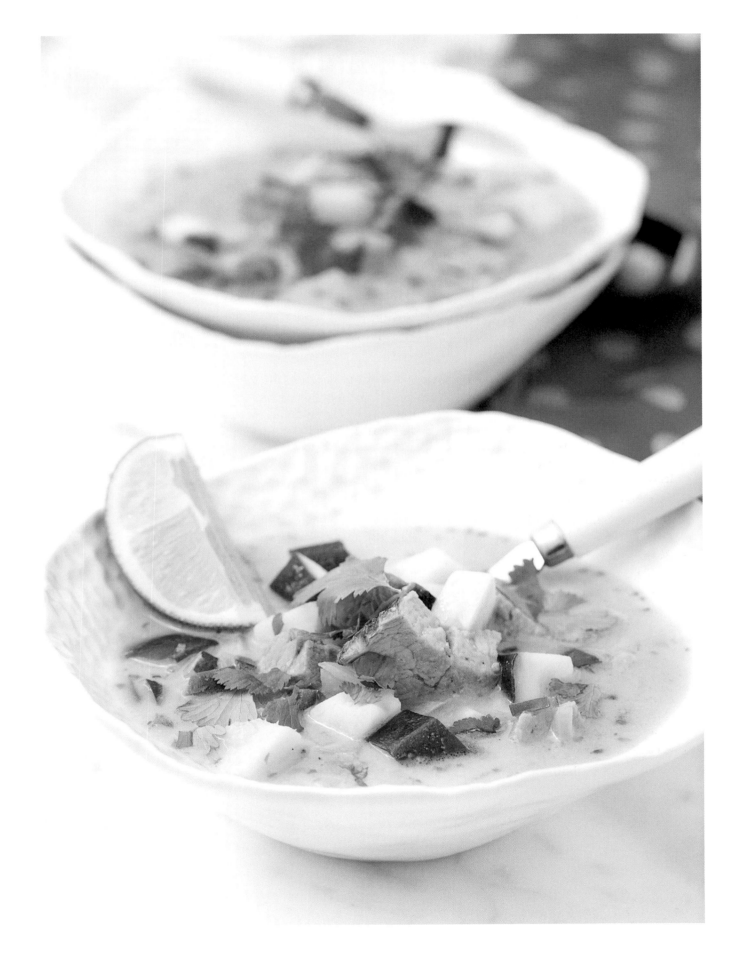

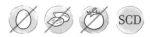

serves: 4 to 6
prep time: 20 minutes
cook time: 35 minutes

I first made this salad on a whim when I had a lot of ingredients to use up. It quickly became a family favorite and is the first salad my husband requests. I think it's the bacon and sweet roasted beets that won him over.

# roasted beet and bacon salad

## ingredients

- 2 medium beets, peeled and thinly sliced
- 6 slices bacon
- ¼ cup raw pecans, chopped*
- 2 red Anjou pears, sliced
- 2 avocados, diced
- 1 head red leaf lettuce, torn into bite-sized pieces
- ¼ cup Champagne Vinaigrette (page 247)

* Omit for nut-free.

## method

1. Place the sliced beets on a rimmed baking sheet. Top with the bacon.

2. Turn the oven on to 400°F and place the tray in the oven without preheating. Roast for 15 minutes, then toss to coat the beets in the rendered bacon fat. Spread everything into a single layer and continue roasting for 15 minutes, until the beets and bacon are slightly crispy.

3. Add the pecans and roast for 5 more minutes. Spoon onto paper towels to drain and set aside to cool. Chop the bacon once cooled.

4. Place the bacon, beets, and pecans in a large salad bowl along with the pears, avocados, and lettuce. Drizzle with the Champagne Vinaigrette, toss to coat, and serve.

tidbits:
If you can tolerate dairy, goat cheese tastes incredible on this salad!

Use whatever fruit is in season: apples, pears, nectarines, and peaches all taste great.

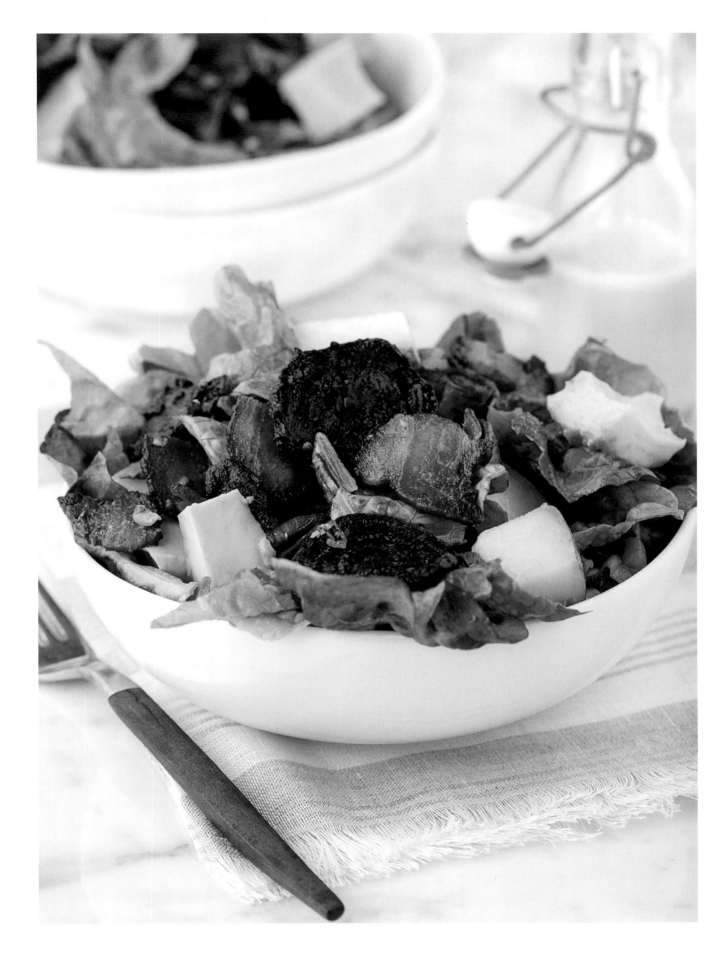

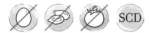

SCD

serves: 4 to 6
prep time: 15 minutes

With an array of fresh fruits and omega-3-rich smoked salmon, this salad will leave you feeling satisfied and replenished.

## 30 minutes or less  spa salad

### ingredients

- 6 cups mixed baby lettuces
- 4 cups chopped butter lettuce, such as Boston or Bibb lettuce
- 1 Bosc pear, cubed
- 3 tangerines, peeled and segmented
- 2 avocados, cubed
- 1 mango, peeled and sliced
- 4 ounces thinly sliced smoked salmon
- ¼ cup pecans*, toasted
- ¼ cup pomegranate seeds
- ¼ cup Champagne Vinaigrette (page 247)

* Omit for nut-free.

### method

Toss all of the ingredients together in a bowl and drizzle with the Champagne Vinaigrette.

make-ahead tip:
Make a double batch of the vinaigrette and use it throughout the week on lunch salads. I often carry a small bottle with me for dining out as well!

This salad travels well for packed lunches. Just leave the dressing separate until ready to eat.

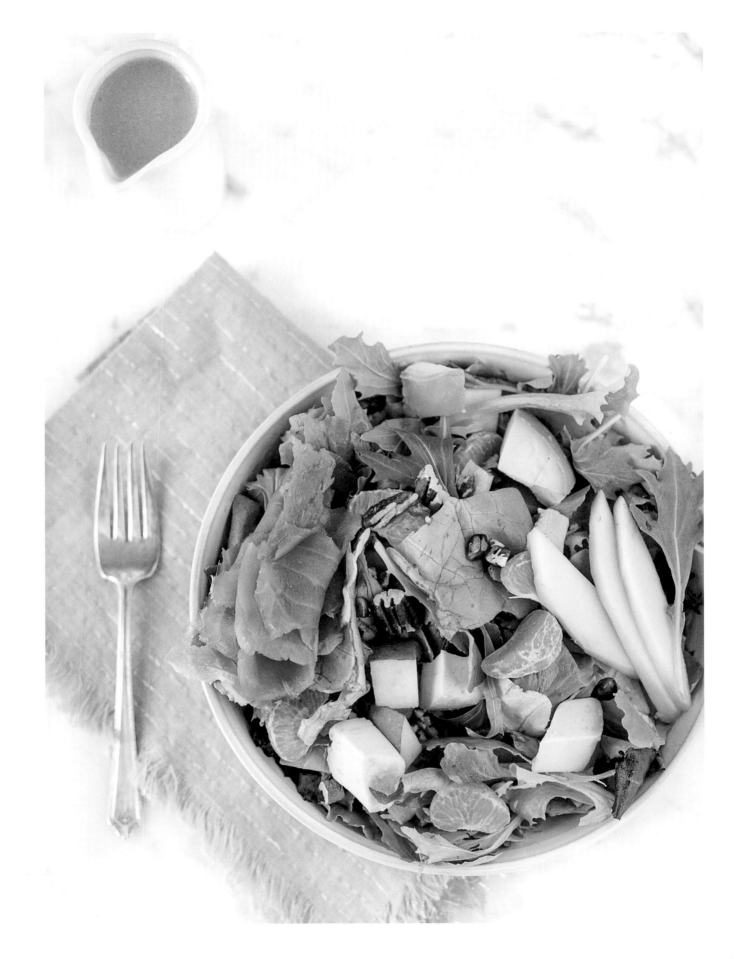

SCD

serves: 6 to 8

prep time: 20 minutes

cook time: 4 hours

The combination of spicy Buffalo sauce and cool Herb Ranch Dressing has always been one of my favorites. I throw the chicken into the slow cooker and let it cook in the sauce for a meal that is stress-free and perfectly flavored.

# buffalo chicken salad

## ingredients

- 3 pounds boneless, skinless chicken breasts
- ¾ cup Buffalo sauce or hot sauce (see Tidbits)
- ¼ cup melted ghee
- 1 tablespoon white vinegar
- 1½ teaspoons sea salt
- ½ teaspoon cayenne pepper
- 3 heads romaine lettuce, torn into bite-sized pieces
- 4 stalks celery, diced
- 3 carrots, peeled and shaved with a vegetable peeler
- ½ cup Herb Ranch Dressing (page 247)

## method

1. Place the chicken, Buffalo sauce, ghee, vinegar, salt, and cayenne pepper in a slow cooker.

2. Cook on high for 3 to 4 hours, flipping the chicken once.

3. Shred the chicken with 2 forks, then stir in ¾ to 1 cup of the sauce from the slow cooker, depending on the spice level desired.

4. Toss the lettuce, celery, carrots, and Herb Ranch Dressing together in a bowl. Divide among plates and serve the shredded chicken over the top.

tidbits:

Want to bulk this salad up even more? Bacon, avocado, and tomatoes are fabulous additions!

Tessemae's hot sauce (aka wing sauce) and the jalapeño pepper sauce from Arizona Pepper's Organic Harvest Foods are both great brands of hot sauce.

make-ahead tip:

Combine the ingredients in Step 1, place in an airtight container, and store in the freezer for up to 6 months. Thaw in the refrigerator the night before, then resume the recipe with Step 2.

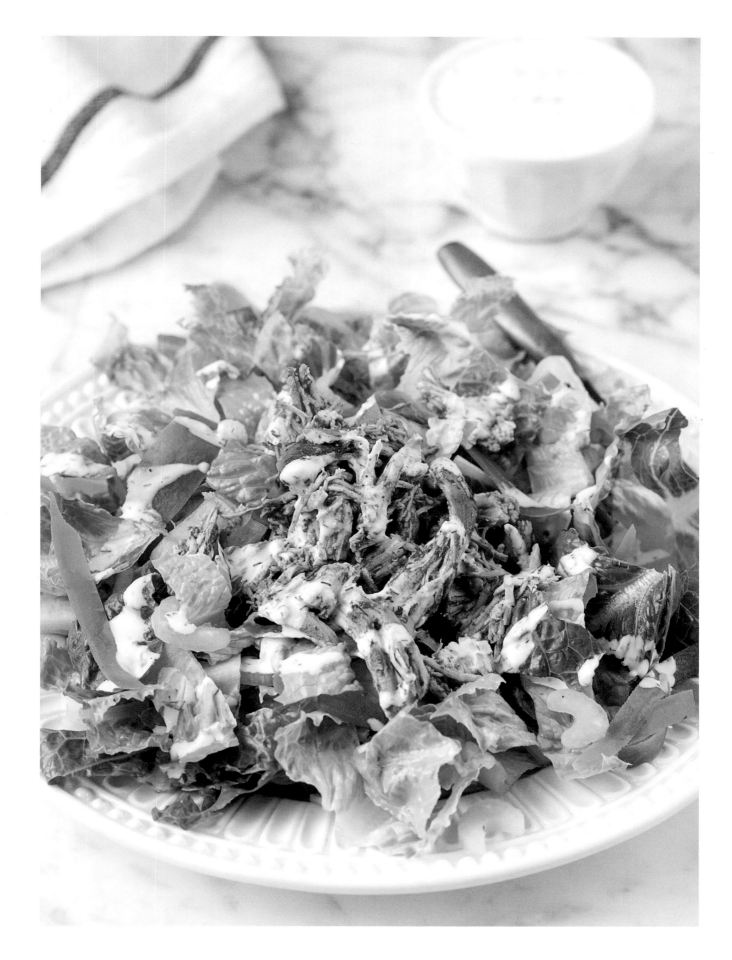

Ø Ø Ø SCD

Use up your leftover roasted chicken in this warm and satisfying salad.

serves: 4 to 6
prep time: 15 minutes
cook time: 15 minutes

30 minutes or less

# roasted chicken, butternut, and apple salad

## ingredients

- 4 ounces prosciutto or bacon, chopped
- ½ cup peeled and cubed butternut squash
- 3 cups shredded cooked chicken
- 2 Fuji apples, julienned
- 1 head escarole, torn into bite-sized pieces
- 1 head butter lettuce, torn into bite-sized pieces
- ½ cup Champagne Vinaigrette (page 247)

## method

1. In a skillet over medium-high heat, cook the prosciutto or bacon until crispy. If using prosciutto, add a teaspoon of bacon fat or ghee to the pan when heating. Remove with a slotted spoon and set aside on paper towels to cool.

2. Add the butternut squash, cover, and cook for 5 minutes. Stir, cover again, and cook for an additional 3 to 5 minutes, until the squash is cooked through and browned.

3. In a bowl, mix together the cooked prosciutto or bacon, chicken, butternut squash, apples, and lettuces.

4. Drizzle the Champagne Vinaigrette over the salad, toss, and serve.

make-ahead tip:
To save time, reserve ½ cup of the cooked butternut squash from the Roasted Chickens with Thyme Gravy (page 118). After completing Step 1, add the squash to the hot pan and cook just long enough to heat through, then continue to Step 3.

tidbits:
Don't have leftover cooked chicken on hand? See the Tidbits tip on page 100 for the quickest way to cook chicken for salads and wraps.

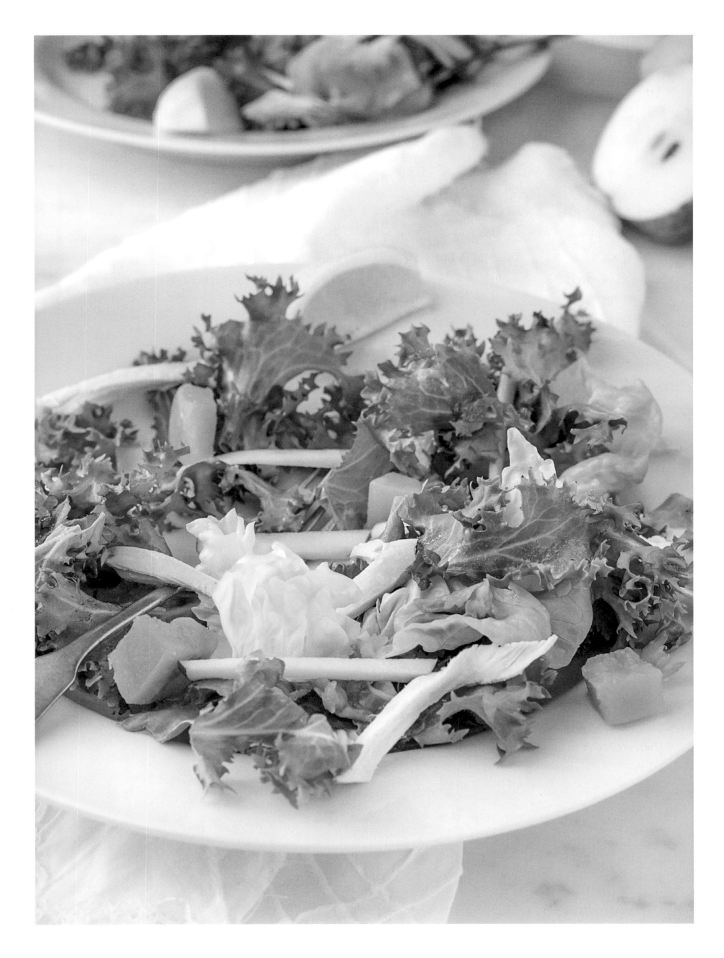

serves: 6

prep time: 15 minutes

This classic salad combines crisp fruit, crunchy walnuts, and tender chicken and is tossed in my dairy-free ranch dressing. The preparation is quick and easy when you have cooked chicken and the dressing on hand. Just toss together and enjoy!

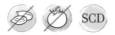

# chicken waldorf salad

## ingredients

- 2 cups red grapes, halved
- 3 stalks celery, thinly sliced
- 2 green apples, diced
- ½ cup raw walnuts*, lightly toasted and chopped
- 12 cups mixed salad greens (about 12 ounces)
- 3 cups shredded cooked chicken breast
- ¾ cup Herb Ranch Dressing (page 247)

*Omit for nut-free.*

## method

In a bowl, toss all of the ingredients together to coat with the dressing, and serve.

make-ahead tip:
This salad is wonderful as a packed lunch. Toss the grapes, celery, apples, walnuts, and chicken in the dressing, cover, and refrigerate for up to 3 days. Add the greens right before serving and toss to coat.

tidbits:
Use leftover Roasted Chicken (page 118) or fresh chicken. The quickest way to cook chicken for a salad is to poach it. Fill a small pot halfway with water and bring to a boil. Add 2 boneless, skinless chicken breasts, then partially cover and simmer on low for 8 minutes. Remove the pan from the heat and let the chicken sit in the hot water, covered, for another 15 minutes. Allow to cool, then shred. (1 pound raw boneless, skinless chicken breasts = about 2½ cups chopped or shredded cooked chicken)

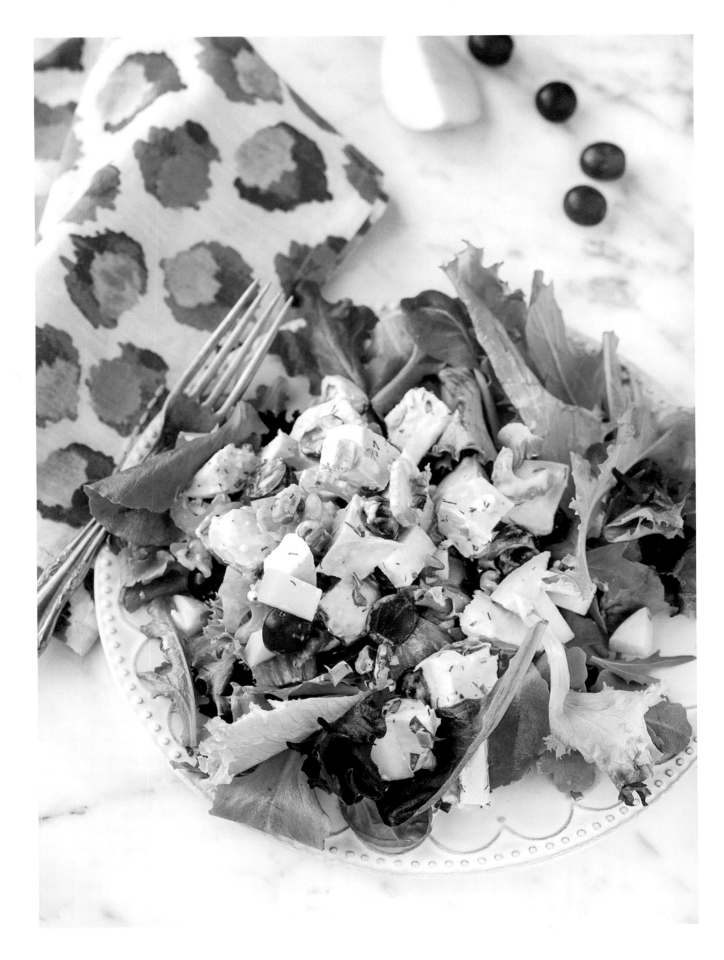

serves: 4
prep time: 15 minutes

Whether you use leftover taco meat from the Beef Tacos recipe (page 146) or make it fresh right before serving, you can have a flavor-packed meal on the table in no time with this taco salad recipe. The dressing will keep for a couple of days and is fabulous for dipping carrots and celery.

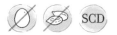 **warm taco salad** with creamy avocado-cilantro vinaigrette

## *ingredients*

DRESSING

- ½ avocado
- ¼ cup fresh cilantro leaves
- ½ small jalapeño, seeded
- 3 tablespoons fresh lime juice
- 1 tablespoon white wine vinegar
- ½ teaspoon sea salt
- ½ cup extra-virgin olive oil

SALAD

- 2 cups Beef Tacos filling (page 146), warmed
- 2 heads romaine lettuce, torn into bite-sized pieces
- 2 medium carrots, peeled and shaved with a vegetable peeler
- 1 tomato, diced
- 2 radishes, thinly sliced

## *method*

1. Make the dressing: In a blender or small food processor, purée the avocado, cilantro, jalapeño, lime juice, vinegar, and salt. With the blender running, slowly drizzle in the olive oil.

2. In a large bowl, mix together the salad ingredients and drizzle with the desired amount of dressing.

make-ahead tip:
Double the recipe for the taco beef (page 146) and store half in the refrigerator for 5 days or in the freezer for up to 3 months. Thaw in the refrigerator, then reheat in a sauté pan over medium heat.

tidbits:
Leftover Chipotle Barbacoa (page 154) also tastes wonderful in this recipe.

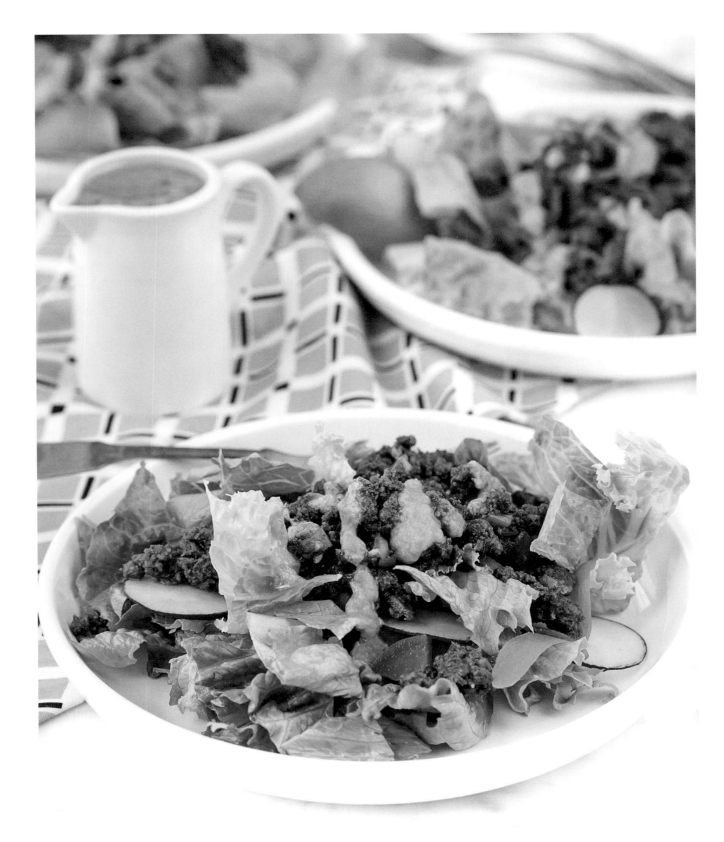

serves: 4 to 6
prep time: 15 minutes

This simple salad has all the flavors of a classic BLT sandwich, but without the bread! Cook an extra portion of bacon with your morning breakfast so you can throw it together quickly at lunchtime or as a dinner salad.

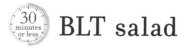 **BLT salad**

*ingredients*

- 12 ounces cooked bacon, chopped
- 2 heads romaine lettuce, torn into bite-sized pieces
- 2 cups cherry tomatoes, halved
- ½ cup Herb Ranch Dressing (page 247)

*method*

Toss all of the ingredients together in a bowl and serve.

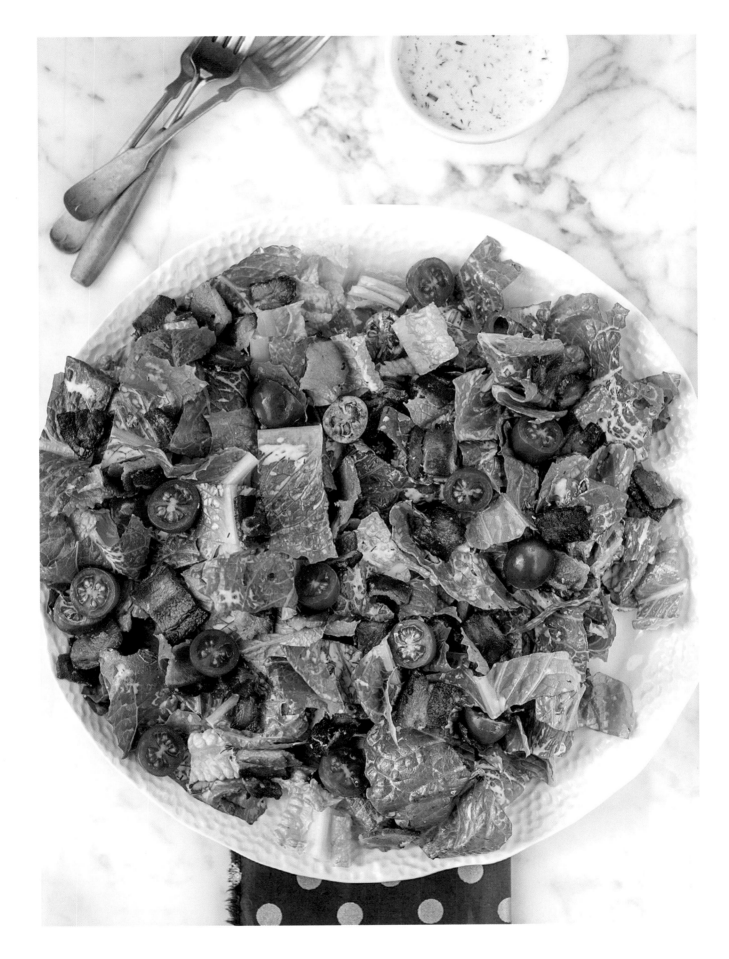

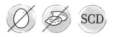

serves: 6

prep time: 10 minutes

cook time: 4 minutes

This crisp summer salad gains flavor from both the dressing and the char on the grilled squash. Light and refreshing, it is the perfect side salad to serve with your favorite grilled meat.

# grilled greek summer squash salad

## ingredients

- 2 medium yellow squash, cut lengthwise into quarters
- 2 medium zucchini, cut lengthwise into quarters
- ¼ cup Greek Dressing (page 247)
- ¼ teaspoon crushed red pepper
- pinch of sea salt and cracked black pepper
- 2 Roma tomatoes, cut into 1-inch pieces

## method

1. Heat a grill or grill pan to medium-high heat.

2. In a large bowl, toss the squash with the Greek Dressing, crushed red pepper, salt, and black pepper.

3. Remove the squash with tongs and place on the grill. Reserve the dressing.

4. Grill the squash, covered, for 2 minutes on each side. Remove and cut into 1-inch pieces.

5. Toss the squash with the tomatoes and a drizzle of the reserved dressing.

make-ahead tip:
Complete Step 2 and refrigerate for up to 2 days before grilling.

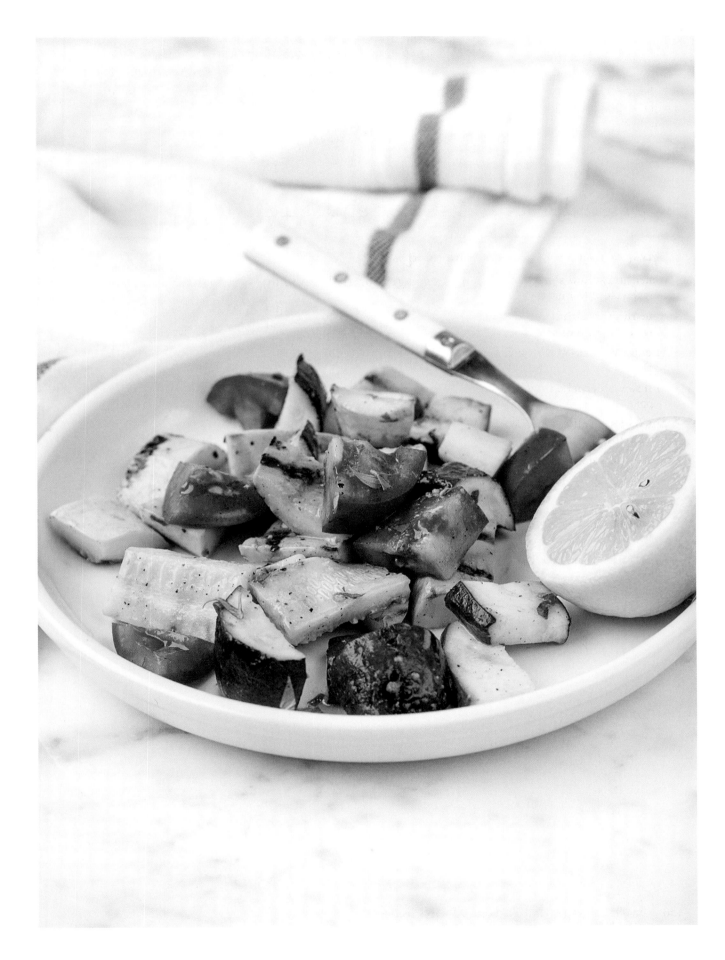

SCD

serves: 4 to 6
prep time: 15 minutes

A smoky and tangy barbecue chicken salad has always been one of my favorites. The contrast between the cool and creamy Herb Ranch Dressing (page 247) and the bold Barbecue Sauce (page 250) pleases the palate, and the crunch of the vegetables brings the dish together seamlessly. I like to use leftover Barbecue Chicken (page 134), but any cooked chicken will do.

# barbecue chicken chopped salad

*(30 minutes or less)*

## ingredients

- 2 heads romaine lettuce, chopped
- ¾ cup peeled and julienned jicama*
- 2 medium tomatoes, diced
- 2 ripe avocados, diced
- ¼ cup chopped fresh basil leaves
- ¼ cup chopped fresh cilantro leaves
- 2 tablespoons chopped scallions
- ¾ cup Herb Ranch Dressing (page 247)
- 2 cups diced cooked chicken
- ¼ cup Barbecue Sauce (page 250)

\* *Omit for SCD.*

## method

1. Toss the first 8 ingredients together in a large bowl. Divide the salad evenly into serving bowls.

2. Toss the chicken with the Barbecue Sauce and divide it among the salads.

make-ahead tip:
You can cook the chicken up to 5 days in advance, making it possible to throw this salad together in a hurry. The Herb Ranch Dressing and Barbecue Sauce can both be made a few days ahead of time as well.

If preparing this salad to pack in lunches, avoid soggy lettuce by keeping the sauces on the side until ready to serve.

tidbits:
You can use leftover Barbecue Chicken (page 134) or fresh chicken. See the Tidbits on page 100 for how to cook chicken quickly.

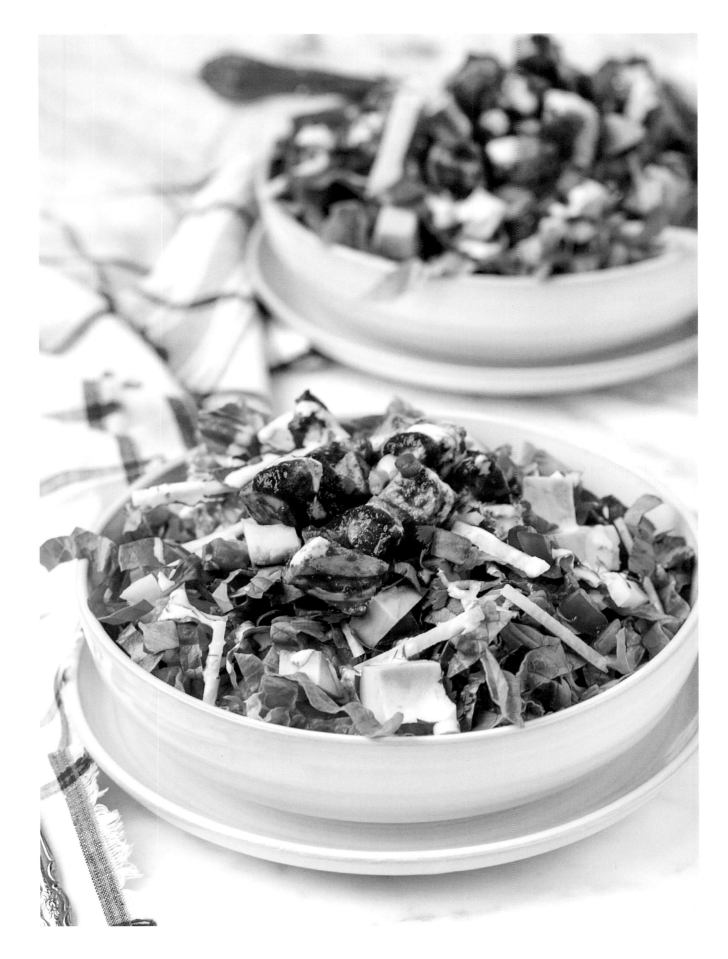

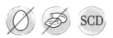

**SCD**

serves: 4 to 6
prep time: 10 minutes
cook time: 10 minutes

Use leftover tender lamb to top this delightfully refreshing and crisp salad inspired by Greek flavors.

## 30 minutes or less greek salad with garlic-oregano lamb

### ingredients

- 2 cups cubed leftover Mediterranean Braised Lamb (page 176)
- 2 heads romaine lettuce, chopped
- 2 Roma tomatoes, diced
- 1 red bell pepper, seeded and diced
- 1 English cucumber, peeled, seeded, and diced
- ½ red onion, thinly sliced
- ¼ cup pitted green olives
- ¼ cup pitted Kalamata olives
- ½ cup Greek Dressing (page 247)
- pepperoncini and lemon wedges, for serving

### method

1. In a covered pan over medium-low heat, reheat the lamb in its juices for 10 minutes. Drain and add the lamb to a large salad or mixing bowl.

2. Add the remaining salad ingredients and Greek Dressing and toss to combine. Serve with pepperoncini and lemon wedges.

tidbits:
Leftover Greek Lamb Burgers (page 178) or Lemon-Oregano Chicken Kabobs (page 138) can be substituted for the Mediterranean Braised Lamb.

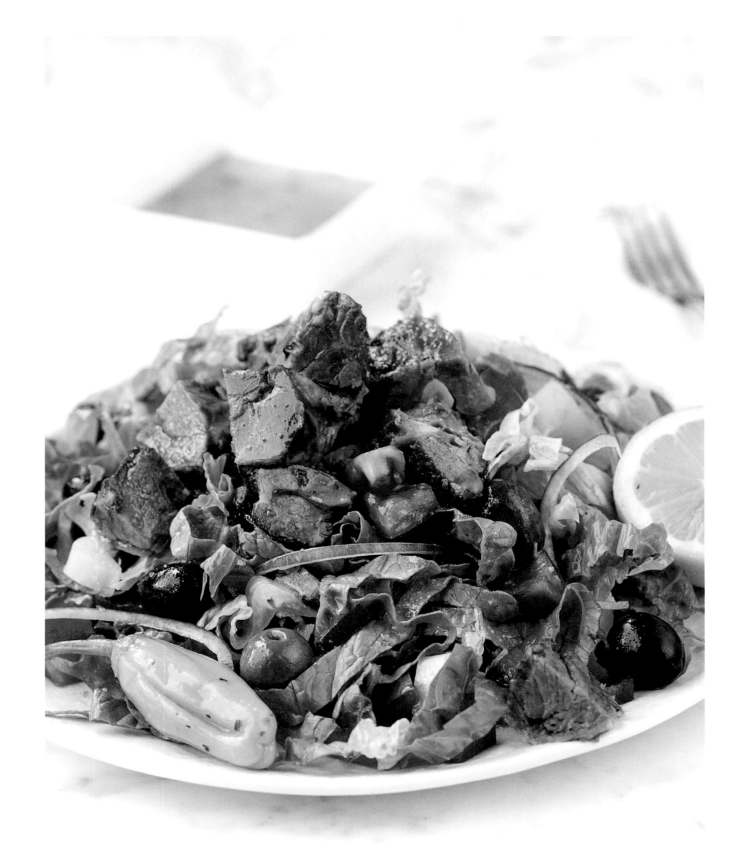

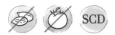

serves: 4 to 6
prep time: 10 minutes

This salad was my go-to lunch while I was writing and editing this book. It is so simple, yet so delicious, so I had to add it to the recipe lineup! It also tastes wonderful rolled in my Wraps (page 262) or on my Sandwich Rolls (page 264) for a packable lunch on the run.

# tuna salad

## ingredients

- 3 (5-ounce) cans tuna, packed in water
- ¾ cup Mayonnaise (page 248)
- 2 tablespoons minced red onion
- 2 tablespoons minced dill pickles
- 1 tablespoon minced fresh dill
- 1 teaspoon yellow mustard
- ½ teaspoon sea salt
- ¼ teaspoon cracked black pepper
- 6 cups baby spinach
- 6 cups arugula
- 2 tart apples, such as Honeycrisp or Pink Lady, thinly sliced
- ½ cup Champagne Vinaigrette (page 247)
- ¼ cup roasted, salted pepitas

## method

1. Drain the tuna and place it in a bowl. Break it apart with a fork and mix in the Mayonnaise, red onion, pickles, dill, mustard, salt, and pepper.

2. Toss the spinach, arugula, apples, Champagne Vinaigrette, and pepitas together in a bowl and divide between plates. Top with scoops of the tuna salad.

make-ahead tip:
Store the prepared tuna mixture in an airtight container for up to 3 days. For packed lunches, keep the tuna and vinaigrette separate from the greens until you're ready to eat.

tidbits:
Wild Planet Foods offers wild and sustainable tuna options. These products can be found online and in health food stores.

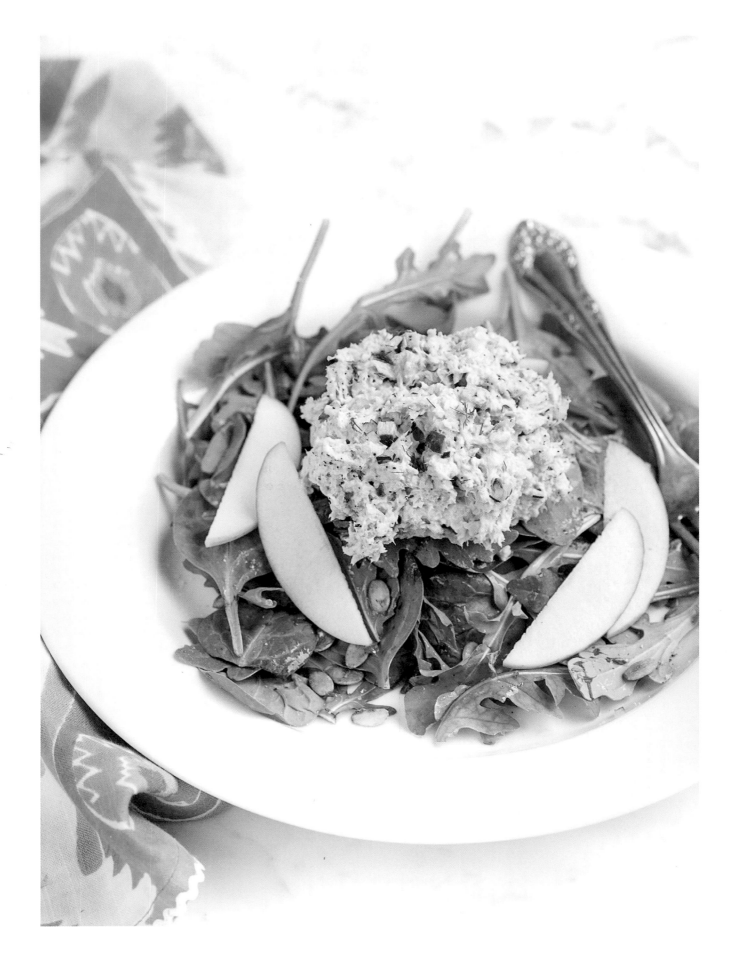

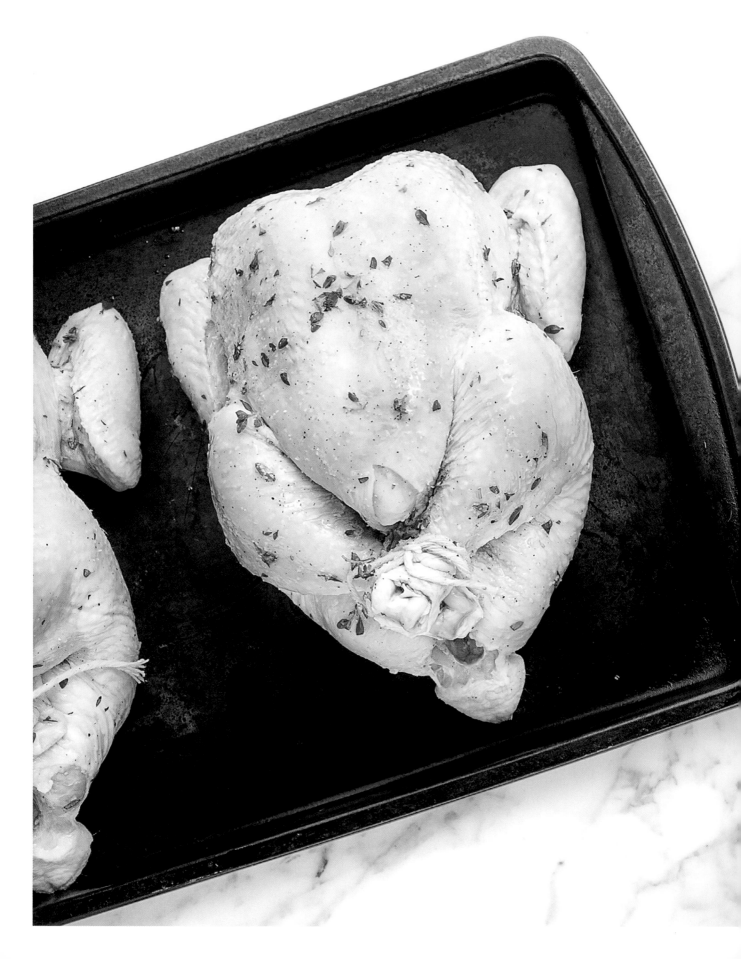

# poultry

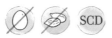

serves: 6 to 8

prep time: 20 minutes

cook time: 45 minutes

Boasting of bold spices, a tangy kick, and crispy skin, this one-pot meal is sure to be a crowd-pleaser. My favorite part is the tender and flavorful sweet potatoes that lie underneath!

# peruvian-style chicken

## ingredients

### PERUVIAN SPICE RUB

- 1 teaspoon melted ghee or extra-virgin olive oil
- 1½ tablespoons paprika
- 1 tablespoon ground cumin
- 2 teaspoons fresh lemon juice
- 1 teaspoon sea salt
- ½ teaspoon cracked black pepper
- ½ teaspoon dried oregano leaves
- 3 cloves garlic, minced
- 2 tablespoons white vinegar

### CHICKEN

- 1 (4-pound) roasting chicken, gizzards removed, cut into 10 parts
- 1½ pounds sweet potatoes, washed and diced*
- 3 small sweet onions, quartered
- 2 yellow bell peppers, seeded and sliced
- 1 clove garlic, minced
- 2 teaspoons melted ghee or extra-virgin olive oil
- ¼ teaspoon sea salt
- ¼ teaspoon cracked black pepper
- 1 lemon, sliced
- handful of fresh cilantro, for garnish

## method

1. Preheat the oven to 425°F.

2. Combine the ingredients for the spice rub in a small bowl.

3. Rinse and dry the chicken pieces, then generously rub them all over with the spice rub.

4. Place the sweet potatoes, onions, bell peppers, and garlic in a roasting pan or 9-by-12-inch baking dish. Drizzle the ghee over the vegetables, season with the salt and pepper, then toss to coat.

5. Arrange the chicken skin side down over the top of the vegetables. Place the lemon slices on top.

6. Roast for 20 minutes, then turn the chicken pieces over and stir the vegetables. Continue roasting for 20 to 25 more minutes, until the chicken skin is crisp and the vegetables are cooked through. Garnish with cilantro.

make-ahead tip:
You can assemble this entire dish in advance and store it in the refrigerator for up to 2 days or in the freezer for 3 months. Bring it to room temperature before roasting by letting it sit out for 20 minutes.

tidbits:
Ask your butcher to break down a whole, bone-in chicken for you to save time and money. Make sure to ask them to keep the back bones so you can make Chicken Stock (page 242)!

*Substitute butternut squash for SCD.

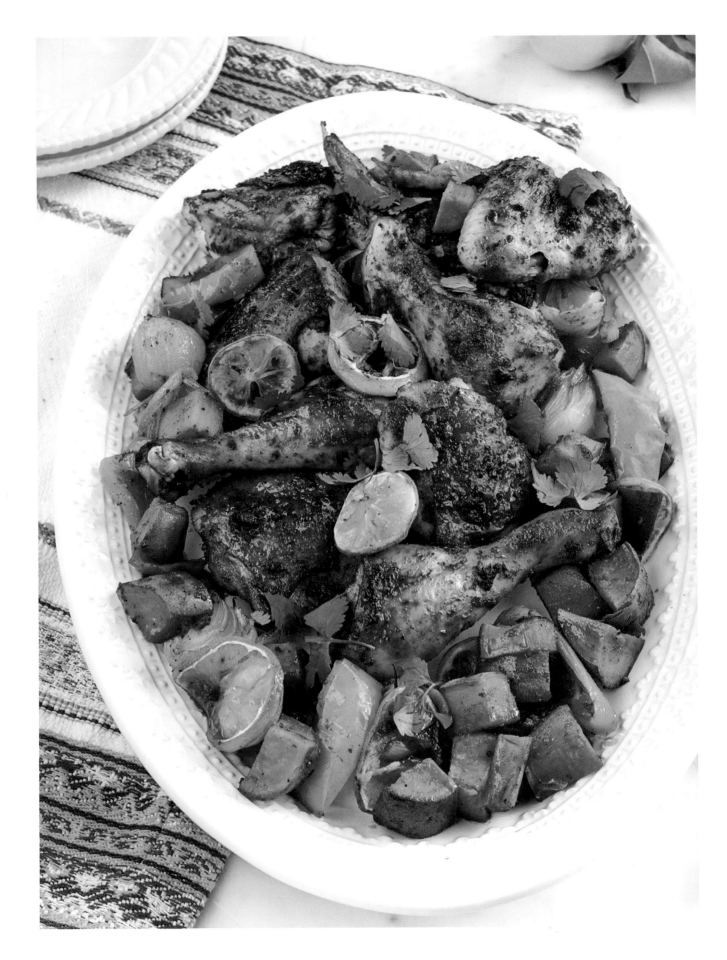

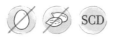

serves: 6 to 8
prep time: 30 minutes
cook time: 50 to 60 minutes

Whole roasted chickens may seem daunting at first, but they are simple to prepare and provide an elegant dinner. I suggest roasting two chickens on a Sunday so you have the additional chicken to use throughout the week when you are shorter on time. Serve one chicken for dinner, then use the leftover chicken in any of the "stretch it" recipes on the next page.

# roasted chickens with thyme gravy

## ingredients

- 5 tablespoons melted ghee or extra-virgin olive oil, divided
- 2 tablespoons fresh thyme leaves
- 3½ teaspoons coarse sea salt, divided
- 1 teaspoon cracked black pepper, divided
- 2 (4-pound) roasting chickens, gizzards removed
- 2 medium yellow onions, quartered, divided
- 7 cloves garlic, peeled, divided
- 2 stalks celery, cut into thirds
- 4 cups peeled and cubed butternut squash (about 1 [2- to 3-pound] squash)
- 3 large carrots, peeled and cut into 1-inch pieces

GRAVY (MAKES 2 CUPS)
- roasted onions, celery, and garlic, reserved from the roasting pan
- 1 cup pan juices
- ¼ to ½ cup Chicken Stock (page 242), warmed
- 1 teaspoon chopped fresh thyme leaves
- sea salt and cracked black pepper to taste

## method

1. Preheat the oven to 450°F.

2. Combine 3 tablespoons of the ghee, the thyme, 2 teaspoons of the salt, and ½ teaspoon of the pepper in a bowl.

3. Rinse the chickens well and pat the outsides and cavities with towels to dry.

4. Rub the thyme mixture all over the outsides of the chickens and under the skin.

5. Stuff each cavity with 2 onion quarters, 2 garlic cloves, ½ teaspoon of the salt, and ¼ teaspoon of the pepper. Tie the legs together with kitchen string. Place the chickens in a roasting pan or on a large rimmed baking sheet.

6. Toss the remaining onion, celery, and garlic with 1 tablespoon of the ghee and spread around the birds. Toss the squash and carrots in the remaining 1 tablespoon of ghee and ½ teaspoon of salt and set aside.

7. Roast for 30 minutes, then reduce the oven temperature to 400°F. Remove the vegetables from the pan and reserve in a bowl for the gravy.

8. Add the squash and carrots to the pan and continue roasting the chickens for 20 to 30 minutes, until a thermometer reads 165°F when inserted into the thickest part of the thigh. Remove from the oven and set the chickens, carrots, and squash aside.

9. Make the gravy: Place the roasted onions, celery, and garlic in a blender.

10. Skim off any fat in the pan and pour 1 cup of the juices and ¼ cup of the Chicken Stock through a sieve into the blender. Purée until very smooth. Stir in the thyme. If the gravy is too thick, slowly add up to ¼ cup more stock until it reaches the desired consistency. Season with salt and pepper if needed.

11. Slice the chicken and serve topped with the hot gravy and vegetables.

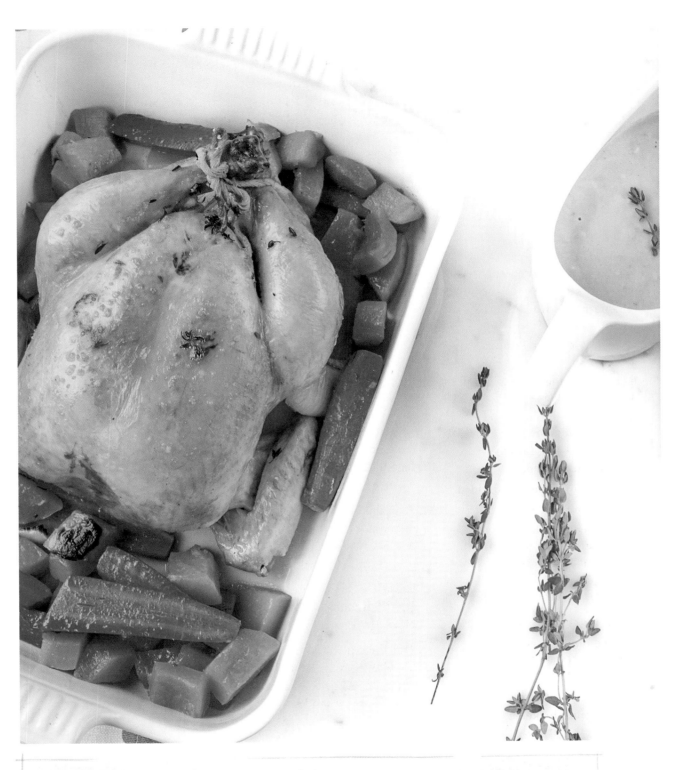

make-ahead tip:

Store the second chicken, tightly wrapped, in the refrigerator for up to 5 days.

stretch it:

· Chicken Stock (page 242)

· Roasted Chicken and Vegetable Soup (page 86)

· Mexican Chicken Soup (page 88)

· Roasted Chicken, Butternut, and Apple Salad (page 98)

· Chicken Waldorf Salad (page 100)

· Barbecue Chicken Chopped Salad (page 108)

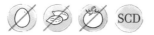

serves: 6

prep time: 5 minutes

cook time: 25 to 30 minutes

These tender chicken thighs are full of flavor and super simple to throw together in a hurry. You likely already have everything for the rub in your fridge, and you can easily substitute your favorite herbs for the sage and parsley. Roasting the vegetables underneath the chicken creates a hearty meal that is all done in one pot!

# garlic-herb chicken thighs

## ingredients

- ⅓ cup ghee or bacon fat, melted, divided
- 1 pound Brussels sprouts, trimmed and halved
- ½ pound carrots, peeled and cut into 2-inch pieces
- pinch of sea salt and pepper
- 4 pounds chicken thighs, bone-in and skin-on
- 3 cloves garlic, minced
- 2 tablespoons chopped fresh parsley
- 1 tablespoon chopped fresh sage
- 1½ teaspoons sea salt

## method

1. Preheat the oven to 375°F. Toss the vegetables with 2 tablespoons of the ghee and sprinkle with a pinch of salt and pepper. Spread the vegetables on a rimmed baking sheet.

2. Trim any excess fat off of the chicken.

3. In a small bowl, combine the remaining ghee, garlic, parsley, sage, and salt. Rub the mixture all over the chicken.

4. Place the chicken skin side up on top of the vegetables and roast for 25 to 30 minutes, until the juices run clear. Turn the oven to broil and brown the skin for 2 minutes before serving.

make-ahead tip:
This dish can be prepared 2 days in advance. Wrap tightly and store in the refrigerator.

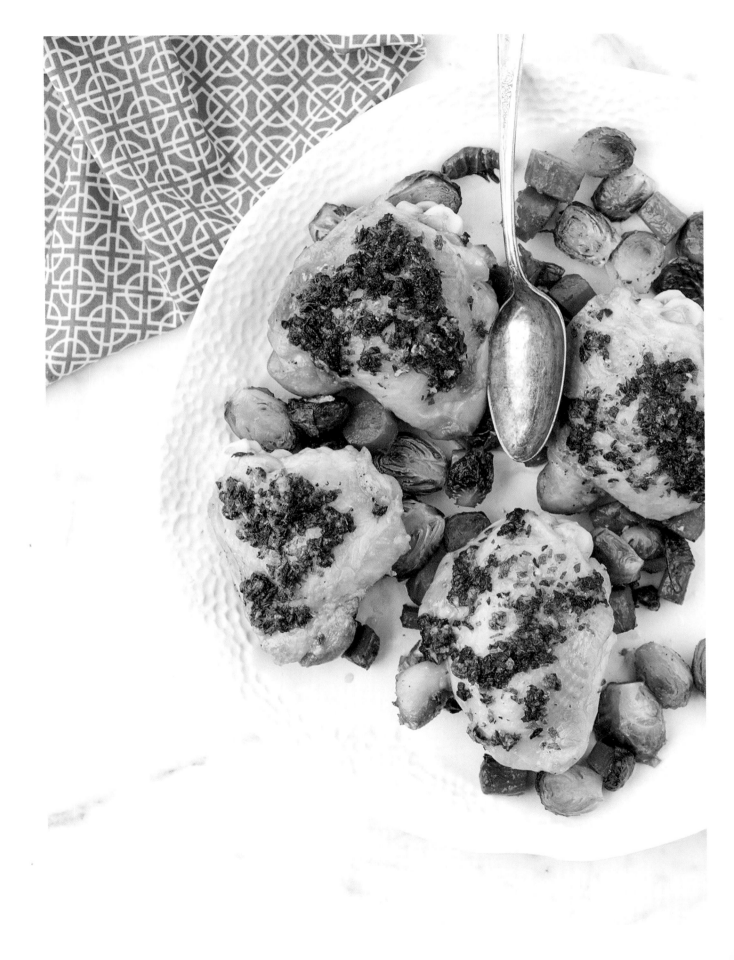

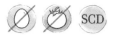

serves: 6

prep time: 20 minutes

cook time: 35 to 40 minutes

An easy baked chicken breast dish is dressed up with a flavorful dairy-free Pesto Sauce (page 256) and a salty prosciutto wrap. This version is purposefully kept tomato-free for those who are allergic to nightshades, but a good marinara sauce on top of this chicken would taste fabulous!

# pesto-stuffed prosciutto chicken

## ingredients

- 1 teaspoon extra-virgin olive oil, ghee, or coconut oil, for greasing the pan

### CHICKEN

- 6 boneless, skinless chicken breast halves (about 3 pounds)
- ¼ teaspoon sea salt
- ¼ teaspoon cracked black pepper
- ¾ cup Pesto Sauce (page 256)
- 12 slices prosciutto, thinly sliced

### CAULIFLOWER

- 1 small head cauliflower, cut into florets
- 2 tablespoons melted ghee or extra-virgin olive oil
- 1 shallot, thinly sliced
- 1 clove garlic, crushed into a paste
- 2 teaspoons fresh lemon juice
- ¾ teaspoon sea salt
- cracked black pepper

## method

1. Preheat the oven to 350°F. Spread the oil on the bottom of a 9-by-12-inch baking dish.

2. Prepare the chicken: With a sharp knife, cut a 1-inch-long slit into the thick side of each chicken breast. Gently use your finger to expand the pocket. Season the chicken with the salt and pepper.

3. Stuff each pocket with 2 tablespoons of Pesto Sauce, then wrap them tightly with slices of prosciutto so that the slits are covered, tucking the ends of the prosciutto under the breasts.

4. Prepare the cauliflower: Toss all of the ingredients together in a bowl. Spread the cauliflower in the bottom of the prepared baking dish.

5. Place the chicken seam side down on top of the cauliflower.

6. Bake for 35 to 40 minutes, until the chicken is cooked through and the cauliflower is tender. After 20 minutes, flip the breasts over and gently stir the vegetables.

make-ahead tip:

The Pesto Sauce can be made up to 3 days in advance and stored tightly covered in the refrigerator.

Prepare the entire dish 2 days in advance and store tightly wrapped in the refrigerator. Bring to room temperature 20 minutes before baking.

tidbits:

Can't find pine nuts for the Pesto Sauce? Sub in chopped macadamia nuts or walnuts. Or, for nut-free, use ¼ cup grated Parmesan cheese.

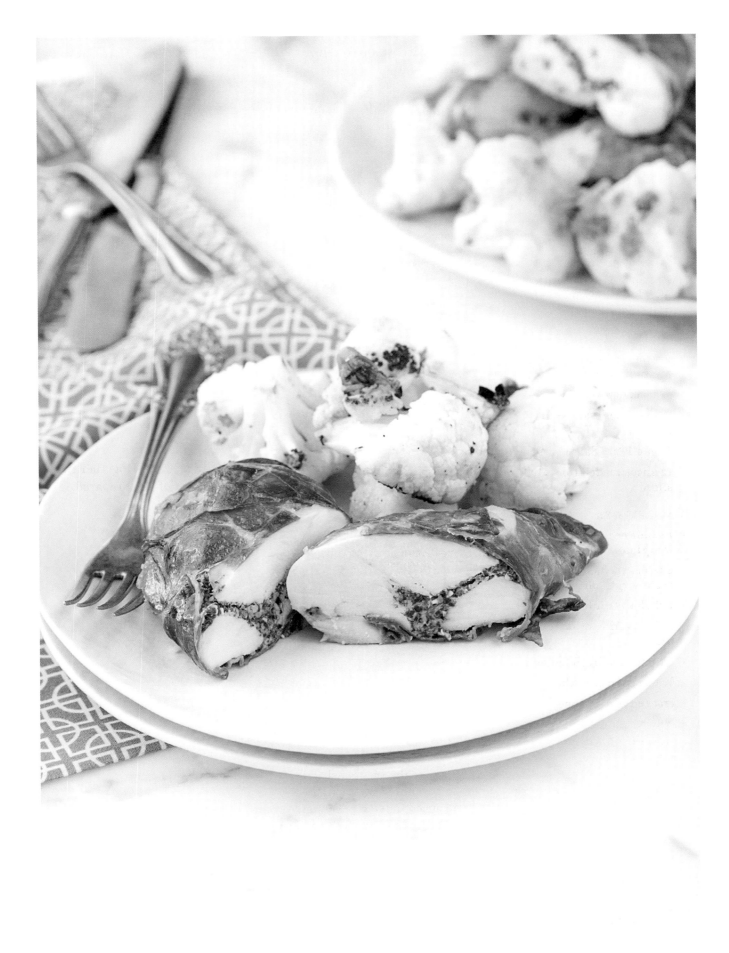

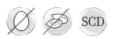

serves: 6

prep time: 20 minutes

cook time: 12 minutes

Enjoy flavors of the islands with these chicken burgers topped with a sweet ring of grilled pineapple. Throw the Grilled Sesame Asparagus and Scallions (page 220) onto the grill at the same time and make your entire meal without the use of a stove!

# hawaiian chicken burgers

## ingredients

### BURGERS

- 2 pounds ground chicken, dark or white meat
- 1 tablespoon coconut aminos*
- 2 teaspoons cold-pressed sesame oil
- 2 cloves garlic, minced
- 1 teaspoon peeled and minced fresh ginger
- 1 teaspoon sea salt
- ¾ teaspoon sesame seeds
- ¼ teaspoon crushed red pepper
- ¼ teaspoon cracked black pepper
- 6 fresh pineapple rings

### SAUCE**

- ¼ cup Mayonnaise (page 248)
- 1 clove garlic, minced
- 2 teaspoons cold-pressed sesame oil
- ¾ teaspoon fresh lime juice
- ¼ teaspoon peeled and minced fresh ginger
- dash of hot sauce

### FIXINGS

- romaine or butter lettuce leaves, for serving
- 1 tomato, sliced
- ½ red onion, thinly sliced

## method

1. Combine all of the burger ingredients except the pineapple in a bowl and form into 6 patties, about 1 inch thick.

2. Whisk together all of the sauce ingredients and refrigerate until ready to use.

3. Heat a grill or grill pan to medium heat and grill the burgers for about 4 minutes on each side, until cooked through.

4. Grill the pineapple rings for 1 minute on each side, then place a ring on top of each burger. Serve between 2 pieces of lettuce, and top with a tomato slice, an onion slice, and sauce.

make-ahead tip:
Store the sauce in the refrigerator for up to 4 days. Prepare the chicken patties up to 2 days in advance and store, tightly wrapped, in the refrigerator.

* Omit for SCD.

** For egg-free, swap the sauce for Guacamole (page 258).

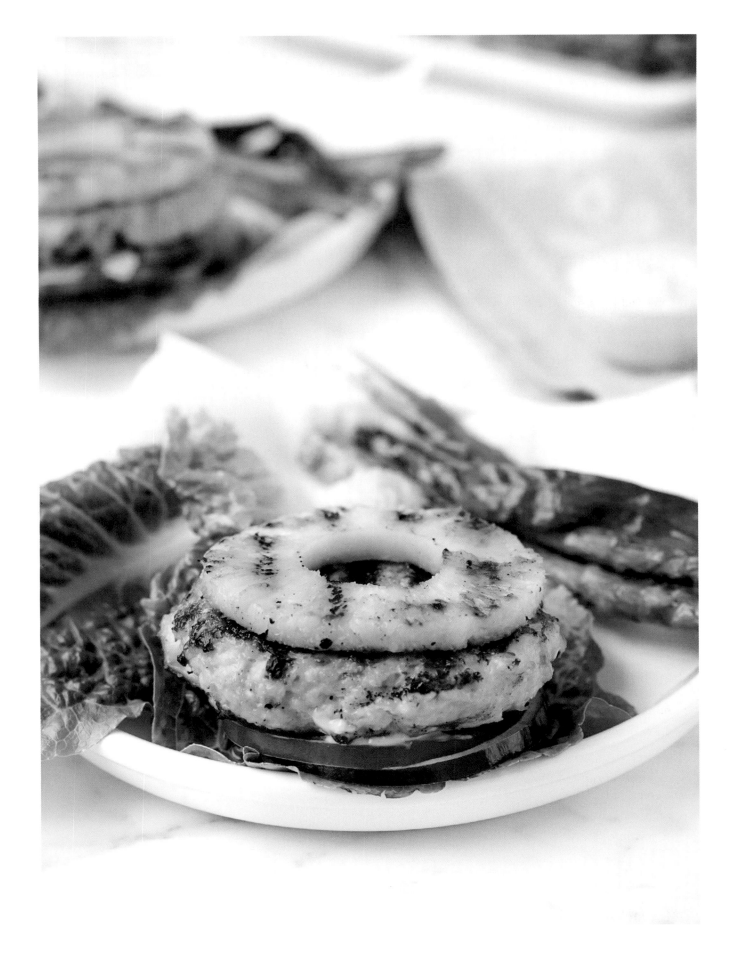

serves: 6
prep time: 20 minutes
cook time: 30 minutes

While traditional Chinese food often uses starches to thicken sauces, this recipe follows a slightly unconventional method of egg yolks to thicken the sauce and make it cling to the meat and vegetables. Feel free to add extra veggies like asparagus and carrots, as this sauce is really versatile and extremely delicious.

# ginger chicken and broccoli

## ingredients

- 3 tablespoons expeller-pressed coconut oil or ghee, divided
- 6 cloves garlic, minced
- 1½ tablespoons peeled and minced fresh ginger
- 6 scallions, white parts only, chopped
- 2 heads broccoli, cut into florets
- 3 pounds boneless, skinless chicken thighs, trimmed of fat and cubed
- 1 cup coconut aminos
- 2 tablespoons toasted (or dark) sesame oil
- 1 teaspoon sea salt
- 2 large egg yolks

## method

1. Heat 2 tablespoons of the coconut oil in a wok or deep skillet over medium-high heat.

2. Add the garlic, ginger, and scallions. Stir constantly for 30 seconds.

3. Add the broccoli florets and continue cooking and stirring for 5 minutes, until the broccoli is bright green.

4. Transfer the vegetables to a plate and return the pan to the burner with the remaining 1 tablespoon of coconut oil.

5. Add the chicken and cook, stirring frequently, for 8 to 10 minutes, until the chicken is browned and cooked through.

6. Using a slotted spoon, transfer the chicken to the plate with the broccoli and return the pan and juices to the burner. If there is less than ¼ cup of liquid in the pan, add water or chicken broth to make ¼ cup.

7. Pour in the coconut aminos, sesame oil, and salt. Bring to a simmer.

8. Beat the egg yolks in a bowl. Temper the yolks by slowly pouring in ½ cup of the hot sauce while whisking constantly.

9. Pour the egg yolk mixture into the hot pan, then stir constantly for 3 minutes to thicken.

10. Add the chicken and vegetables back into the pan and stir to coat. Cook for an additional 7 to 10 minutes, until the chicken and broccoli are fully cooked.

tidbits:
Tempering eggs before adding them to a hot pan helps to ensure that they don't curdle or scramble when they hit the heat.

Stir-fry some different vegetables and chicken the next day and use any leftover sauce!

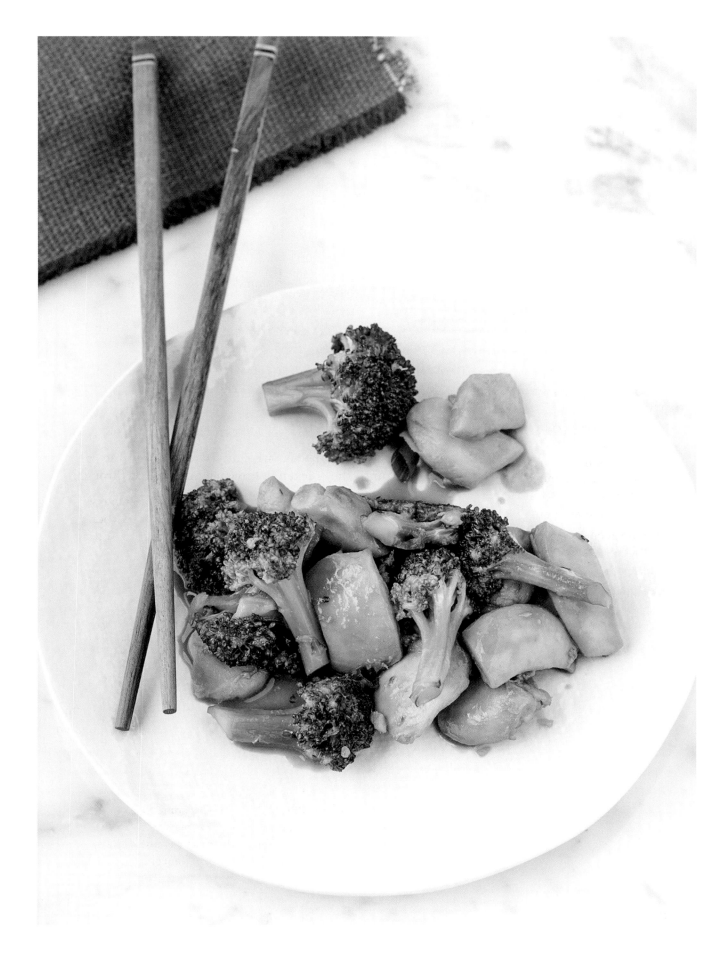

serves: 4 to 6

prep time: 15 minutes

cook time: 14 minutes

I used to order a sandwich similar to this at one of my favorite burger joints as a kid. In this lightened-up version, my grain-free Wraps (page 262) replace the buns and homemade dairy-free Herb Ranch Dressing (page 247) provides a little tang.

# california chicken wraps

## ingredients

- 10 Wraps (page 262)
- 2 pounds boneless, skinless chicken breasts
- sea salt and cracked black pepper
- 3 tablespoons Dijon mustard
- 1 tablespoon honey
- 12 slices bacon
- 2 avocados, sliced
- 2 cups chopped romaine lettuce
- ½ cup Herb Ranch Dressing (page 247)

## method

1. If the Wraps are frozen, allow them to sit at room temperature for 30 minutes.

2. Season the chicken liberally with salt and pepper.

3. Mix together the Dijon mustard and honey and spread half all over the chicken, reserving the other half for basting. Allow the chicken to marinate at room temperature while the grill heats.

4. Heat a grill to medium-high heat, then reduce the heat to medium. Grill the chicken, covered, until cooked through, about 7 minutes on each side. Brush the remaining honey mustard sauce on the chicken during the last minute of grilling.

5. Meanwhile, cook the bacon to your desired crispiness. Set on paper towels to drain. Strain the fat and save for later use.

6. Allow the chicken to rest for 10 minutes, then slice it thinly on the diagonal.

7. Assemble the wraps with the chicken, bacon, avocado slices, lettuce, and a drizzle of the dressing.

tidbits:

Don't overstuff the wraps or they may tear.

Swap the avocado slices for fresh Guacamole (page 258) for a little kick!

make-ahead tip:

We prepare the components for these wraps at the beginning of the week and throw them together like sandwiches at lunchtime. Have a dozen Wraps ready to go in the freezer and the dressing made ahead of time. For packing in lunches, avoid a soggy wrap by keeping the sauces separate until you're ready to eat. If you don't have any Wraps on hand in the freezer, use lettuce wraps or the Pure Wraps brand. They work great for this recipe and can be found online.

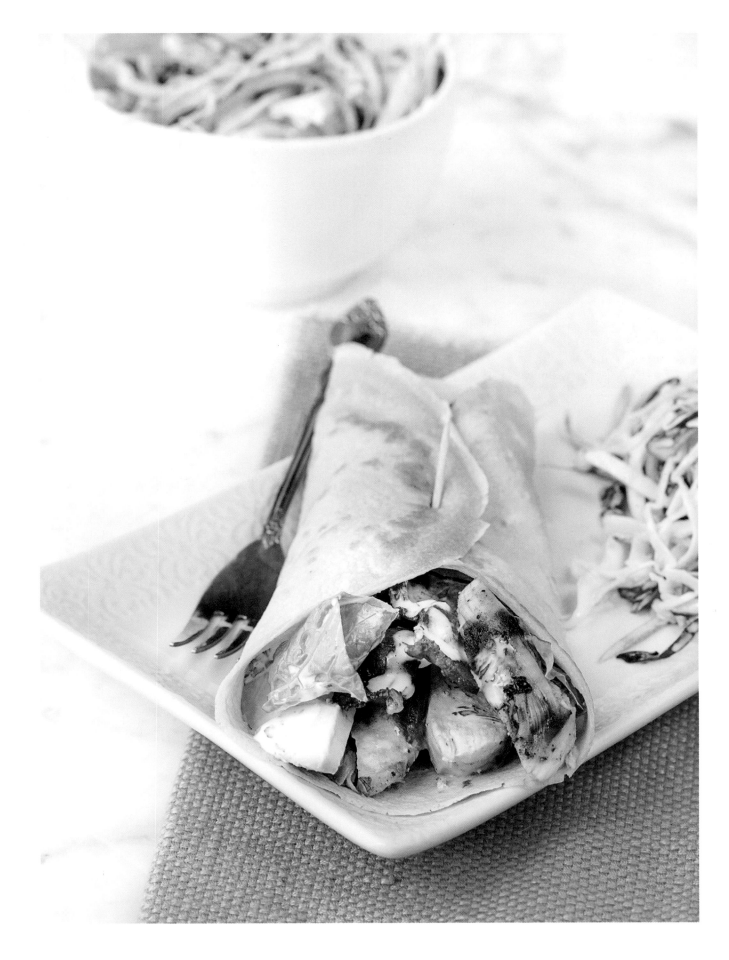

serves: 6
prep time: 15 minutes
cook time: 6 hours

This dish is typically marinated, roasted, and then simmered on the stove, but my recipe simplifies everything with the use of a slow cooker. The flavors of the Indian spices intensify throughout the day, and the traditional heavy cream is replaced with a dairy-free substitute, cashew cream. Serve over Vegetable Biryani (page 216) or steamed vegetables.

# chicken tikka masala

## ingredients

- ½ cup raw cashews
- 2½ pounds boneless, skinless chicken thighs, cut into 2-inch cubes
- 2 cups tomato puree
- ½ medium yellow onion, chopped
- 2 cloves garlic, minced
- 2½ tablespoons garam masala
- 2 teaspoons sea salt
- 1 teaspoon ground ginger
- ½ teaspoon paprika
- ¼ teaspoon cayenne pepper
- ¼ cup chopped fresh cilantro, for garnish

## method

1. Place the cashews in a bowl and cover with water. Cover with a towel or plastic wrap and set aside.

2. Place the chicken, tomato puree, onion, garlic, garam masala, salt, ginger, paprika, and cayenne pepper in a slow cooker. Toss to coat the chicken.

3. Cover and cook on low for 6 hours.

4. When the chicken is just about done cooking, drain the cashews and place them in a blender. Add ¼ cup of fresh water and blend the cashews into a smooth cream. Stir the cashew cream into the chicken right before serving and garnish with the cilantro.

make-ahead tip:
Complete Step 2 and place the contents in an airtight container or resealable bag. Refrigerate for 2 days, or freeze for up to 3 months and thaw overnight in the refrigerator before continuing to Step 3.

Alternatively, freeze the completed dish for up to 3 months, then thaw in the refrigerator overnight and rewarm on the stovetop over medium-low heat or in a slow cooker on the warm setting until heated through.

tidbits:
If dairy is tolerated, ½ cup grass-fed heavy cream can be substituted for the cashew cream.

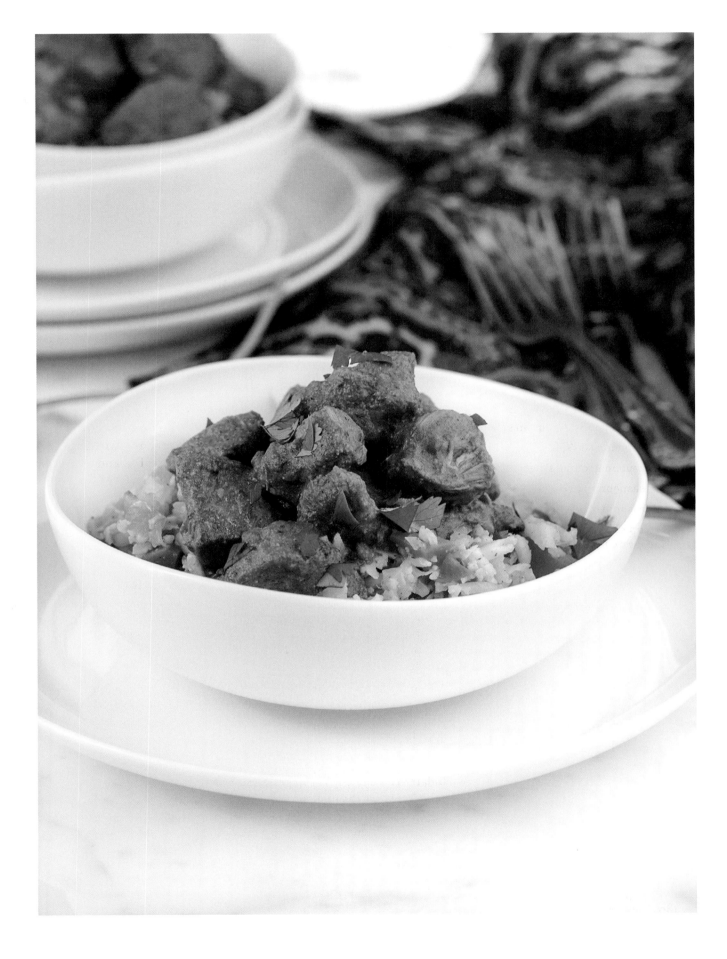

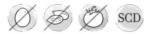

serves: 10

prep time: 20 minutes

cook time: 3 to 6 hours

This flavorful curry caters to those who cannot tolerate nightshade vegetables. If that doesn't describe you, feel free to add some cayenne pepper. Serve it over Basic Cauli-Rice or Coconut, Cilantro, & Lime Cauli-Rice (page 218).

# chicken curry

## ingredients

- 3 pounds boneless, skinless chicken breasts or thighs
- 1 medium yellow onion, sliced
- 6 cloves garlic, sliced
- 1 (1-ounce) piece ginger, peeled and sliced into discs
- 2 teaspoons coconut aminos*
- 1½ teaspoons fish sauce
- 2½ teaspoons sea salt
- 2½ teaspoons ground cumin
- 2½ teaspoons ground turmeric
- 1½ teaspoons ground coriander
- ¾ teaspoon ground nutmeg
- ¼ teaspoon ground allspice
- 2 cups full-fat coconut milk
- 5 large carrots, peeled and julienned
- 2 cups broccoli florets (about 10 ounces)
- ½ cup frozen peas, thawed
- ½ cup raw cashew pieces, toasted** (optional)
- chopped fresh cilantro, for garnish (optional)

*Omit for SCD.*
**Omit for nut-free.*

## method

1. Toss the chicken with the onion, garlic, ginger, coconut aminos, fish sauce, salt, and all of the spices.

2. Add to a slow cooker, cover, and cook on high for 2 hours or on low for 4 hours.

3. Discard the ginger pieces and liquid, remove the chicken, and shred with 2 forks. Return the chicken to the slow cooker.

4. Add the coconut milk, carrots, broccoli, and peas and continue cooking for 1 hour on high or 2 hours on low, until the vegetables are crisp-tender.

5. Serve with toasted cashew pieces sprinkled over the top and cilantro, if desired.

make-ahead tip:
Complete Step 1 and place the contents in an airtight container or resealable bag. Refrigerate for 2 days, or freeze for up to 3 months and thaw overnight in the refrigerator, before continuing to Step 2.

Alternatively, freeze the completed dish for up to 3 months, then thaw in the refrigerator overnight and warm on the stovetop over medium-low heat or in a slow cooker on the warm setting until heated through.

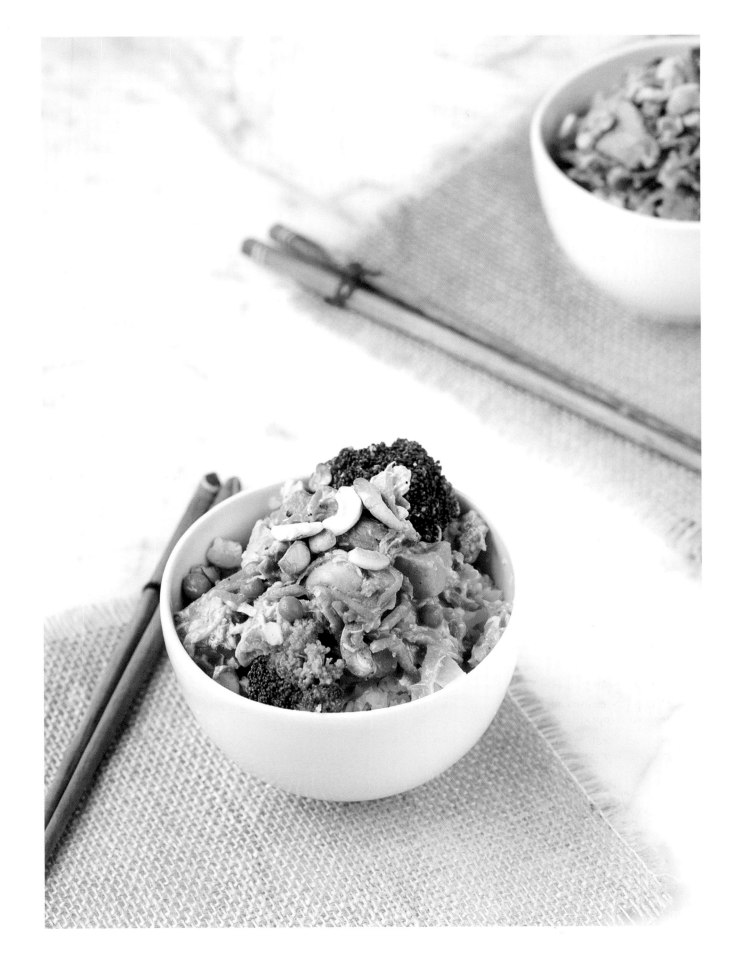

serves: 6

prep time: 5 minutes

cook time: 30 minutes

With a quick dry rub prior to grilling and a basting of homemade Barbecue Sauce (page 250) at the end, this chicken gets a double dose of iconic barbecue flavor. Serve with Jicama Apple Bacon Slaw (page 230) or simply with a green salad and crisp watermelon for a quintessential summertime meal.

# barbecue chicken

## ingredients

- 5 pounds chicken parts, bone-in and skin-on
- ¼ cup Barbecue Dry Rub (page 244)
- ½ cup Barbecue Sauce (page 250)

## method

1. Preheat a grill to medium-high heat. If using a charcoal grill, set it up with 2 heat zones: medium-high and low.

2. Rub the chicken all over with the Barbecue Dry Rub. Set aside while the grill heats.

3. Place the chicken skin side down on the grill. Sear the pieces for 5 minutes, then lower the heat to medium and flip the chicken over. If using a charcoal grill, move the chicken away from the heat source to the cooler side of the grill. Cover and leave undisturbed for 15 minutes.

4. Brush the skin sides of the chicken with the Barbecue Sauce, then turn them skin side down and brush the bottoms. Cook for 5 minutes, then flip again and cook for 5 minutes more.

tidbits:
Tessemae's and Paleo Chef are two Paleo-friendly brands of barbecue sauce that can be purchased online or in some health food stores for convenience.

make-ahead tip:
The rub will keep for 6 months, and the sauce can be stored in the refrigerator for 1 week or the freezer for 6 months. Coat the chicken in the rub the night before and store in the refrigerator to speed up dinnertime even more. Allow the chicken to come to room temperature while the grill is preheating.

stretch it:
Save 2 cups diced leftover chicken and any additional Barbecue Sauce to use in Barbecue Chicken Chopped Salad (page 108). Many of the leftover ingredients from the Jicama Apple Bacon Slaw can also be used for the Barbecue Chicken Chopped Salad.

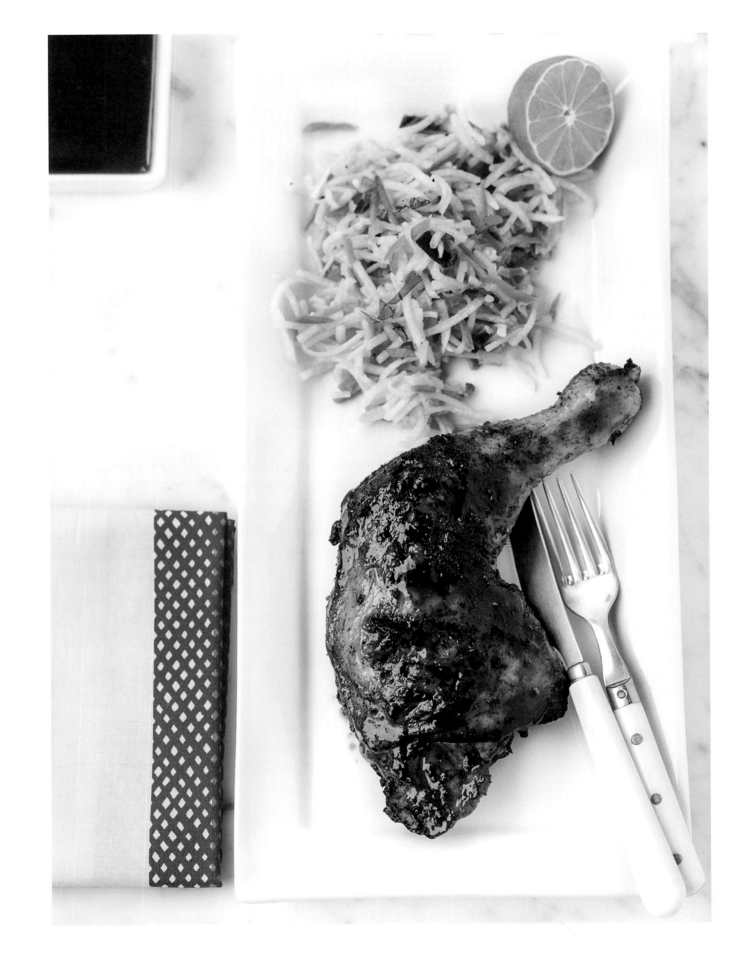

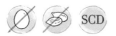

⊘ 🚫 SCD

serves: 4 to 6
prep time: 10 minutes
cook time: 3 or 8 hours

With only ten minutes to prep and five main ingredients, you will be surprised at the incredible flavors of this dish. It can be made in a slow cooker or on the stovetop. Serve it over Coconut, Cilantro, & Lime Cauli-Rice (page 218) with sautéed Cumin-Garlic Summer Squash (page 236) or a simple green salad to complete the meal.

# chicken verde

## ingredients

- 1 tablespoon ghee or coconut oil
- 6 chicken legs, bone-in and skin-on
- sea salt and cracked black pepper
- 2 cloves garlic, crushed into a paste
- 2 teaspoons ground cumin
- 1 teaspoon ground coriander
- 2 cups Roasted Tomatillo Salsa (page 258), divided

## method

1. Heat the ghee in a heavy-bottomed pot or Dutch oven over medium-high heat.

2. Season the chicken generously with salt and pepper. Mix the garlic, cumin, and coriander in a small bowl, and rub it all over the chicken. Working in batches, brown the chicken on all sides, about 2 minutes per side.

3. For the slow cooker: Pour 1 cup of the salsa into the slow cooker and arrange the browned legs on top. Cover and cook on low for 8 hours.

   For the stovetop: Keep the legs in the pot and pour in 1 cup of the salsa. Simmer, covered, over medium-low heat for 3 hours.

4. Serve the chicken with the remaining 1 cup of the salsa.

make-ahead tip:
If using homemade salsa, make it up to 5 days in advance to save prep time.

tidbits:
For convenience, store-bought salsa verde or roasted tomatillo salsa may be purchased. Look for fresh brands if possible, or jarred varieties that do not contain sugar or additives.

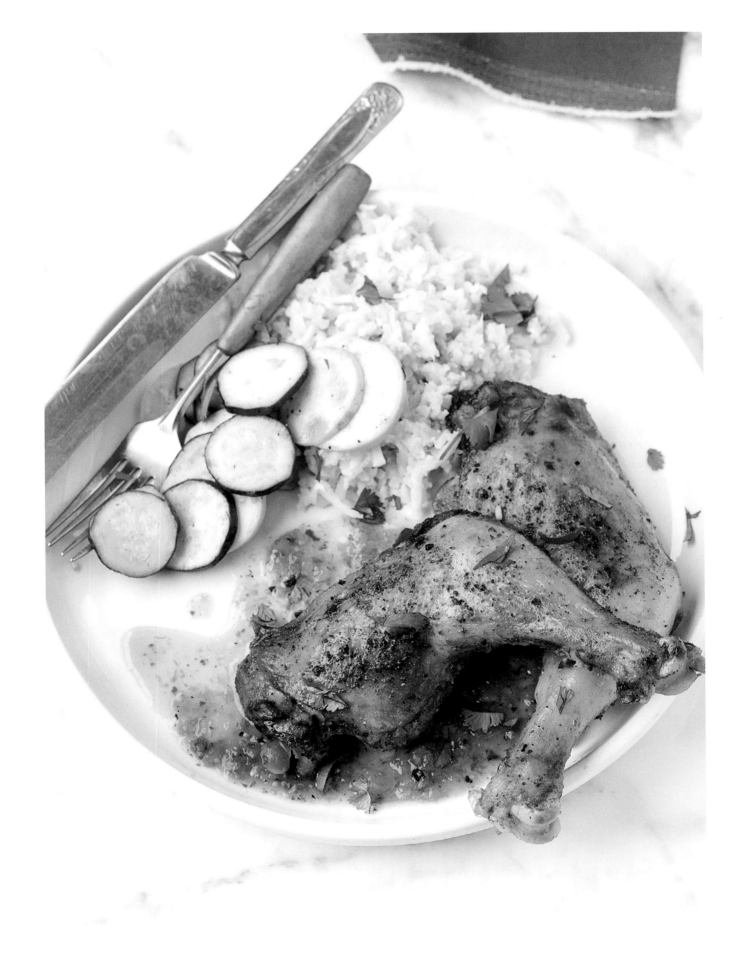

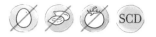

serves: 6

prep time: 10 minutes, plus at least 30 minutes marinating time

cook time: 8 to 10 minutes

I use my Greek Dressing (page 247) to marinate these Mediterranean-inspired chicken kabobs. Serve with Grilled Greek Summer Squash Salad (page 106) or over Greek Salad (page 110).

# lemon-oregano chicken kabobs

## ingredients

- 2 pounds boneless, skinless chicken breasts, cut into 1-inch pieces
- ½ cup Greek Dressing (page 247)
- sea salt and cracked black pepper

## method

1. Soak 8 to 10 wooden skewers in water for at least 1 hour, or use metal skewers.

2. Marinate the chicken in the Greek Dressing for at least 2 hours in the refrigerator, or for 30 minutes at room temperature.

3. Preheat a grill or grill pan to medium-high heat.

4. Thread the chicken onto the skewers and discard the marinade. Season each skewer with salt and pepper to taste. Grill for 8 to 10 minutes, turning occasionally, until all sides are browned and the center is cooked through.

make-ahead tip:
The chicken can marinate in the refrigerator for up to 48 hours.

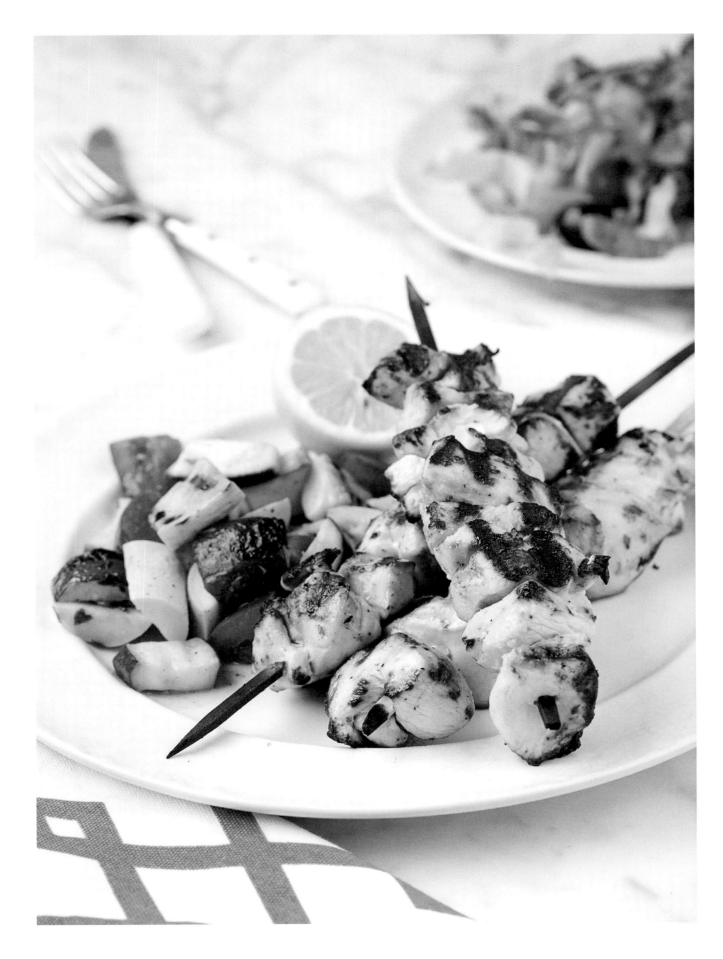

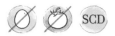

serves: 6
prep time: 30 minutes
cook time: 35 to 38 minutes

Casseroles are a little tricky when it comes to Paleo because cheeses and the standard canned and creamy soups cannot be used for binding and moisture. I use a cashew sauce in this dish that is reminiscent of all the flavors of casseroles I remember growing up, making this a true comfort food.

# chicken and rice casserole

## ingredients

### SAUCE

- 1 cup raw whole cashews
- ¾ cup Chicken Stock (page 242)
- 2 teaspoons dried thyme leaves
- 1 teaspoon sea salt
- ½ teaspoon fresh lemon juice

### CASSEROLE

- 3 tablespoons ghee or extra-virgin olive oil, divided
- 3 cloves garlic, minced
- 2 shallots, minced
- 4 ounces cremini mushrooms, minced
- 3 cups riced cauliflower (see Tidbits)
- 8 ounces broccoli florets, roughly chopped
- 1½ teaspoons sea salt
- ¾ teaspoon cracked black pepper
- 2 cups shredded cooked chicken

## method

1. Fill a bowl with boiling water and place the cashews in the water. Soak for 30 minutes.

2. Preheat the oven to 375°F and lightly grease a 3-quart casserole dish with 1 teaspoon of the ghee.

3. Heat the remaining 2 tablespoons of ghee in a sauté pan over medium-high heat. Sauté the garlic, shallots, and mushrooms for 3 minutes. Add the cauliflower, broccoli, salt, and pepper and continue cooking for 7 to 10 minutes, until the vegetables are crisp-tender. Stir in the chicken, then remove from the heat and set aside.

4. Drain the soaked cashews and place them in a blender with the remaining sauce ingredients. Blend on high for 30 to 45 seconds, until very smooth. Stir the sauce into the chicken and vegetable mixture, then turn the entire mixture into the prepared casserole dish.

5. Bake, covered, for 15 minutes. Uncover and continue baking for 10 minutes.

### tidbits:

To rice cauliflower, run florets through a food processor with a grating attachment or use a box grater to create ricelike pieces. Pick out any large fragments that didn't get shredded and save for another use.

Store-bought rotisserie chicken made with clean ingredients makes this dish especially quick and easy, but leftover Roasted Chicken (page 118) or any cooked chicken will work. To quickly prepare fresh chicken, see the Tidbits on page 100.

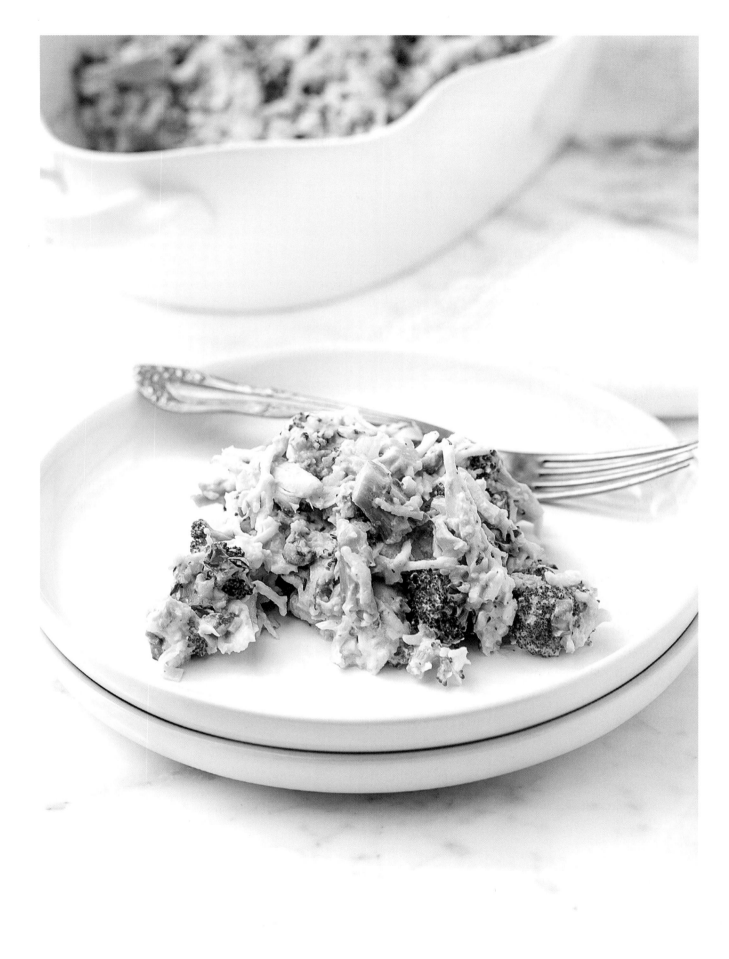

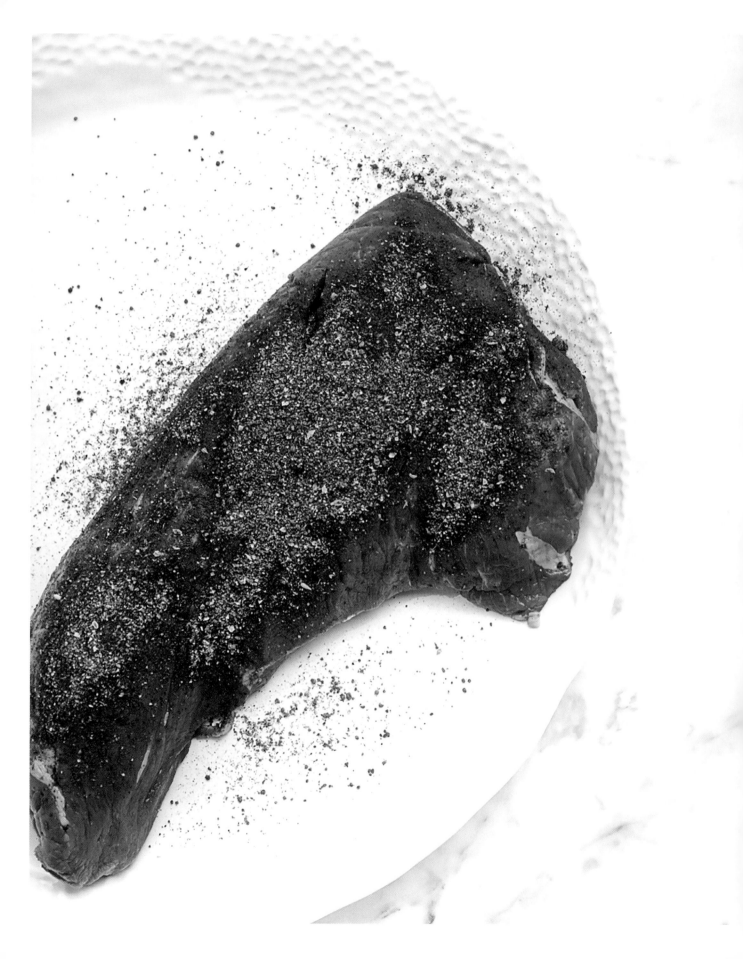

# beef, pork, and lamb

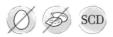

serves: 6 to 8
prep time: 20 minutes
cook time: 6 to 8 hours

Short ribs are one of my favorite cuts of meat, and anything slathered in my smoky Barbecue Sauce (page 250) instantly becomes a favorite, so this dish was destined to be winner. With all the work being done in a slow cooker, your stovetop and time are free to make Creamy Mashed Root Vegetables (page 214) to soak up all the delicious sauce, and a side of crisp Green Beans Almondine (page 212).

# barbecue beef short ribs

## ingredients

- 2 tablespoons bacon fat or ghee
- 5 pounds bone-in short ribs, cut into 3-inch pieces
- 2 teaspoons sea salt, divided
- ½ teaspoon cracked black pepper, divided
- 1 small yellow onion, roughly chopped
- 1½ cups Barbecue Sauce (page 250), plus more for serving (optional)
- 1 tablespoon Dijon mustard
- ½ teaspoon natural liquid smoke
- ½ teaspoon cayenne pepper

## method

1. Heat the bacon fat in a large pot over medium-high heat.

2. Trim the ribs of excess fat, then rinse and pat them dry with paper towels. Season all over with 1 teaspoon of the salt and ¼ teaspoon of the pepper.

3. Working in batches, brown the ribs on all sides, then place them in the bottom of a slow cooker.

4. Add the onion, Barbecue Sauce, Dijon mustard, liquid smoke, cayenne pepper, remaining 1 teaspoon of salt, and remaining ¼ teaspoon of pepper to the slow cooker.

5. Toss to coat, cover, and cook on high for 6 hours or on low for 8 hours. Stir the ribs once or twice during the cooking time to ensure even coating and cooking.

6. Transfer the ribs to a platter, skim off any fat from the top of the liquid in the slow cooker, and serve the liquid over the top of the meat. Serve with additional Barbecue Sauce, if desired.

make-ahead tip:
To save time in the morning, brown the meat and put everything into the slow cooker insert the night before. Keep it in the fridge, then pop the insert into the base the next morning, and it will be ready to devour at dinnertime.

tidbits:
Store any leftovers with the sauce spooned over the top in the refrigerator for 3 days or freezer for 3 months. Reheat in a covered saucepan over medium-low heat until warmed through.

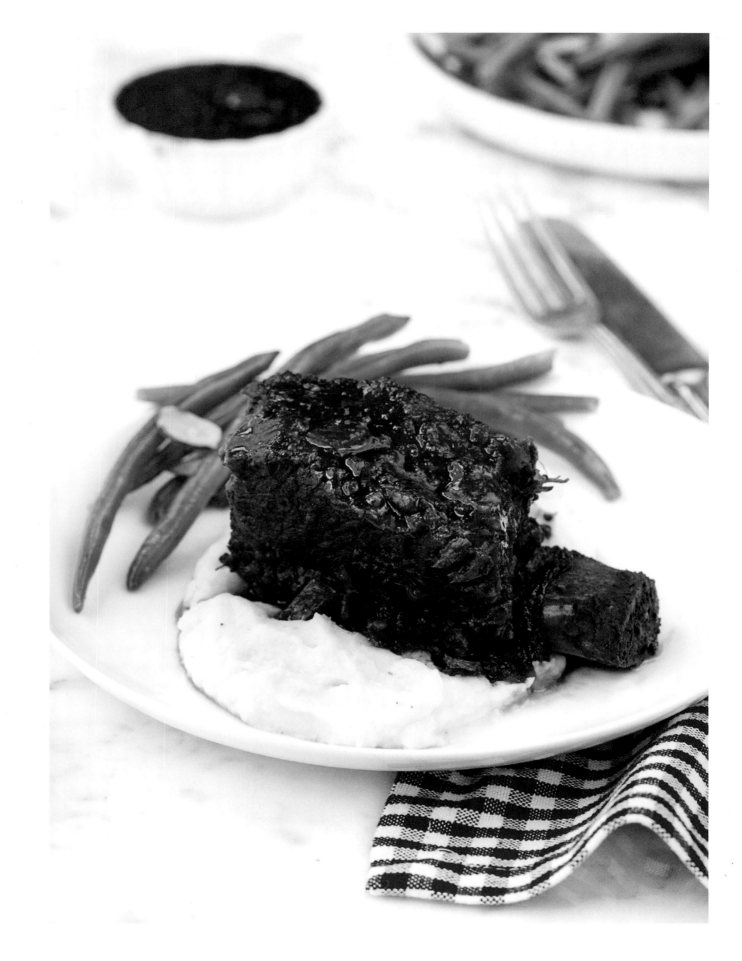

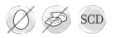

serves: 6
prep time: 10 minutes
cook time: 20 minutes

Beef tacos are my go-to meal when I'm running short on time or forget to plan dinner. I always keep a jar of my Taco Seasoning (page 244) in the pantry and a few pounds of grass-fed ground beef in the freezer so I can throw this meal together anytime and get dinner on the table in 30 minutes.

# beef tacos

## ingredients

- 3 pounds ground beef
- ¾ cup diced yellow onion
- 3 cloves garlic, minced
- ¾ cup water
- 2 cups tomato puree
- 4 to 5 tablespoons Taco Seasoning (page 244)

### SERVING SUGGESTIONS

- large romaine, butter, or iceberg lettuce leaves, for wrapping the filling
- sliced avocado
- Guacamole (page 258)
- sliced red onion
- diced tomatoes
- chopped fresh cilantro
- lime quarters

## method

1. Heat a deep sauté pan over medium heat.

2. Brown the beef, onion, and garlic until the beef is cooked through, about 5 minutes.

3. Drain the excess fat if necessary, and add the remaining ingredients.

4. Simmer for 15 minutes, until ready to serve.

make-ahead tip:
Store the filling in the refrigerator for 5 days or freezer for 3 months. Thaw in the refrigerator and reheat, uncovered, in a sauté pan over medium heat.

stretch it:
Double the recipe and save 2 cups of the meat to make my Warm Taco Salad with Creamy Avocado-Cilantro Vinaigrette (page 102) and 2 cups to make my Breakfast Burritos (page 54).

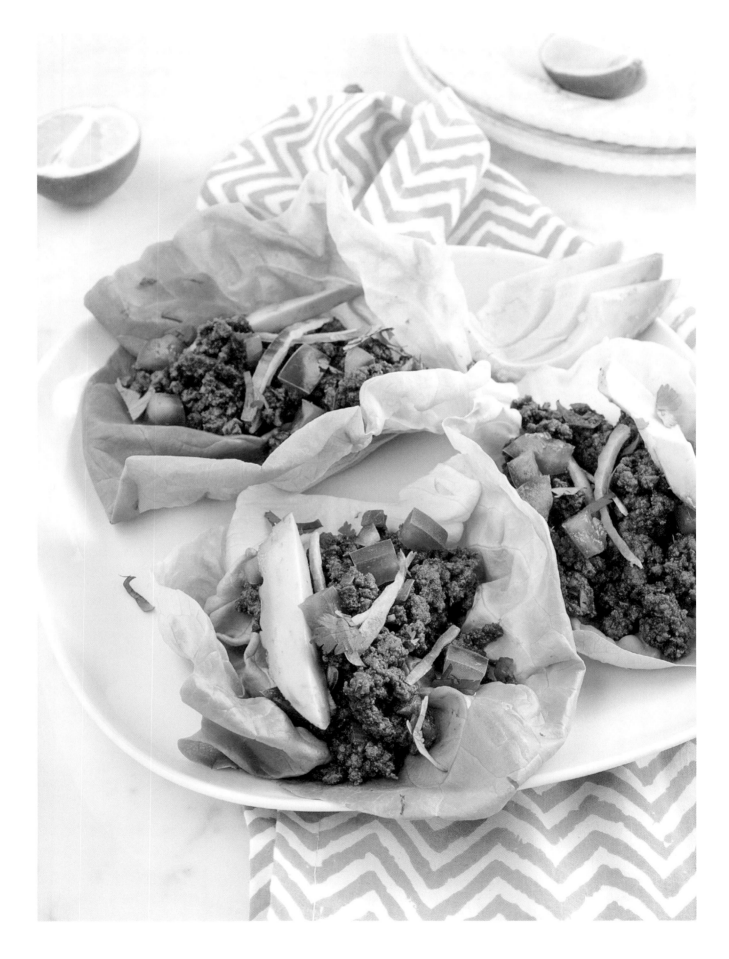

serves: 6

prep time: 25 minutes

cook time: 20 minutes, or
6 hours in a slow cooker

Meatloaf is made into bite-sized meatballs and topped with a quick homemade ketchup sauce. Serve with Creamy Mashed Root Vegetables (page 214). These meatballs are so versatile and convenient—they can also be used in spaghetti sauce or even substituted for the ground beef in Beef Stroganoff (page 150) for a Swedish meatball–style dinner!

# meatloaf meatballs

## ingredients

### SAUCE

- 2 cups tomato puree
- ¼ cup tomato paste
- ¼ cup honey
- ¼ cup coconut aminos
- 1½ tablespoons apple cider vinegar
- 1 tablespoon plus 1 teaspoon Dijon mustard
- 1 teaspoon sea salt
- 1 teaspoon onion powder
- ½ teaspoon allspice

### MEATBALLS

- 2 small Vidalia onions
- 2 large carrots, quartered
- 1 clove garlic, peeled
- 2 large eggs, whisked
- 2 tablespoons coconut flour or ½ cup almond meal
- ¾ teaspoon sea salt
- 1 teaspoon ground dried oregano
- ¼ teaspoon cracked black pepper
- 1½ pounds ground beef
- ½ pound lean ground pork

## method

1. In a bowl, whisk together all of the sauce ingredients. Reserve ¾ cup of the sauce and place the rest in a skillet.

2. Bring the sauce to a boil, then simmer uncovered on medium-low heat to thicken while the meatballs cook.

3. Preheat the oven to 375°F.

4. Place the onions, carrots, and garlic in a food processor. Process until the vegetables are coarsely chopped.

5. Add the eggs, flour, salt, oregano, pepper, and reserved ¾ cup of sauce and pulse until everything is combined.

6. Add the meats and pulse a few times more to combine.

7. Use your hands or a 1-tablespoon cookie scoop to form golf ball–sized meatballs. Place them on a rimmed baking sheet.

8. Bake the meatballs for 20 minutes, turning once halfway through.

9. Serve hot with the thickened sauce over the top.

10. *Slow Cooker Instructions:* Place the uncooked meatballs in a slow cooker and cover with the sauce. Cook on high for 2 hours, then reduce to low and cook for 4 hours more.

### make-ahead tip:

Store the sauce for up to 3 days in the refrigerator. Prepare the meatballs the night before and store in the refrigerator. Bring to room temperature for 20 minutes before baking or slow cooking.

Freeze uncooked meatballs on a rimmed baking sheet lined with parchment paper. Once frozen, transfer the meatballs to a freezer-safe bag or container. Pull out the desired number of meatballs the night before and thaw in the refrigerator, or place the entire sealed bag in the sink and run warm water over it until thawed. Bake or cook in a slow cooker.

beef, pork, and lamb

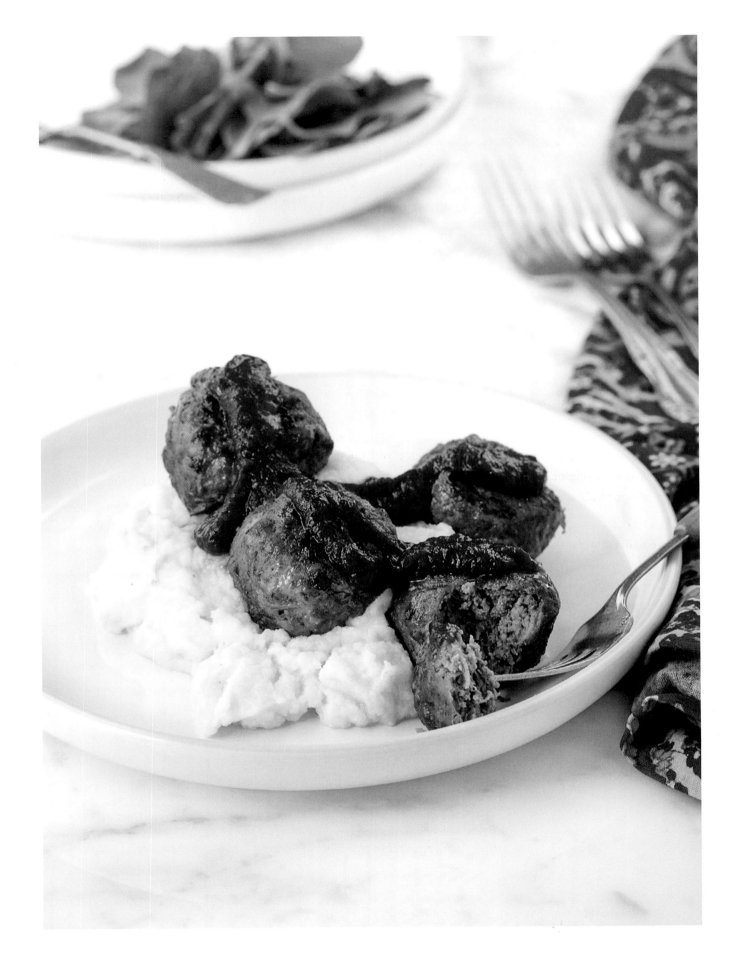

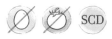

serves: 6
prep time: 20 minutes
cook time: 35 minutes

While most stroganoff recipes use strips of beef, I grew up eating the ground beef version, probably because it was much cheaper. I remember using a can of cream of mushroom soup and sour cream, but this version is dairy-free and on par with the memories I have of the flavors. My mom always served it over egg noodles or rice. Here, yellow squash ribbons are the vessel for the sauce.

# beef stroganoff

## ingredients

- 3½ cups water, divided
- 3 ounces raw cashew pieces (about ¾ cup)
- 2 tablespoons ghee or extra-virgin olive oil, divided
- 2 pounds ground chuck
- 1¼ teaspoons sea salt, divided
- ¼ teaspoon cracked black pepper
- ½ large yellow onion, diced
- 2 pounds yellow squash
- 8 ounces cremini mushrooms, sliced
- ½ cup dry sherry*
- 1 cup low-sodium beef stock
- 2¼ teaspoons fresh lemon juice
- 1¾ teaspoons apple cider vinegar
- ¼ cup chopped fresh parsley, packed

*Use dry white wine for SCD.*

## method

1. Boil 3 cups of the water, then remove from the heat. Pour the cashew pieces into the hot water and set aside.

2. Melt 1 tablespoon of the ghee in a large pot over medium-high heat. Brown the ground chuck with ½ teaspoon of the salt and the pepper for 8 minutes, until cooked through. Remove the browned meat with a slotted spoon, set aside, and return the pot to the stove.

3. Add the remaining 1 tablespoon of ghee, onion, and ½ teaspoon of the salt. Sauté for 5 to 7 minutes, until the onion is translucent.

4. Meanwhile, make the squash noodles. Cut off the ends, then use a vegetable peeler to create long ribbons. Stop at the middle when the seeds are visible and switch to the other side. Discard the seeded portion.

5. Add the mushrooms to the pot with the onion and continue cooking until the mushrooms are soft, 3 to 5 minutes.

6. Pour the sherry into the pot and stir constantly to remove the browned bits from the bottom. Simmer for 5 minutes.

7. Add the beef stock and meat to the pot and reduce the heat to medium-low. Allow to simmer while making the cashew cream.

8. Drain the cashews and place them in a blender with ¼ cup of the water, the lemon juice, and the apple cider vinegar. Blend until very smooth and creamy.

> make-ahead tip:
> The cashew cream will keep for 2 days in the refrigerator, and the vegetables can be prepped the night before.

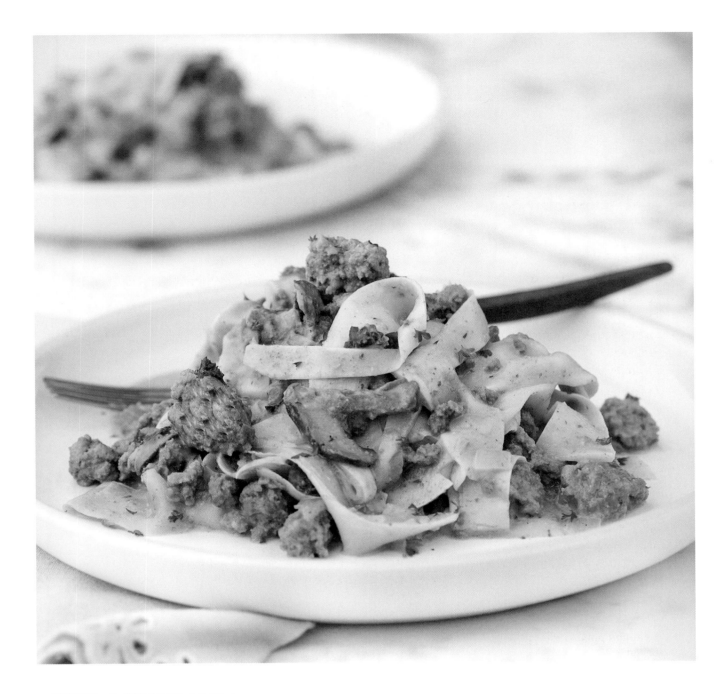

tidbits:
Make this dish into Swedish meatballs by using the meatballs from page 148 instead of the ground chuck! Follow the same steps, but brown the meatballs for 15 minutes, until cooked through.

9. Spoon the cashew cream into the pot and add the parsley. Stir to combine, then let simmer for 10 minutes.

10. Bring the remaining ¼ cup of water to a boil in a shallow skillet. Add the squash ribbons and the remaining ¼ teaspoon of sea salt. Cover and steam for 8 minutes, until tender. Drain the noodles.

11. Season the sauce to taste with salt and pepper, then serve atop the squash noodles.

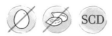

serves: 6 to 8

prep time: 20 minutes,
plus 25 minutes if making
homemade salsa

cook time: 45 minutes

Mild peppers are stuffed with a hearty mix of meat and vegetables
and smothered and baked in a tangy and smoky chile verde sauce.

# enchilada stuffed peppers

## ingredients

- 3 cups Roasted Tomatillo Salsa (page 258) or store-bought salsa verde
- 2 pounds ground bison or beef
- 1½ cups peeled and diced sweet potatoes*
- ½ cup diced yellow onion
- 1 cup peeled and diced carrots
- 3 cups baby spinach, roughly chopped
- 2½ teaspoons sea salt
- 2 teaspoons ground cumin
- 1½ teaspoons chili powder
- 1½ teaspoon ground coriander
- 8 large poblano or pasilla peppers
- sliced avocado or Guacamole (page 258), for serving

*Substitute butternut squash for SCD.*

## method

1. Make the homemade Roasted Tomatillo Salsa, if using.

2. Preheat the oven to 375°F.

3. Brown the bison in a deep sauté pan over medium heat until cooked through. Drain the grease from the pan, then add the sweet potatoes, onion, carrots, spinach, salt, and spices. Sauté for 10 minutes, until the vegetables have softened slightly.

4. Leaving the stems on, cut a Y-shaped slit down the top and center of each pepper. Gently scrape out and discard the seeds.

5. Stuff each pepper generously with the bison mixture, being careful not to tear the pepper.

6. Spread a thin layer of salsa on the bottom of a baking dish, then arrange the peppers on top. Spoon the remaining salsa over each pepper.

7. Bake, covered, for 20 minutes, then uncover and bake for 15 more minutes, until the peppers are soft and the salsa is hot.

8. Serve with avocado slices or Guacamole.

stretch it:
Extra filling and salsa taste delicious stuffed into the Breakfast Burritos on page 54 instead of the taco meat and vegetables called for.

tidbits:
If purchasing store-bought salsa verde, refrigerated fresh salsa is preferable to jarred. Look for organic brands that do not contain added sugar or preservatives.

make-ahead tip:
Prepare through Step 5, allow to cool to room temperature, then freeze for up to 3 months. Thaw in the refrigerator for 24 hours prior to baking.

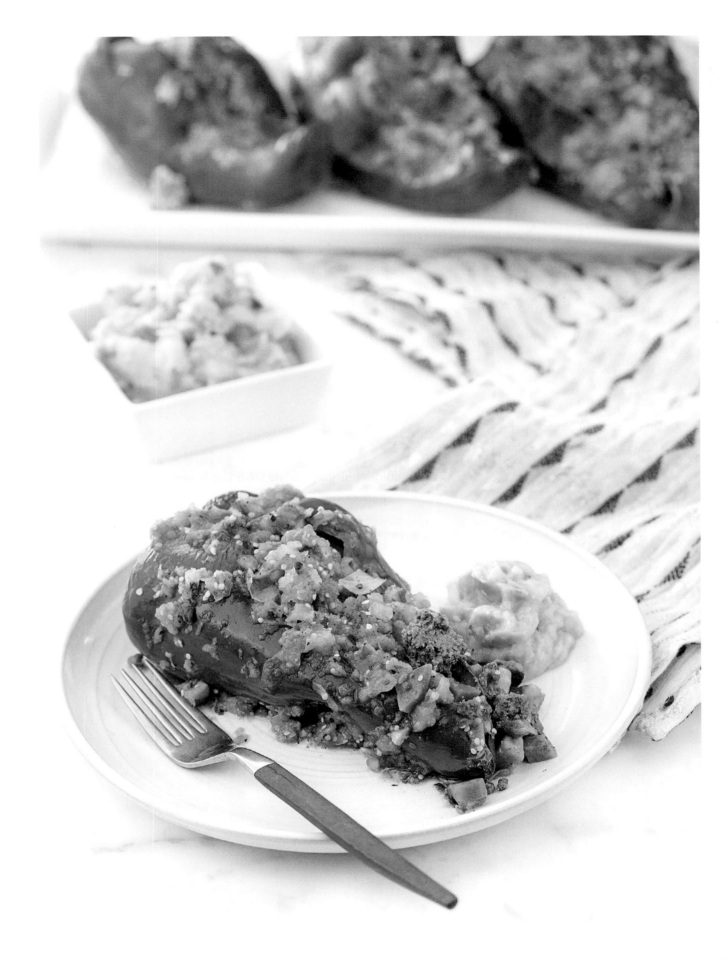

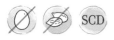

serves: 6

prep time: 20 minutes

cook time: 8 to 9 hours

Whole sheep, fire pits, and holes in the ground are not an option for us, so I use a slow cooker and a beef center shoulder roast for my barbacoa. This version is so easy to make and tastes incredible on my Wraps (page 262) or thrown on top of a big taco salad.

# chipotle barbacoa

## ingredients

- 1 (3-pound) center-cut beef shoulder roast
- 3 to 5 large dried chipotle peppers, seeds removed
- 1 small yellow onion, quartered
- ¼ cup fresh lime juice
- ¼ cup tomato paste
- 4 cloves garlic, peeled
- 1½ tablespoons apple cider vinegar
- 2 teaspoons ground cumin
- 2 teaspoons sea salt
- 1 teaspoon ground dried oregano
- ½ teaspoon ground cloves
- ¾ cup low-sodium beef stock or Chicken Stock (page 242)
- 3 bay leaves

FOR SERVING
- lettuce
- salsa of choice
- Guacamole (page 258)
- chopped fresh cilantro

## method

1. Cut the roast into 2 pieces and trim any fat. Place in a slow cooker.

2. Combine the chipotle peppers, onion, lime juice, tomato paste, garlic, vinegar, cumin, salt, oregano, and cloves in a food processor or blender. Process until smooth.

3. Pour the puréed pepper mixture over the roast and add the stock and bay leaves.

4. Cover and cook on low for 7 hours.

5. Remove the beef and shred with 2 forks. Return the meat to the slow cooker and continue cooking for 1 to 2 hours, until very tender.

6. Serve over a bed of lettuce with salsa, Guacamole, and cilantro.

make-ahead tip:
Prepare Steps 1 through 3 and store in an airtight bag or container. Freeze for up to 3 months or refrigerate for up to 3 days before cooking.

tidbits:
A pork or lamb roast also works wonderfully for this recipe.

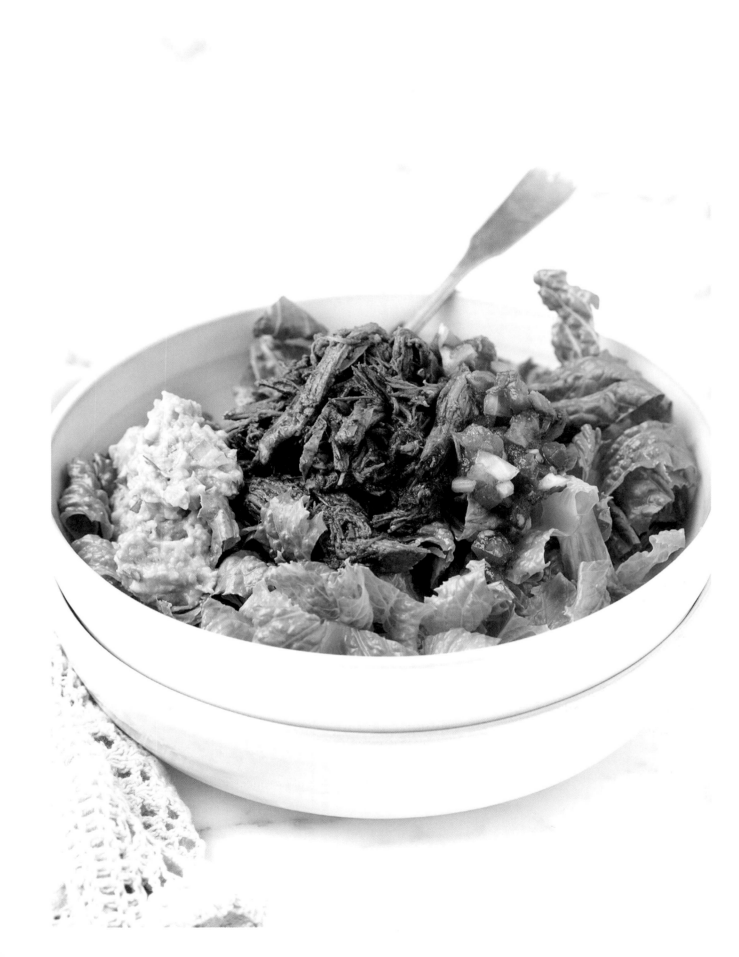

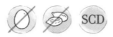

serves: 6 to 8

prep time: 20 minutes

cook time: 40 minutes, or 4 to 6 hours in a slow cooker

The word *arrabbiata* translates to "angry" in Italian and is the name of a popular pasta dish in a spicy red sauce. I personally am not a huge lover of chili heat, but my husband is, so this one is for his tastes and for all of you who love a little kick in your food! To cut the spice level, use mild sausage and reduce the crushed red pepper.

# sausage and peppers arrabbiata

## ingredients

- 2 pounds spicy Italian sausage, casings removed, crumbled
- 1 medium yellow onion, quartered and thinly sliced crosswise
- 3 cloves garlic, minced
- ½ cup dry white wine, such as Sauvignon Blanc
- 1 red bell pepper, seeded and sliced
- 1 yellow bell pepper, seeded and sliced
- 8 ounces cremini mushrooms, sliced
- 1½ teaspoons Italian seasoning
- 1 teaspoon sea salt, plus more if needed
- 1 teaspoon crushed red pepper
- 1 (18-ounce) jar diced tomatoes
- 3 pounds sweet potatoes*
- ¼ cup chopped fresh basil
- ¼ cup chopped fresh parsley

---

* *Use butternut squash or zucchini noodles for SCD.*

## method

1. Brown the sausage with the onion and garlic in a large skillet over medium-high heat, until cooked through.

2. Using a slotted spoon, transfer the meat to a slow cooker. Leave the grease in the pan and return it to the stove.

3. Pour in the wine and scrape the bottom of the pan to deglaze, then simmer for 5 minutes to reduce the liquid.

4. Pour the contents of the skillet into the slow cooker and add the bell peppers, mushrooms, Italian seasoning, salt, crushed red pepper, and tomatoes.

5. Cover and cook on high for 4 hours or on low for 6 hours. Alternatively, cover the skillet and cook on the stovetop for 30 minutes.

6. Peel the sweet potatoes, cut off the narrow ends, then slice them in half crosswise. Use a spiral slicer to create noodles. Alternatively, leave the sweet potatoes whole and julienne them.

7. Steam the noodles in a covered pot filled with 1 inch of water for 1 to 2 minutes, until crisp-tender. Drain in a colander.

8. Stir the fresh basil and parsley into the sauce right before serving and adjust the seasoning if necessary. Serve the sauce over the steamed noodles.

> **make-ahead tip:**
> Complete Steps 1 through 4, let cool to room temperature, and store in the refrigerator overnight, or freeze for up to 3 months for later use. Bring to room temperature before continuing to Step 5. The noodles can be kept in the refrigerator for 2 days prior to cooking.
>
> **tidbits:**
> Check the sausage ingredients carefully. Look for one that has a natural pork casing and contains no additives or sugar.

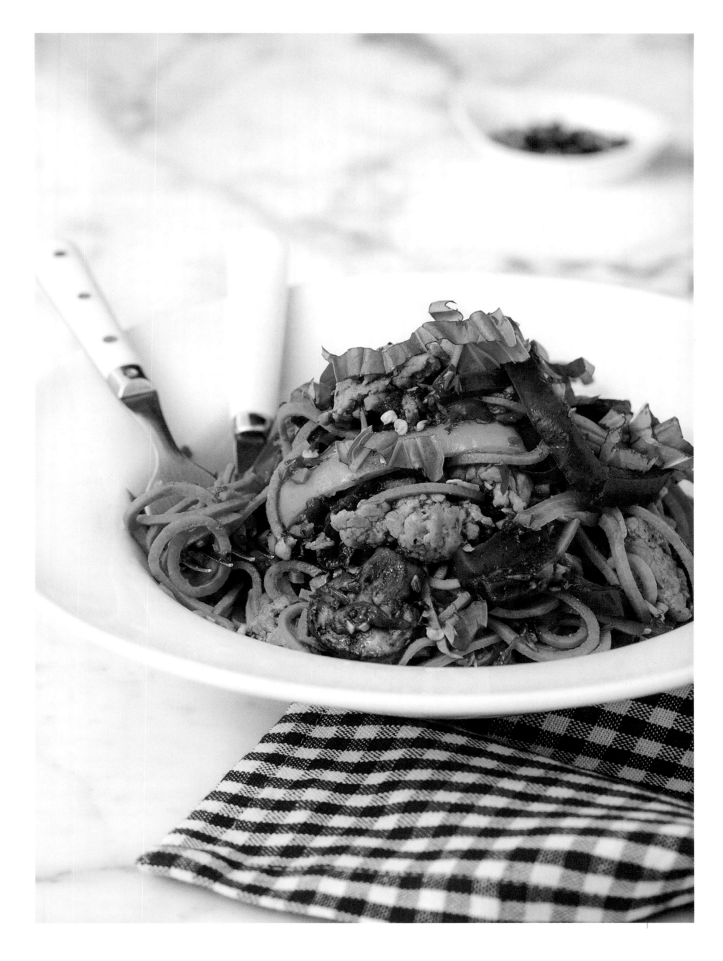

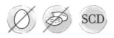

Ø 🚫 SCD

serves: 6

prep time: 15 minutes

cook time: 8 hours

This Cuban favorite is made of tender shredded beef that cooks slowly all day in a slightly tangy and spicy tomato sauce. Serve over a bed of salad greens, with Pan-Fried Plantains or Coconut, Cilantro, & Lime Cauli-Rice (page 218), or simply on its own!

# ropa vieja

## ingredients

- 2 pounds flank steak, cut into 4 pieces
- 1 red bell pepper, seeded and sliced
- 1 yellow bell pepper, seeded and sliced
- 1 yellow onion, sliced
- 2 jalapeños, seeded and sliced
- 2 cloves garlic, minced
- 1 (18-ounce) jar diced tomatoes
- 1 tablespoon apple cider vinegar
- 1 teaspoon dried oregano leaves
- 2 teaspoons ground cumin
- 1 bay leaf
- 2½ teaspoons sea salt
- ¼ cup pimento-stuffed green olives, halved
- fresh cilantro, for garnish
- Pan-Fried Plantains, for serving (optional)

## method

1. Place all of the ingredients except the olives in a slow cooker, with the beef on the bottom.

2. Cover and cook, undisturbed, on low for 7 hours. Add the olives and cook for an additional hour.

3. Skim any fat off the top of the sauce, then shred the meat with 2 forks and return it to the sauce before serving. Garnish with fresh cilantro and serve with Pan-Fried Plantains, if desired.

## pan-fried plantains

- coconut oil
- 2 very ripe plantains
- coarse sea salt
- fresh lime juice

Heat ¼ inch of coconut oil in a skillet over medium-high heat. Peel the plantains, then cut them in half lengthwise and again crosswise. Working in batches, fry the slices on each side until they are golden brown, about 2 minutes. Drain on paper towels and sprinkle with sea salt and a drizzle of lime juice.

**make-ahead tip:**
Put all the ingredients in an airtight container. Refrigerate for 3 days or freeze for up to 3 months and defrost in the refrigerator overnight before placing in the slow cooker.

**stretch it:**
Double the recipe and remove half before adding the olives. Store it for up to 3 days and use it in Enchilada Stuffed Peppers (page 152) in place of the ground bison, or for tacos throughout the week!

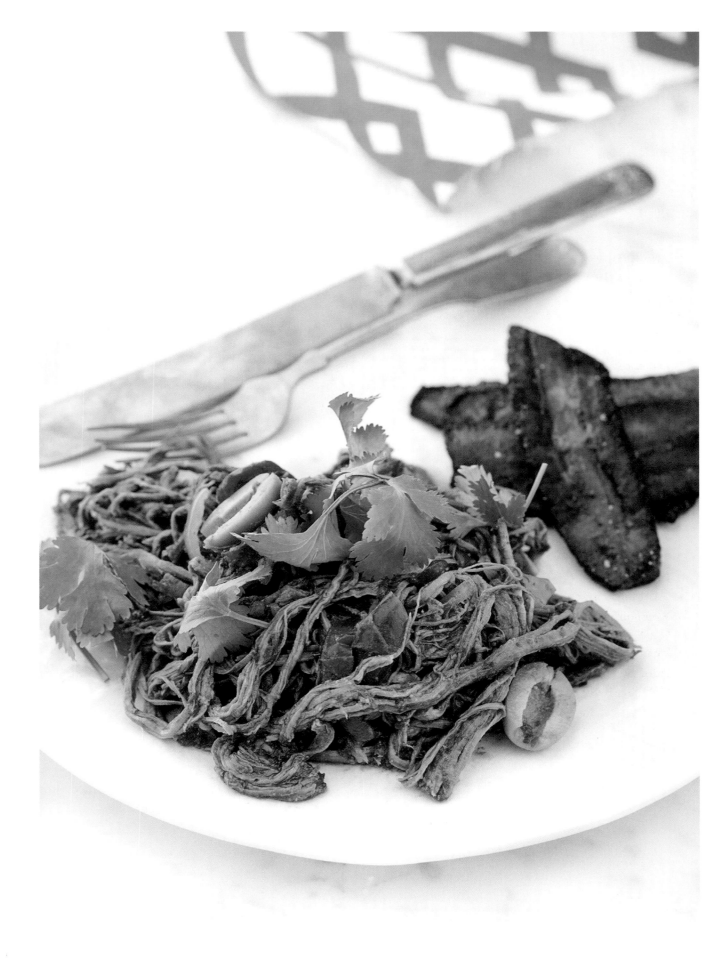

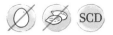

serves: 6 to 8

prep time: 20 minutes

cook time: 5 to 8 hours

Jicama may seem like a strange ingredient to add to this dish, but it provides a slight crunch similar to that of water chestnuts or bamboo shoots and adds a mildly sweet flavor. Serve this stew over any of the cauliflower rice recipes (pages 218–219).

# slow cooker thai beef stew

## ingredients

- 2 tablespoons coconut oil, divided
- 3 pounds beef stew meat, trimmed of fat
- 1 medium yellow onion, thinly sliced
- 2 cloves garlic, minced
- 2 teaspoons peeled and minced fresh ginger
- 1 (13½-ounce) can full-fat coconut milk
- ⅓ cup tomato paste
- ½ cup Thai red curry paste
- 2 tablespoons fish sauce
- 2 teaspoons fresh lime juice
- 2 teaspoons sea salt
- 2 cups broccoli florets
- 2 cups julienned carrots
- 1 cup peeled and julienned jicama*
- fresh cilantro, for garnish

\* Omit for SCD.

## method

1. Heat 1 tablespoon of the coconut oil in a large skillet over medium-high heat. Working in batches, brown the meat on all sides.

2. Use a slotted spoon to transfer each batch of browned meat directly to the slow cooker, then continue browning. Wipe out the skillet between batches if a lot of liquid has accumulated at the bottom to ensure even browning.

3. Wipe out the skillet and add the remaining 1 tablespoon of coconut oil. Sauté the onion, garlic, and ginger over medium-high heat for 5 minutes.

4. Pour in the coconut milk and stir continuously to release the browned bits on the bottom of the pan.

5. Add the tomato paste, curry paste, fish sauce, lime juice, and salt, then pour the mixture over the beef in the slow cooker.

6. Cook on high for 5 hours or low for 8 hours. Add the broccoli, carrots, and jicama during the last 30 minutes if cooking on high, or the last hour if cooking on low. Serve garnished with cilantro.

stretch it:
The leftover meat tastes fabulous in scrambled eggs!

make-ahead tip:
Prepare Steps 1 through 5, then place the contents in an airtight container or bag. Freeze for up to 3 months, then thaw overnight in the refrigerator before continuing to Step 6.

tidbits:
Thai Kitchen makes a great red curry paste with good-quality ingredients.

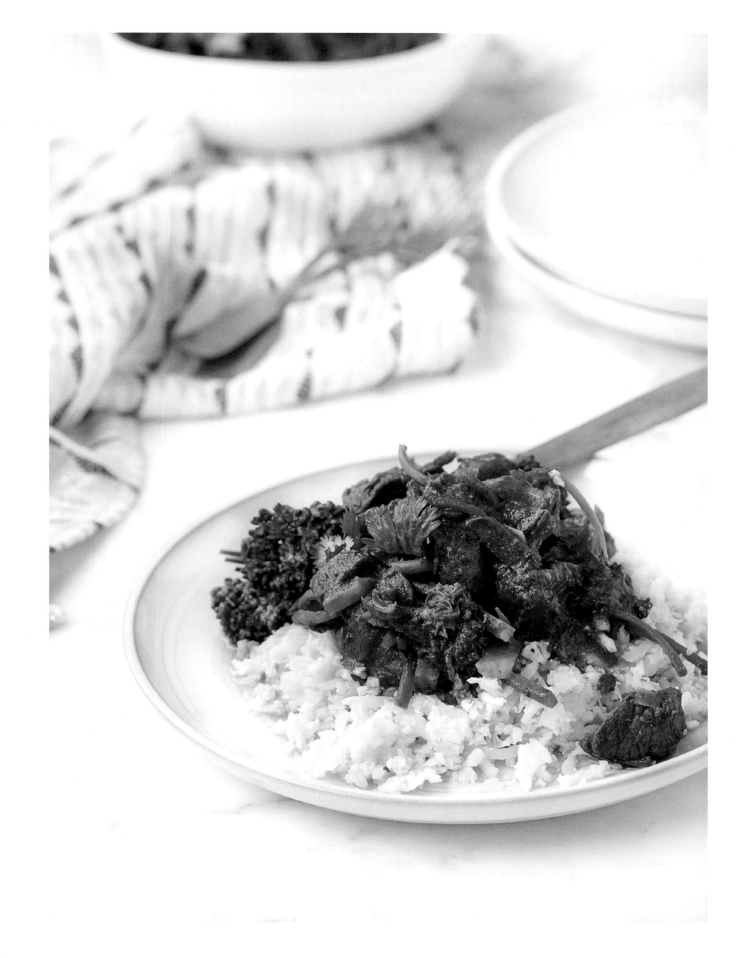

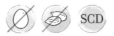

serves: 6 to 8

prep time: 1 hour

cook time: 8 to 10 minutes

I love kabobs because the entire meal is on one skewer. The marinated beef melts in your mouth, and you have free time while it marinates since the "side dish" is grilled right along with the meat!

# pineapple beef kabobs

## ingredients

- ¼ cup coconut aminos*
- ⅓ cup unsweetened pineapple juice
- 1 scallion, minced
- 2 cloves garlic, crushed into a paste
- 1 tablespoon cold-pressed sesame oil
- 1 tablespoon peeled and grated fresh ginger
- ½ teaspoon sea salt
- ¼ teaspoon crushed red pepper
- 2 pounds sirloin steak, trimmed and cut into 1-inch cubes
- 3 large zucchini or yellow squash, cubed
- 2 red bell peppers, seeded and cut into 1-inch pieces
- 1 large red onion, cut into thick 1-inch pieces
- 1 small pineapple, peeled, cored, and cut into 1-inch cubes

*For SCD, omit the coconut aminos and add an additional ½ teaspoon sea salt.*

## method

1. If using wooden skewers, soak 12 skewers in a dish of water for 1 hour.

2. In a small bowl, combine the coconut aminos, pineapple juice, scallion, garlic, sesame oil, ginger, salt, and crushed red pepper.

3. Place the beef in a large baking dish and pour half of the marinade over it. Toss to coat. Cover and refrigerate for 45 minutes (see Tidbits). Reserve the other half of the marinade for basting.

4. Preheat a grill or grill pan to medium-high heat.

5. Drain the meat and discard the juices. Thread the meat, vegetables, and pineapple onto the soaked skewers or metal skewers.

6. Grill, covered, for 8 to 10 minutes, turning occasionally and basting with the reserved marinade.

tidbits:

Because grass-fed beef is already lean compared with conventional beef, the enzymes in the pineapple juice will break through the muscle tissue quickly. Do not marinate longer than 45 minutes if using grass-fed meat. Conventional beef can be marinated for up to 4 hours.

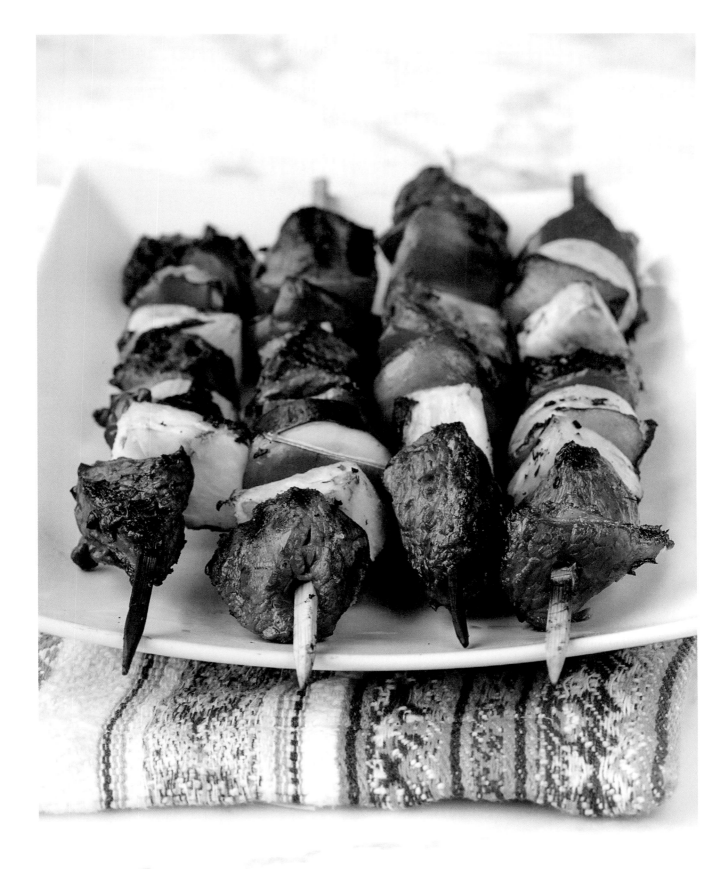

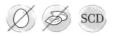

serves: 8
prep time: 10 minutes
cook time: 16 minutes

These juicy burgers are seasoned with Mexican flavors before being grilled to perfection and topped with fresh Guacamole and salsa. Serve with Smoky Roasted Sweet Potatoes (page 222) for a lively summertime dinner.

# mexican burgers

## ingredients

- 3 pounds ground beef
- ⅓ cup minced red onion
- ¼ cup chopped fresh cilantro
- 2 cloves garlic, minced
- 1½ teaspoon ground cumin
- ¾ teaspoon sea salt
- ½ teaspoon ground coriander
- ¼ teaspoon cracked black pepper
- ½ cup salsa of choice
- ½ cup Guacamole (page 258)
- 1 head romaine lettuce

## method

1. Preheat a grill or grill pan to medium heat.

2. Combine the beef, onion, cilantro, garlic, cumin, salt, coriander, and pepper in a bowl. Mix until just combined, then form into 8 (¾-inch-thick) patties.

3. Grill, covered, for 6 to 8 minutes on each side for medium doneness.

4. Top the burgers with salsa and Guacamole and wrap with large lettuce leaves.

tidbits:
My favorite store-bought salsa is the Organic Tomatillo & Roasted Yellow Chili Salsa from Trader Joe's. Grab your favorite jar or make a batch of any of the homemade salsas (page 258) to make these burgers your own.

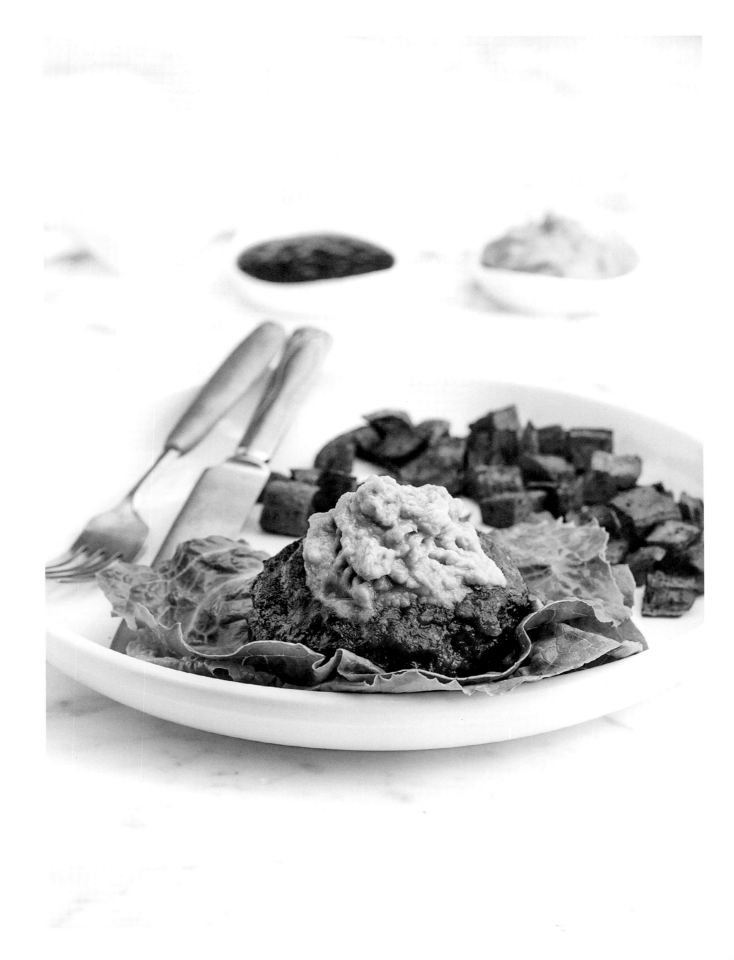

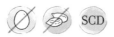

∅ 🐟 SCD

serves: 6
prep time: 15 minutes
cook time: 25 minutes

I love a good pizza, but sometimes making the crust from scratch is too time-consuming. This simple pasta combines all my favorite pizza flavors in a one-pot meal. I love to throw kale or other power greens into this dish, where they are concealed from my son, Asher, by the delicious pepperoni and sauce.

# pepperoni pizza pasta

## ingredients

- 4 ounces pepperoni, cut into wedges and sliced crosswise
- ¾ pound mild Italian sausage, casings removed
- 3 cups stemmed and coarsely chopped kale
- ¾ teaspoon sea salt
- 3 pounds yellow squash
- ¾ cup tomato paste
- 1 to 3 tablespoons water
- 1 tablespoon nutritional yeast*
- 2 teaspoons dried oregano leaves

*Substitute Parmesan cheese for SCD.*

## method

1. Heat a large pot over medium-high heat. Add the pepperoni and cook for 2 minutes on each side, until browned. Remove with a slotted spoon and set aside.

2. Crumble the sausage and add it to the pot along with the kale and salt. Cook for 5 to 7 minutes, until the sausage is cooked through.

3. Meanwhile, trim the ends off of the squash and use a spiral slicer or julienne slicer to create noodles.

4. Add the noodles to the pot and sauté for 5 minutes, until crisp-tender.

5. Stir in the tomato paste, 1 tablespoon of the water, nutritional yeast, and oregano. Cover and continue cooking for 8 minutes, until the sauce is simmering and the noodles are soft. Add up to 2 more tablespoons of water if the sauce needs to be thinned further.

tidbits:
Check the sausage and pepperoni ingredients carefully to avoid sugars, nitrates, and other additives. Applegate brand makes a wonderful pepperoni, and bulk organic sausage can be found at most health food stores.

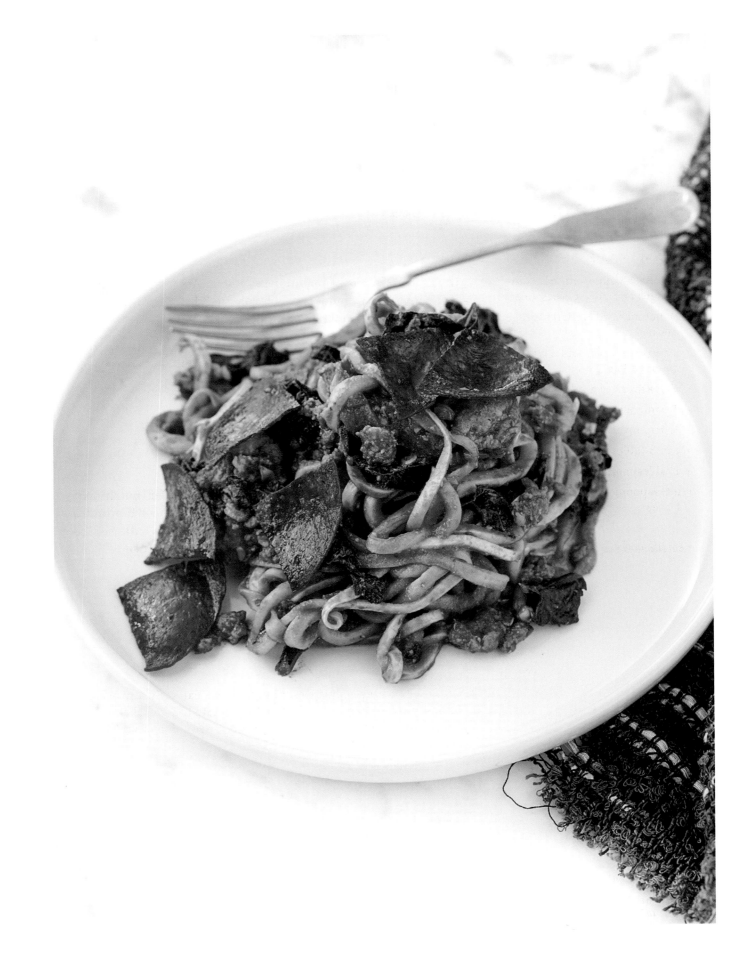

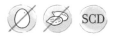

serves: 6
prep time: 5 minutes
cook time: 22 minutes

This is another of my go-to shortcut meals when the day is almost over and I've forgotten to plan dinner. A quality spaghetti sauce can take hours to simmer down and obtain the flavor it deserves, so I turn to the jar in a pinch and spruce it up with my own seasonings from the pantry and extra garlic! I keep ground beef in the freezer at all times for this purpose and throw whatever vegetables I have into the spiral slicer if I don't have spaghetti squash on hand.

# shortcut spaghetti with meat sauce

## ingredients

- 2 teaspoons ghee or extra-virgin olive oil
- 4 cloves garlic, minced
- 2 pounds ground beef
- 1 tablespoon Italian seasoning
- 1 tablespoon dried parsley
- 2 teaspoons onion powder
- 1½ teaspoons sea salt
- ½ teaspoon cracked black pepper
- ½ teaspoon crushed red pepper
- 5 cups store-bought spaghetti sauce (see Tidbits)
- pasta alternative of your choice (see Serving Suggestions)

## method

1. Heat the ghee in a saucepan over medium-high heat. Sauté the garlic for 1 minute, until fragrant. Add the beef and seasonings, reduce the heat to medium, and cook for 10 minutes, until the beef is cooked through. Drain any grease.

2. Pour in the spaghetti sauce and simmer for 10 minutes. Serve over the pasta substitute of your choice.

Serving Suggestions
Roasted spaghetti squash is a wonderful spaghetti substitute. Follow the method on page 204, omitting the Roma tomatoes.

Spiral-sliced or julienned yellow squash or zucchini noodles (see the Tidbits on page 194) or sweet potato noodles (page 156) also work well.

For a change from noodles, steamed broccoli also serves as a wonderful bed to hold this hearty sauce.

> tidbits:
> Check the labels closely when buying jarred spaghetti sauce. Look for a short list of ingredients that does not include sugar, soybean or canola oil, or citric acid. The ingredients should be simple: tomatoes, extra-virgin olive oil, garlic, herbs, salt, spices, and sometimes vegetables such as carrots, mushrooms, or celery. My favorite brands are Middle Earth Organics and Eden Organics.

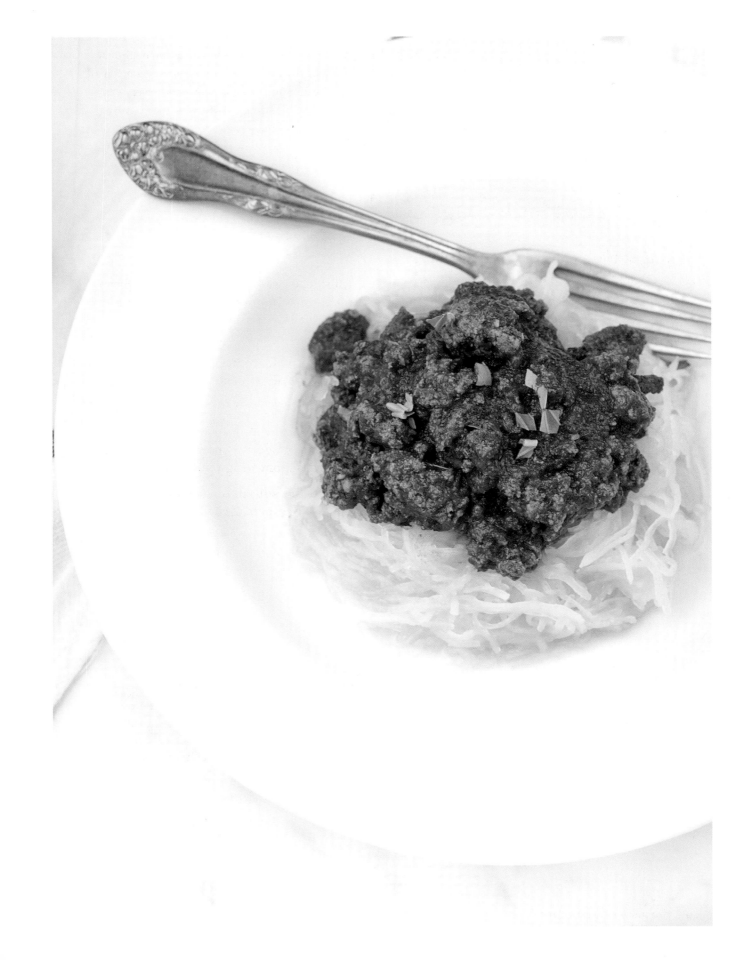

serves: 4 to 6

prep time: 15 minutes plus
30 minutes marinating time

cook time: 30 minutes

For a quick and easy grilled dinner, this combo of barbecue-rubbed steak and watermelon salad is a crowd-pleaser and hits the spot on a hot summer night.

# barbecue tri-tip with grilled watermelon salad

## ingredients

### STEAK

- 1 tri-tip roast, about 2½ to 3 pounds
- ¼ cup Barbecue Dry Rub (page 244)
- 1 teaspoon sea salt

### SALAD

- 2 cups cubed seedless watermelon
- 1 teaspoon melted coconut oil
- ½ cup balsamic vinegar
- 1 tablespoon honey
- 6 cups arugula
- 1 radish, thinly sliced
- 2 tablespoons roasted and salted pepitas
- 2 tablespoons extra-virgin olive oil
- sea salt and cracked black pepper

## method

1. Prepare the steak: Rub the steak all over with the dry rub and salt and let sit at room temperature for 30 minutes.

2. Preheat a grill or grill pan to medium-high heat, then sear the steak on all sides. Reduce the heat to medium-low or move the steak away from the coals, and continue to grill, covered, for 20 minutes for medium-rare (140°F) or 30 minutes for medium-well (160°F), turning occasionally.

3. Remove the steak from the grill and tent with foil. Allow to rest for 15 minutes.

4. Prepare the salad: Toss the watermelon in the oil and place it in a grill basket. Grill on both sides for 2 minutes, until light grill marks are present.

5. Meanwhile, heat the balsamic vinegar in a saucepan over medium-high heat. Once simmering, decrease the heat to medium-low and simmer until reduced by half, about 8 minutes. Remove from the heat and whisk in the honey.

6. Toss the grilled watermelon with the balsamic reduction, arugula, radish, pepitas, olive oil, and a pinch of salt and pepper.

7. Slice the steak against the grain on a diagonal and serve with the salad.

| make-ahead tip: | tidbits: | stretch it: |
|---|---|---|
| The steak can marinate in the rub, covered in the refrigerator, for up to 24 hours. | If watermelon isn't in season, peaches or nectarines are a great variation for the salad. | Use any leftover steak in Balsamic Steak Pizza (page 172). |

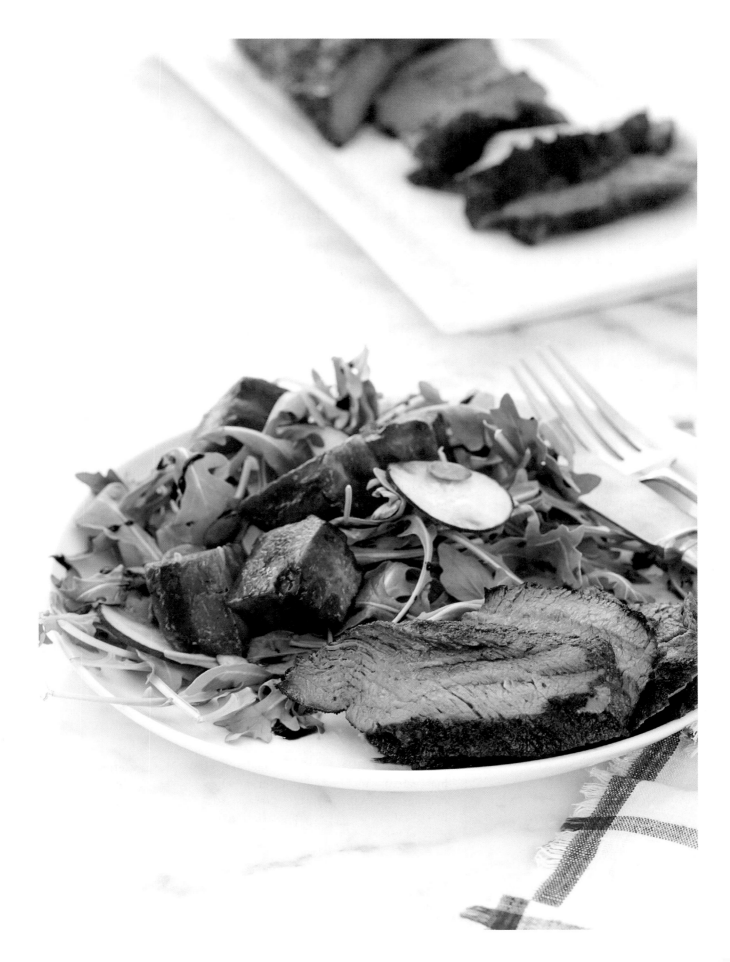

serves: 4

prep time: 20 minutes

cook time: 35 minutes

This nut-free flatbread-style pizza is a great way to use up leftover steak or other barbecued meat from the night before. The balsamic reduction is sweet and robust and stands in for a traditional tomato sauce.

# balsamic steak pizza

## ingredients

### TOPPING

- 1 tablespoon extra-virgin olive oil
- ½ red onion, thinly sliced
- ½ teaspoon sea salt
- ¼ teaspoon cracked black pepper
- ½ cup balsamic vinegar
- 2 teaspoons honey
- ¾ cup cubed leftover Barbecue Tri-Tip (page 170)
- 1 cup arugula
- ¼ cup chopped fresh basil

### CRUST

- 1½ cup arrowroot powder
- ½ cup coconut flour
- ½ cup melted ghee
- 3 large eggs
- 2 tablespoons warm water
- ½ teaspoon sea salt
- ½ teaspoon baking soda

## method

1. Preheat the oven to 400°F.

2. Heat the olive oil in a skillet over medium-high heat. Add the onion, salt, and pepper and sauté for 3 minutes. Reduce the heat to medium-low and continue cooking for 15 minutes while preparing the crust.

3. Make the crust: Combine the ingredients in the bowl of a food processor or stand mixer. Mix for 15 seconds, until a loose dough forms. Allow the dough to sit for 5 minutes, then mix again until a ball of dough forms. Divide the dough into two balls and place them between 2 sheets of parchment paper. Flatten them into discs, then roll into ¼-inch-thick circles, smoothing any rough edges to make them round. Transfer the bottom sheet of parchment and the crusts to a baking sheet and bake the crust for 15 minutes. Allow to cool for 10 minutes.

4. Increase the heat on the onions to medium-high and pour in the balsamic vinegar, stirring to release any browned bits from the bottom of the skillet. Bring to a boil, then decrease the heat to medium-low and let the vinegar simmer and reduce for 5 minutes. Remove from the heat and stir in the honey.

5. Spread the reduced balsamic and onion mixture on the crusts and arrange the steak on top. Place the pizzas back in the oven for 2 minutes to warm the steak. Remove from the oven and top with the arugula and basil.

tidbits:

If you do not have leftover tri-tip, any cooked steak or chicken will work for this pizza, or simply serve it as a vegetarian dish.

make-ahead tip:

Bake the crust 3 days in advance and store in the refrigerator, or freeze for 6 months. Thaw at room temperature for 20 minutes before adding the onions and steak.

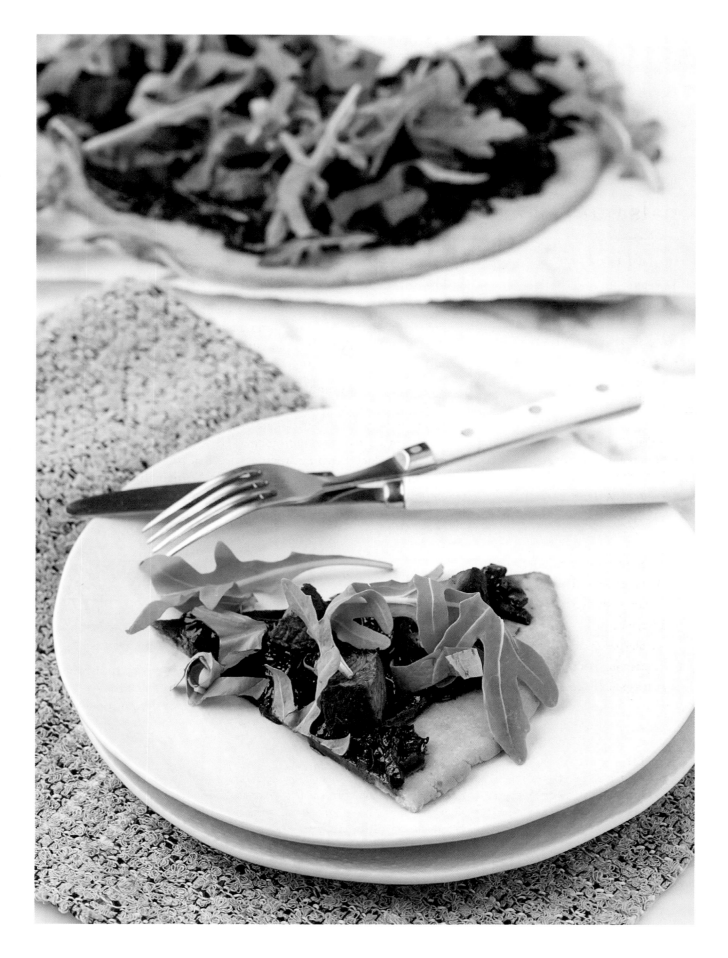

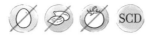

serves: 4 to 6

prep time: 10 minutes

cook time: 10 to 15 minutes

I often think of pork chops as being tough or dry, but this recipe produces chops that are perfectly seasoned and moist. They pair wonderfully with Lemon-Roasted Asparagus and Brussels Sprouts (page 224). I use thin pork chops because they are quicker to cook and help ensure that I can get dinner on the table in less than 30 minutes.

# rosemary-lemon pork chops

## ingredients

- 6 bone-in, thin-cut pork chops (about 6 ounces each)
- sea salt and cracked black pepper
- 2 tablespoons ghee or bacon fat, divided
- 3 sprigs fresh rosemary
- 3 cloves garlic, halved
- 2 teaspoons fresh lemon juice

## method

1. Place a roasting pan in the oven and preheat it to 400°F.

2. Generously season both sides of the pork chops with salt and pepper.

3. Heat 1 tablespoon of the ghee, the rosemary, and the garlic in a large skillet over medium-high heat.

4. Working in batches, sear the chops for 1 minute on each side, basting with the ghee from the pan as they brown. Add the remaining tablespoon of ghee after half of the chops have been browned.

5. Add the browned pork chops, liquid from the skillet, and lemon juice to the hot roasting pan and place it in the preheated oven. Roast for 5 minutes, until the pork chops are cooked through or register 140°F to 145°F at the thickest part.

6. Remove the pan from the oven and transfer the pork chops and juices to a plate. Tent loosely with foil and allow to rest for 5 minutes before serving.

tidbits:
If making the Lemon-Roasted Asparagus and Brussels Sprouts (page 224), begin cooking the dish while you sear the pork chops. The tray can stay in the oven while you roast the pork chops and continue cooking while the pork rests.

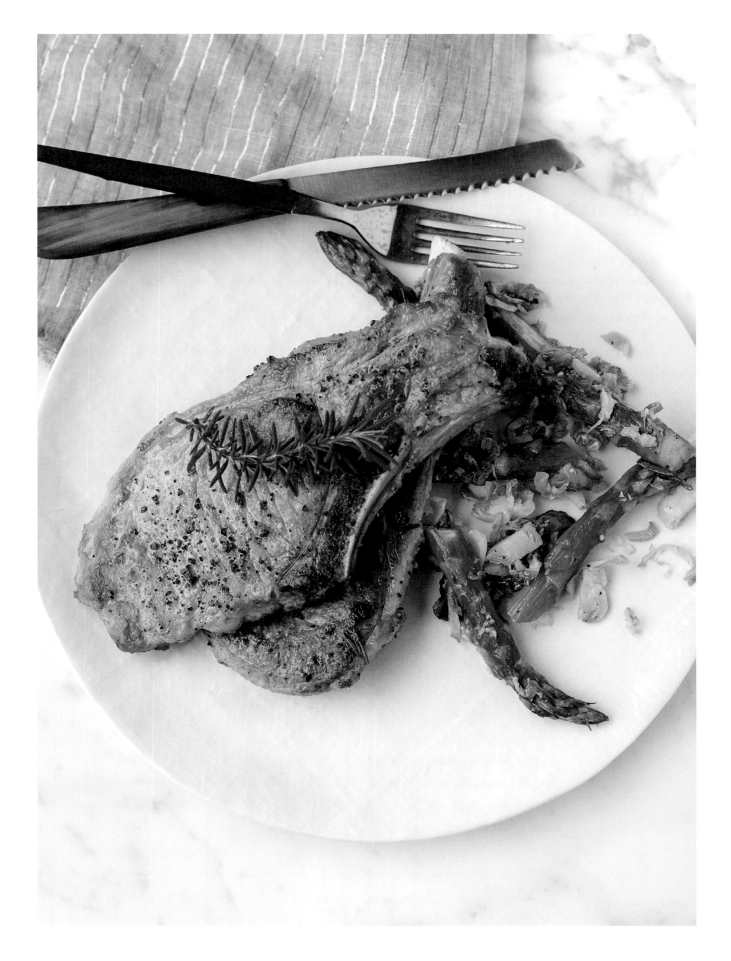

serves: 8

prep time: 10 minutes

cook time: 8 hours

This lamb shoulder cooks slowly all day with a few simple herbs and seasonings to produce a tender and flavorful meal. While the slow cooker does the work, you can complete the meal quickly by making my Roasted Squash and Beets in Tahini Sauce (page 234) or Grilled Greek Summer Squash Salad (page 106).

# mediterranean braised lamb

## ingredients

- 2 tablespoons ghee, bacon fat, or olive oil
- 1 (5-pound) lamb shoulder roast, trimmed and tied
- 10 cloves garlic, peeled
- sea salt and cracked black pepper
- ¼ cup extra-virgin olive oil
- ½ cup chopped fresh oregano leaves or 3 tablespoons dried
- zest of 1 lemon, grated
- juice of 1 lemon
- 2 teaspoons arrowroot powder*, for gravy, if desired

* Omit for SCD.

## method

1. Heat the ghee in a large skillet over medium-high heat.

2. Pierce 10 holes all around the lamb and insert the whole garlic cloves. Season the meat generously with salt and pepper.

3. Sear the meat for about 45 seconds on each side, then transfer it to a slow cooker.

4. Pour the olive oil over the top and add the oregano, lemon zest, and lemon juice.

5. Cover and cook on low for 8 hours, basting and turning the roast occasionally.

6. Slice the roast on the diagonal and serve with the juices over the top. The juices may be simmered on the stove to reduce into a thicker gravy or whisked with 2 teaspoons arrowroot powder, if desired.

tidbits:
A lamb leg roast may be substituted for the shoulder.

make-ahead tip:
Cook the meat and store in its juices, tightly covered, for up to 5 days in the refrigerator or 3 months in the freezer. Reheat the meat and juices in a covered pot on the stove over medium-low heat until warmed through.

stretch it:
Use leftover meat to make Greek Salad with Garlic-Oregano Lamb (page 110).

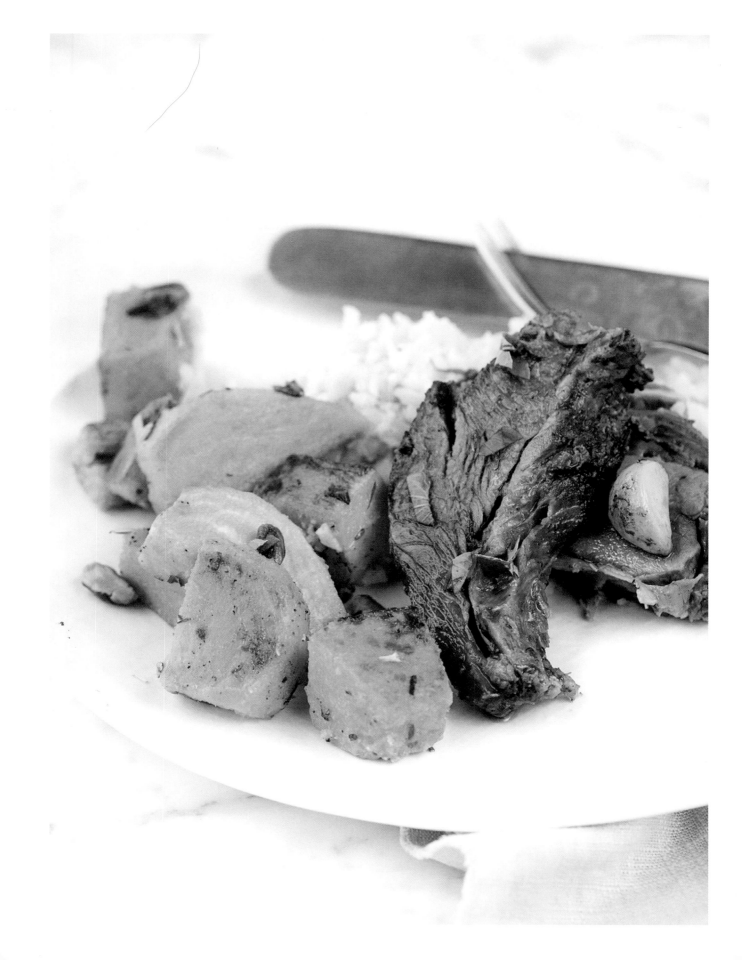

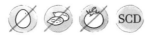

serves: 6 to 8

prep time: 20 minutes

cook time: 8 minutes

The flavor of these burgers is reminiscent of a gyro, but without all the work or the pita. While they are filling all on their own, they go really well with Grilled Greek Summer Squash Salad (page 106).

# greek lamb burgers with tzatziki sauce

## ingredients

- 3 pounds ground lamb
- 1 tablespoon chopped fresh rosemary
- 1 tablespoon chopped fresh oregano leaves
- 3 tablespoons fresh lemon juice
- 5 cloves garlic, minced
- 3 tablespoons extra-virgin olive oil
- ¾ teaspoon sea salt
- ¼ teaspoon cracked black pepper

### Tzatziki sauce

- 1½ cups dairy-free plain yogurt
- ¾ cup peeled, seeded, and diced cucumber
- 2 tablespoons extra-virgin olive oil
- 1 tablespoon fresh lemon juice
- 2 cloves garlic, minced
- 2 teaspoons red wine vinegar
- 2 teaspoons chopped fresh dill
- sea salt and cracked black pepper to taste

### For serving

- 1 head romaine lettuce, leaves separated
- 1 red onion, thinly sliced
- 2 tomatoes, sliced*

## method

1. In a large bowl, mix the meat with the rosemary, oregano, lemon juice, garlic, olive oil, salt, and pepper. Cover and let sit at room temperature while the grill heats.

2. Preheat a grill or grill pan to medium-high heat.

3. Meanwhile, mix all of the ingredients for the tzatziki sauce in a medium bowl. Cover and place in the fridge until ready to serve.

4. Form the ground lamb mixture into 8 (¾-inch-thick) burger patties.

5. Grill the patties for 4 minutes on each side, with the grill lid closed, until the internal temperature reaches 160°F for medium doneness.

6. Assemble the burgers on top of lettuce leaves with onion and tomato slices and a generous tablespoon of tzatziki sauce. Serve the extra sauce on the side.

make-ahead tip:
Prepare the patties 2 days in advance and store, tightly covered, in the refrigerator. The sauce will keep for 3 days in the refrigerator.

tidbits:
Plain Greek yogurt may be used for the sauce if dairy is tolerated.

stretch it:
If there are extra burgers, serve them atop Greek Salad with Garlic-Oregano Lamb (page 110) instead of braised lamb.

* Omit for nightshade-free.

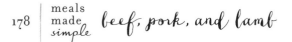

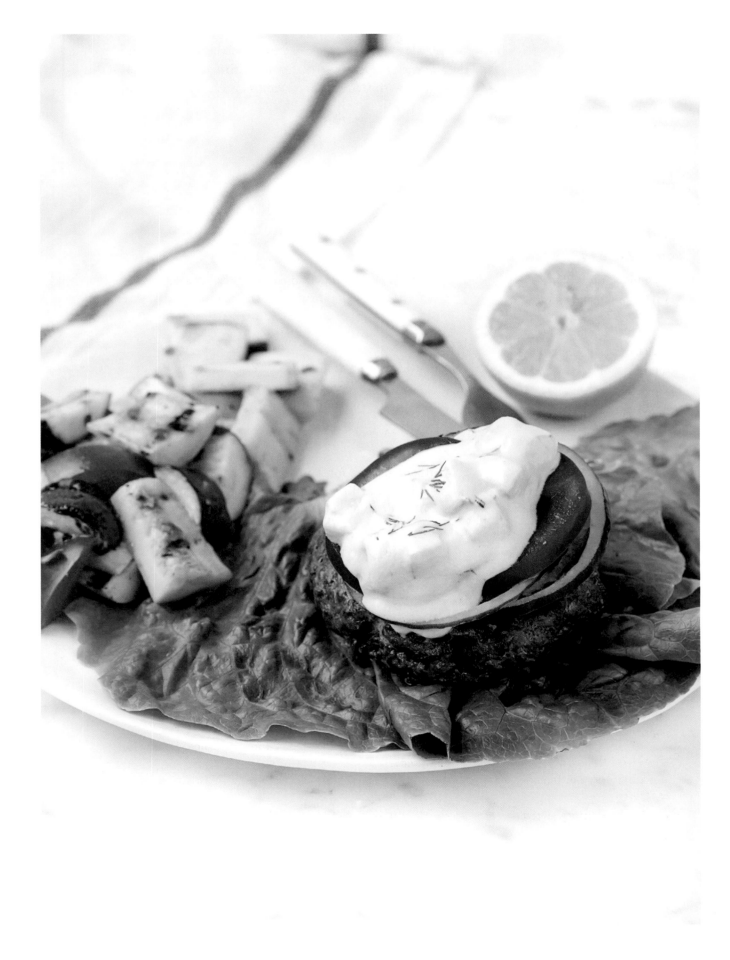

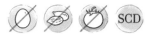

serves: 4 to 6 (per tenderloin)
prep time: 15 minutes plus
30 minutes marinating time
cook time: 25 minutes

Grilling two tenderloins at once saves time—you can enjoy one for dinner and repurpose the other in meals throughout the week, such as my White Pork Chili (page 90) and Pork Stir-Fry (page 182).

# maple-dijon pork tenderloin

## ingredients

- 4 cloves garlic, crushed into a paste
- 3 tablespoons chopped fresh tarragon
- ⅓ cup grade B maple syrup or honey*
- ¼ cup apple cider vinegar
- 3 tablespoons Dijon mustard
- ½ teaspoon sea salt
- ¼ teaspoon cracked black pepper
- 2 pork tenderloins, trimmed (1½ to 2 pounds each)
- 4 ounces prosciutto, chopped
- ½ cup extra-virgin olive oil
- 6 cups baby greens
- 2 pears, sliced

*Use honey for SCD.*

## method

1. In a small bowl, mix together the garlic, tarragon, maple syrup, vinegar, mustard, salt, and pepper. Place the tenderloins in a resealable bag and pour the marinade over them. Toss to coat, then leave at room temperature for 30 minutes.

2. Preheat a grill or grill pan to medium-high heat. Remove the pork from the bag and reserve the marinade. Sear the pork on all sides, then reduce the heat to medium and grill, covered, for an additional 15 minutes, until the pork reaches an internal temperature of 140°F. Turn the pork occasionally while it cooks.

3. Meanwhile, cook the prosciutto in a skillet over medium heat for 5 minutes, until crisp. Pour in the reserved marinade and cook over medium-high heat until boiling to ensure that any traces of raw pork are cooked. Reduce the heat to low and simmer for 10 minutes. Remove from the heat and slowly drizzle in the olive oil, whisking continuously. Set aside to cool.

4. Remove the pork from the grill and tent with foil. Let rest for 10 minutes. Remove 1 tenderloin to a cutting board and slice on a slight diagonal. Allow the other tenderloin to cool completely before wrapping and storing in the refrigerator.

5. Toss the lettuce and pears with half of the sauce and serve the salad with the sliced pork. Serve the extra sauce on the side to drizzle over the pork.

**stretch it:**
Use the second pork tenderloin in White Pork Chili (page 90) or Pork Stir-Fry (page 182).

**make-ahead tip:**
The pork can marinate, covered, in the refrigerator for up to 24 hours, so you can prepare it the night before and throw it on the grill right before dinner. Allow to sit at room temperature for 30 minutes before grilling.

**tidbits:**
The recipe can easily be cut in half and grilled for the same amount of time if serving for only one meal.

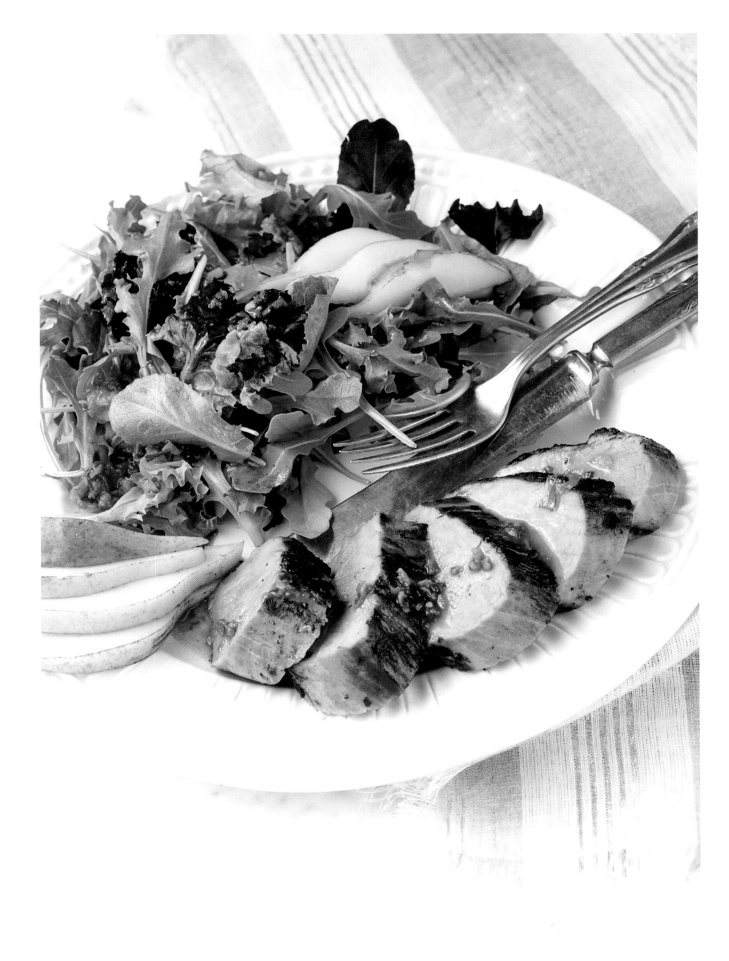

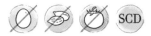

Use up the last of your Maple-Dijon Pork Tenderloin (page 180) in this light stir-fry filled with lots of fresh vegetables.

serves: 6

prep time: 15 minutes

cook time: 14 minutes

## pork stir-fry

### ingredients

- 1 tablespoon ghee or coconut oil
- 1 tablespoon toasted sesame oil
- 3 cloves garlic, minced
- 2 scallions, white and green parts, minced
- 1 teaspoon peeled and grated fresh ginger
- 1 pound broccolini, cut into florets and stalks trimmed to 2 inches
- 1 pound baby bok choy, tough bottom portion of stalk trimmed to about 2 inches
- ½ pound snow peas
- 1 cup sliced cremini mushrooms
- 2½ cups sliced leftover Maple-Dijon Pork Tenderloin (page 180) or other leftover pork
- 3 tablespoons coconut aminos*
- ¼ teaspoon sea salt

*Substitute Chicken Stock (page 242) for SCD.*

### method

1. Heat the ghee and sesame oil in a large skillet or wok over medium-high heat. Sauté the garlic, scallions, and ginger for 1 minute, until fragrant. Add the remaining vegetables and sauté for 8 minutes more, until the vegetables are crisp-tender.

2. Stir in the pork, coconut aminos, and salt and cook for 5 minutes more, until the pork is warmed through.

tidbits:
Leftover Roasted Chicken (page 118) works equally well in this recipe!

meals made simple *beef, pork, and lamb*

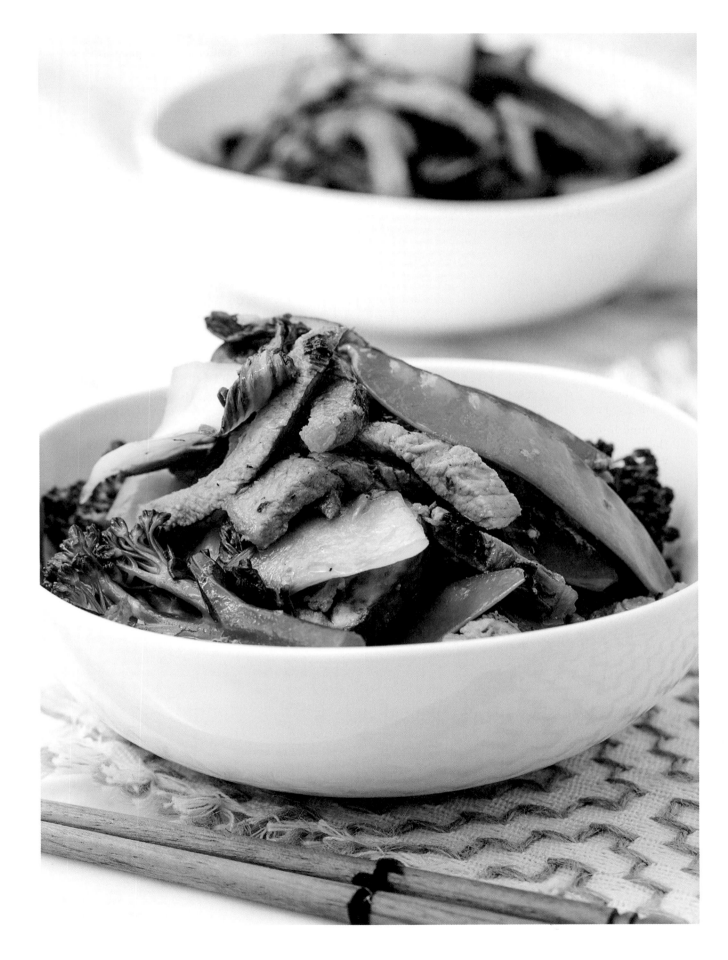

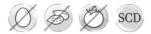

serves: 8 to 10

prep time: 20 minutes

cook time: 4 hours 20 minutes to 8 hours 20 minutes

A pork shoulder cooks slowly in a slow cooker to produce extremely tender and flavorful shredded meat. Serve it with Catalan-Style Spinach (page 226) and the flavorful carrots that cook alongside the meat. Save the leftover pork to use in one of the "stretch it" recipes below, or serve it over salads throughout the week!

# slow cooker braised pork shoulder

## ingredients

- 1 tablespoon ghee or bacon fat
- 1 (5-pound) boneless pork shoulder roast, trimmed of fat and cut into 4 large chunks
- sea salt and cracked black pepper
- 6 ounces pancetta, diced
- 2 small yellow onions, diced
- 5 cloves garlic, minced
- 1½ teaspoons fennel seeds*
- ¾ cup dry red wine
- 1 cup Chicken Stock (page 242)
- 1 pound carrots, peeled and cut into 3-inch pieces

*Fennel seeds are SCD legal if you have been symptom free.*

## method

1. Melt the ghee in a large Dutch oven or deep skillet over medium-high heat.

2. Generously season the shoulder pieces with salt and pepper.

3. Brown the pieces in batches, then place them in the slow cooker.

4. In the same pan that you browned the pork, sauté the pancetta, onions, garlic, and fennel seeds over medium heat for 5 to 7 minutes, until the onions are soft. Pour the mixture on top of the pork.

5. While the pan is still hot, pour in the wine and stir continuously to release any browned bits from the bottom. Pour it into the slow cooker and add the Chicken Stock.

6. Cover and cook on low for 8 hours or on high for 4 hours. Add the carrots during the last 2 hours of cooking.

7. Skim off any fat from the surface, then slice or shred the meat and ladle a bit of the sauce over the top.

tidbits:
Take the time to brown the meat and onions before adding them to the slow cooker. It gives the dish a more robust and deep flavor overall and helps render some of the fat from the pork so it doesn't all end up floating to the top of the sauce!

make-ahead tip:
Complete Steps 1 through 5 up to 3 months in advance. Let cool, then place in an airtight container or resealable bag and store in the freezer. Thaw overnight in the refrigerator before completing Step 6.

Store the leftover meat with ½ cup of the juices in the refrigerator for up to 5 days total, whether for use on its own or in one of the "stretch it" recipes.

stretch it:
Pork Ragu (page 186)—save 1½ cups of the juices and 3 cups of the shredded meat for this dish.

Cuban Pork Panini (page 188)—save ½ cup of the juices and 1 cup of the shredded meat for this dish.

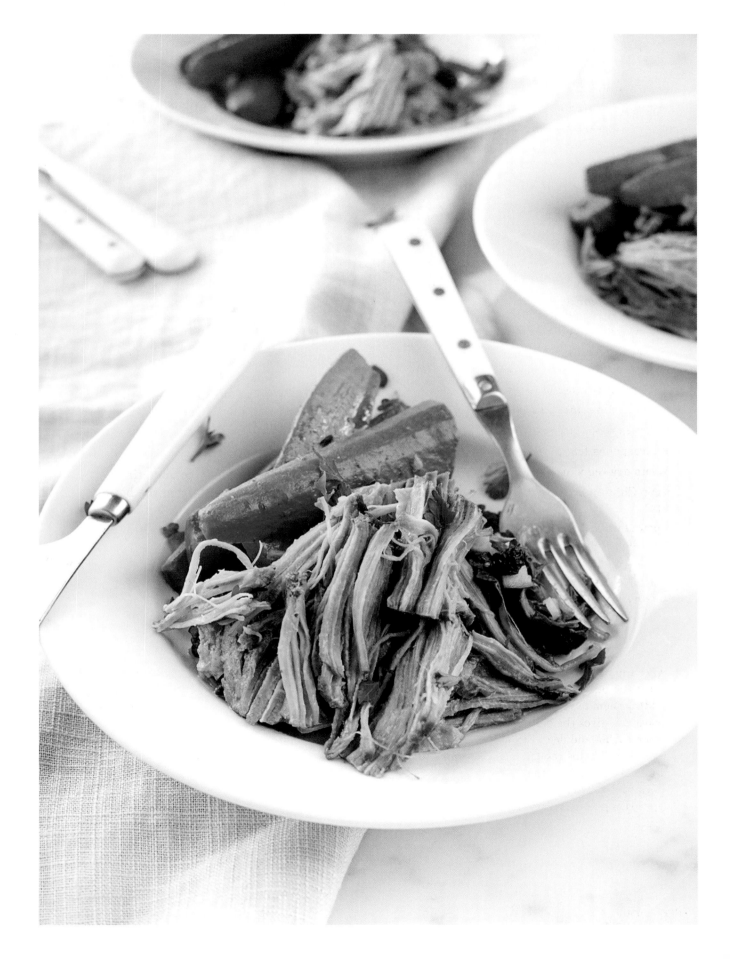

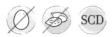

serves: 4 to 6
prep time: 15 minutes
cook time: 33 to 35 minutes

Meal prep is a cinch when you use your leftover Slow Cooker Braised Pork Shoulder (page 184) in this delectable tomato ragu served over butternut squash noodles.

# pork ragu

## ingredients

- 1½ cups reserved juices from Slow Cooker Braised Pork Shoulder (page 184)
- ½ cup minced carrots
- ½ cup minced fennel bulb
- 2 cloves garlic, minced
- 1 cup tomato puree
- 1 tablespoon tomato paste
- 1 (4-pound) butternut squash
- ¼ cup chopped fresh parsley
- 1 tablespoon chopped fresh sage
- 3 cups leftover shredded pork from Slow Cooker Braised Pork Shoulder (page 184)
- sea salt and cracked black pepper

## method

1. Heat the reserved pork juices in a saucepan over medium-high heat. Simmer for 15 minutes, until the liquid has reduced by about half.

2. Add the carrots, fennel, garlic, tomato puree, and tomato paste and simmer, covered, for 10 minutes, until the vegetables are soft.

3. Meanwhile, cut the long neck off the squash and reserve the bulb-shaped part with the seeds for another use. Peel the neck section and cut it in half crosswise.

4. Use a spiral slicer to cut the squash into noodles. Alternatively, use a julienne slicer and run it along the entire neck of the squash to create noodles.

5. Stir the herbs and pork into the sauce and cook for 5 minutes more, until the pork is warmed through.

6. Season with salt and pepper to taste, then reduce the heat to medium-low and keep warm while the noodles cook.

7. Heat about ½ inch of water in a deep skillet over medium-high heat. Add the noodles, cover, and steam for 3 to 5 minutes, until crisp-tender. Drain and top with the ragu sauce.

tidbits:
Cooked ground beef or pork and a good-quality beef or pork stock may be substituted for the shredded pork and juices, although the flavors will change and additional salt will likely be needed.

make-ahead tip:
Slow Cooker Braised Pork Shoulder can be kept in the fridge for up to 5 days, whether stored in its juices or used to make this recipe. For example, you can prepare the pork 3 days in advance of making the ragu and then store the ragu for up to 2 days in the fridge; or you can make the pork 2 days in advance and store the ragu for up to 3 days. The ragu can be frozen for up to 3 months. Thaw in the refrigerator overnight before reheating on the stove.

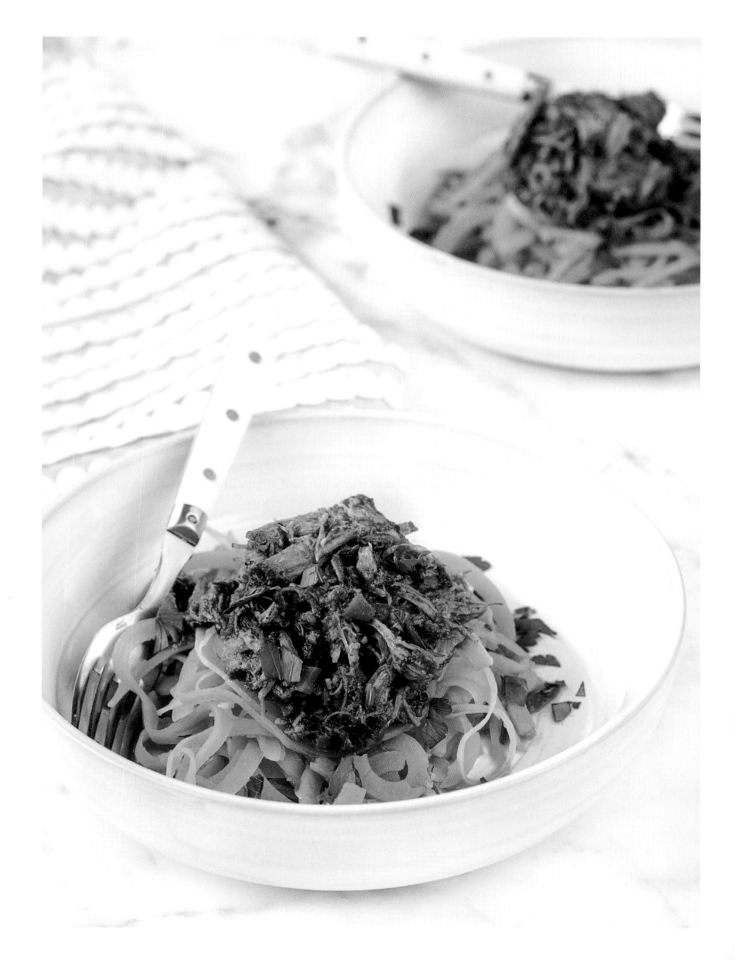

yield: 6 paninis

prep time: 10 minutes

cook time: 5 minutes, or 15 minutes with fresh Wraps

Use up your leftover Slow Cooker Braised Pork (page 184) in this quick and easy panini recipe inspired by the traditional Cuban pork sandwich. With tender braised pork, prosciutto, pickles, and a Dijon spread, you will be surprised at how much flavor can come from such a simple dish.

# 30 minutes or less cuban pork panini

## ingredients

- 12 Wraps (page 262)
- 1 cup leftover shredded pork from Slow Cooker Braised Pork Shoulder (page 184)
- ½ cup reserved juices from Slow Cooker Braised Pork Shoulder (page 184)
- 6 slices prosciutto or 12 slices bacon, cooked
- 12 dill pickle slices

DIJON AIOLI
- ¼ cup Mayonnaise (page 248)
- 1 tablespoon plus 1 teaspoon Dijon mustard
- 1 tablespoon fresh orange juice
- ¼ teaspoon ground cumin
- ⅛ teaspoon ground dried oregano

## method

1. If the Wraps are frozen, allow them to sit at room temperature for 30 minutes.

2. In a small saucepan over medium heat, reheat the shredded pork in its juices until warmed through.

3. While the pork is heating, make the Dijon Aioli: In a small bowl, whisk together the Mayonnaise, Dijon mustard, orange juice, cumin, and oregano.

4. Heat a panini press to medium heat or a grill pan or skillet to medium-high heat.

5. Assemble each panini with 2 Wraps, a spoonful of shredded pork, a slice of prosciutto or 2 slices cooked bacon, 2 pickle slices, and a tablespoon of the Dijon Aioli.

6. Grill in the panini press for 2 minutes, until the outside is toasted and the contents are hot. If using a grill pan or skillet, cook for 2 minutes on one side, then flip and cook for an additional 2 minutes.

tidbits:
Want to make these but don't have the shredded pork prepared? Any leftover thinly sliced roasted pork will do.

make-ahead tip:
The Dijon Aioli can be made up to 3 days in advance and stored, covered, in the refrigerator. Prepare the Wraps ahead of time and keep them in the freezer to make these paninis a quick meal.

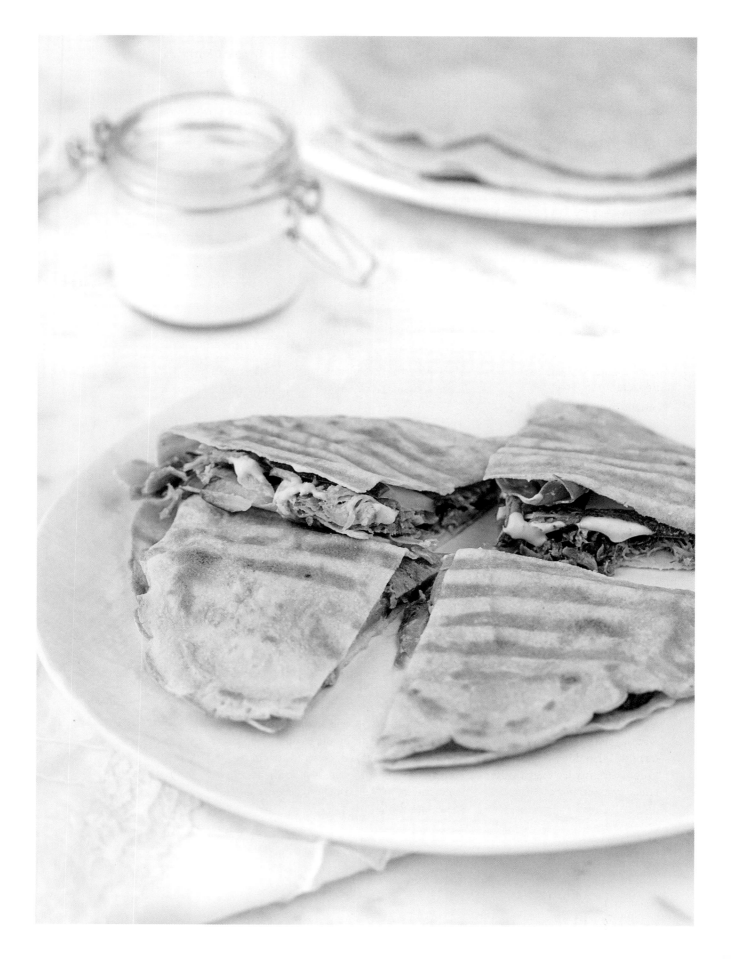

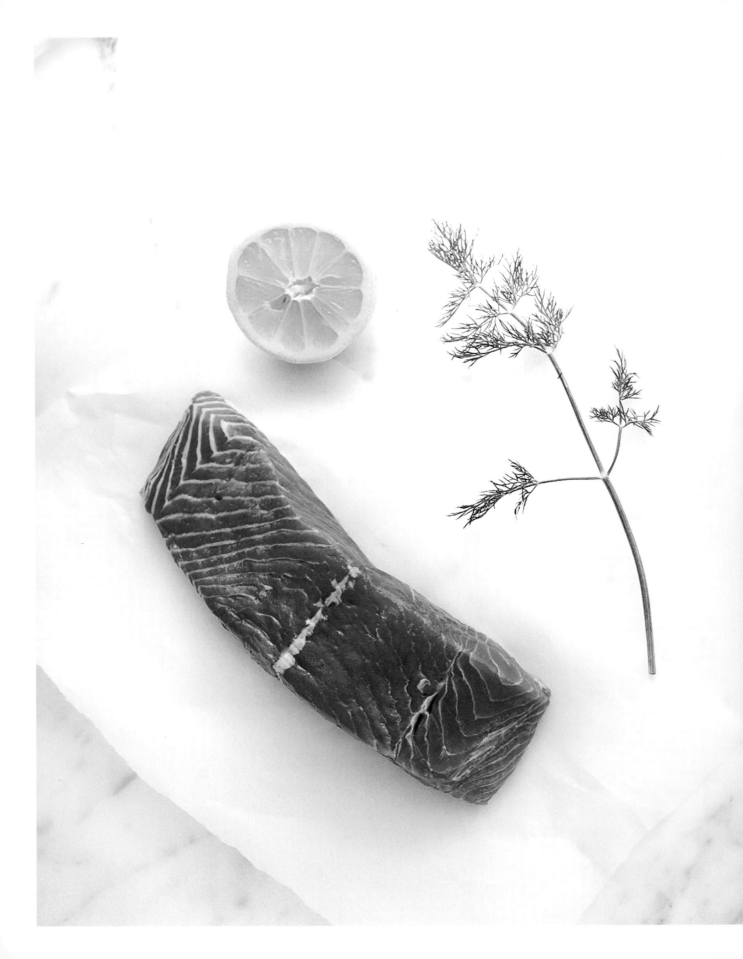

# seafood

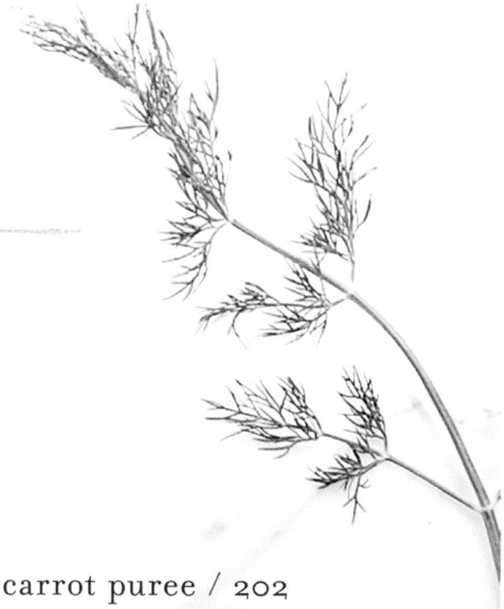

fish tacos / 192

pesto pasta with scallops / 194

summer shrimp rolls / 196

creamy dill salmon / 198

crab and asparagus linguine / 200

poached cod with butternut squash and carrot puree / 202

roasted tomato and shrimp pasta / 204

pesto orange roughy / 206

barbecue salmon with grilled peach salsa / 208

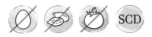

serves: 6

prep time: 20 minutes

cook time: 6 minutes

These fish tacos are bursting with flavor and will leave you feeling satisfied but not heavy afterward. Seasoned with a nightshade-free marinade, this dish is perfect for those who are intolerant of peppers and tomatoes but still want a Mexican flair to their meals.

## fish tacos

### ingredients

- 3 tablespoons macadamia nut oil or extra-virgin olive oil
- 1½ tablespoons fresh lime juice
- 2 cloves garlic, crushed into a paste
- ¾ teaspoon ground cumin
- ¾ teaspoon sea salt
- 1½ pounds white flaky fish, such as tilapia, cod, or mahi mahi
- 1 head butter lettuce, leaves separated
- 2 cups shredded cabbage
- Mango-Pineapple Salsa (page 258), for serving

### method

1. In a small bowl, whisk together the oil, lime juice, garlic, cumin, and salt. Place the fish in a shallow glass dish, pour the marinade over the top, and turn the fish in the marinade to coat.

2. Cover and marinate at room temperature for 15 minutes.

3. Meanwhile, heat a grill or grill pan to medium heat.

4. Grill the fish, covered, for 3 minutes on each side, until it just starts to flake in the center.

5. Serve the grilled fish atop the butter lettuce leaves with cabbage and salsa.

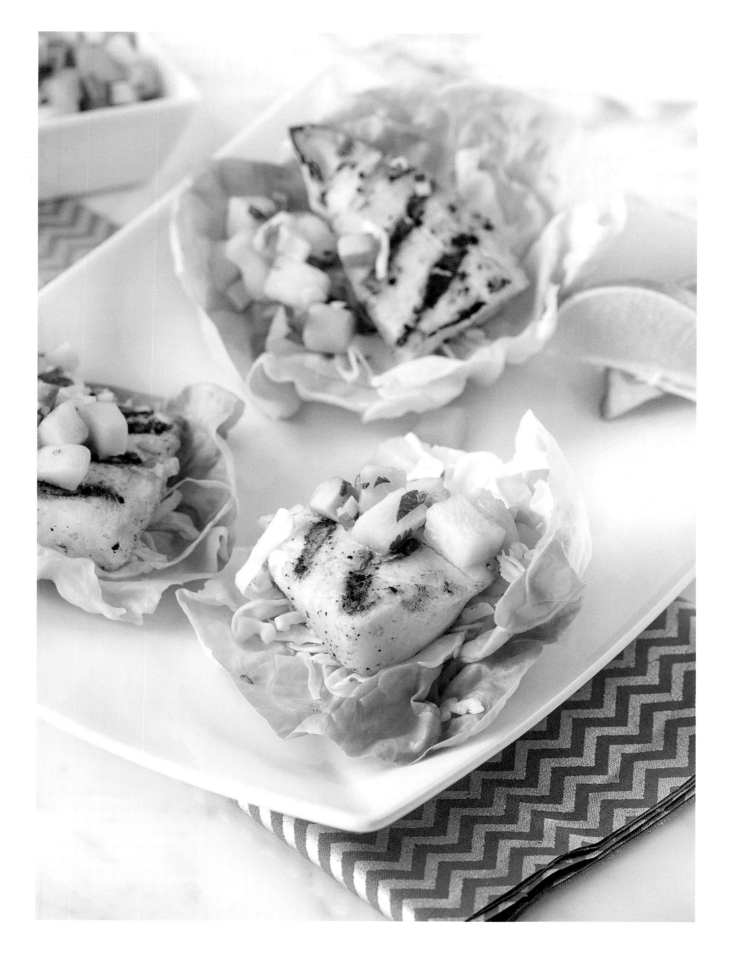

serves: 6
prep time: 35 minutes
cook time: 15 minutes

White sweet potatoes, or the Hannah variety, are much less sweet than their orange cousins and make wonderful noodles. My grandmother always put boiled white potatoes in her pesto pasta dish when I was growing up, so these noodles were the natural choice for a pasta alternative in this pesto dish. Shrimp or chicken can easily be substituted for the scallops, or the pasta can be served as a hearty vegetarian side dish.

# pesto pasta with scallops

## ingredients

- 2 pounds white sweet potatoes, peeled and halved crosswise*
- 1 tablespoon ghee or extra-virgin olive oil, divided
- 1 pound bay scallops
- 2 cloves garlic, minced
- 1 bunch broccoli rabe, tough non-leafy stems removed
- ½ teaspoon sea salt
- ¼ teaspoon cracked black pepper
- ½ cup Pesto Sauce (page 256)
- ¼ cup pine nuts**, toasted, for serving

* Use squash or celeriac noodles for SCD.
** Omit for nut-free.

## method

1. Using a spiral slicer or julienne peeler, cut the sweet potatoes into noodles. Place the noodles in a bowl of ice water for 30 minutes to remove some of the starch.

2. Heat 1 teaspoon of the ghee in a heavy-bottomed pot over medium-high heat.

3. Sear the scallops for 30 seconds on each side. Remove and set aside. Wipe the pot down quickly with a towel to remove any excess liquid.

4. Drain the noodles and pat them dry with a paper towel.

5. Heat the remaining 2 teaspoons of the ghee in the pot over medium heat. Add the garlic, broccoli rabe, noodles, salt, and pepper and sauté for 10 minutes.

6. Stir in the Pesto Sauce, cover, and steam for 3 minutes, until the noodles are tender but not mushy. Gently toss the scallops with the pasta and divide among 6 bowls. Garnish with toasted pine nuts.

make-ahead tip:
The sweet potatoes can be stored in ice water in the refrigerator for up to 2 days to eliminate a step at mealtime.

The Pesto Sauce can be stored in the refrigerator for up to 3 days.

tidbits:
Zucchini or yellow squash noodles are great in this dish as well. They do not need to soak in an ice water bath, and they take about half the cooking time as sweet potato noodles.

Sea scallops, prawns, or shrimp work as a substitute for the bay scallops. Go with whatever is fresh and wild!

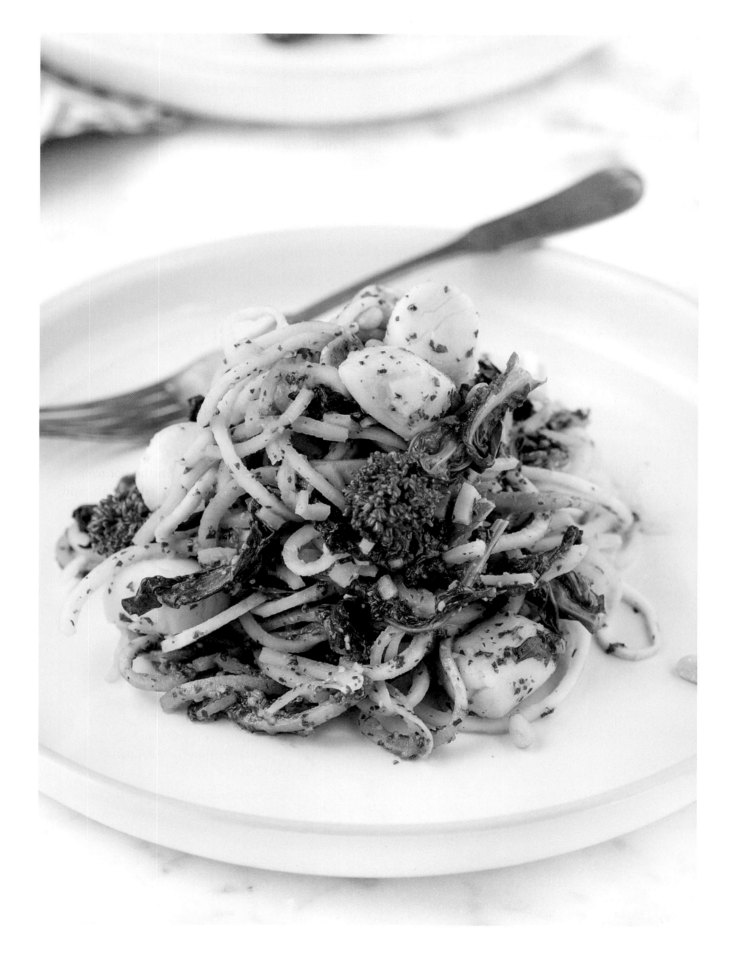

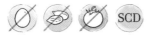

SCD

serves: 6

prep time: 20 minutes

cook time: 4 minutes

Refreshing and perfect on a hot summer day, these summer shrimp lettuce wraps can be on the table in less than 30 minutes.

# (30 minutes or less) summer shrimp rolls

## ingredients

- 1 large cucumber, seeded and julienned (about 1½ cups)
- 2 large carrots, peeled and julienned (about 1½ cups)
- 1 cup strawberries, sliced
- ¼ cup fresh lemon juice
- 2 teaspoons honey
- 3 tablespoons chopped fresh cilantro
- 3 tablespoons chopped fresh mint
- 2 tablespoons chopped scallions, green and white parts
- 1 teaspoon coarse sea salt, divided
- 1½ pounds large wild-caught shrimp, peeled, deveined, and tails removed
- 3 tablespoons extra-virgin olive oil
- ½ teaspoon cracked black pepper
- 6 large butter lettuce leaves, such as Boston lettuce

## method

1. Toss the cucumber, carrots, strawberries, lemon juice, honey, herbs, scallions, and ¼ teaspoon of the salt together in a bowl. Cover and refrigerate.

2. Preheat a grill or grill pan to medium-high heat.

3. Rinse and pat dry the shrimp, then toss them with the olive oil, remaining ¾ teaspoon of the salt, and pepper.

4. Grill the shrimp for 2 minutes on each side, until they're pink. Remove from the grill and coarsely chop.

5. Spoon the shrimp, vegetable mix, and a small drizzle of the juices from the bowl onto each lettuce leaf and roll up gently.

> **make-ahead tip:**
> Make everything up to 3 days in advance and store in the refrigerator. Keep the lettuce separate until ready to serve.
>
> **tidbits:**
> The shrimp can also be sautéed over medium heat until cooked through if a grill is not accessible.

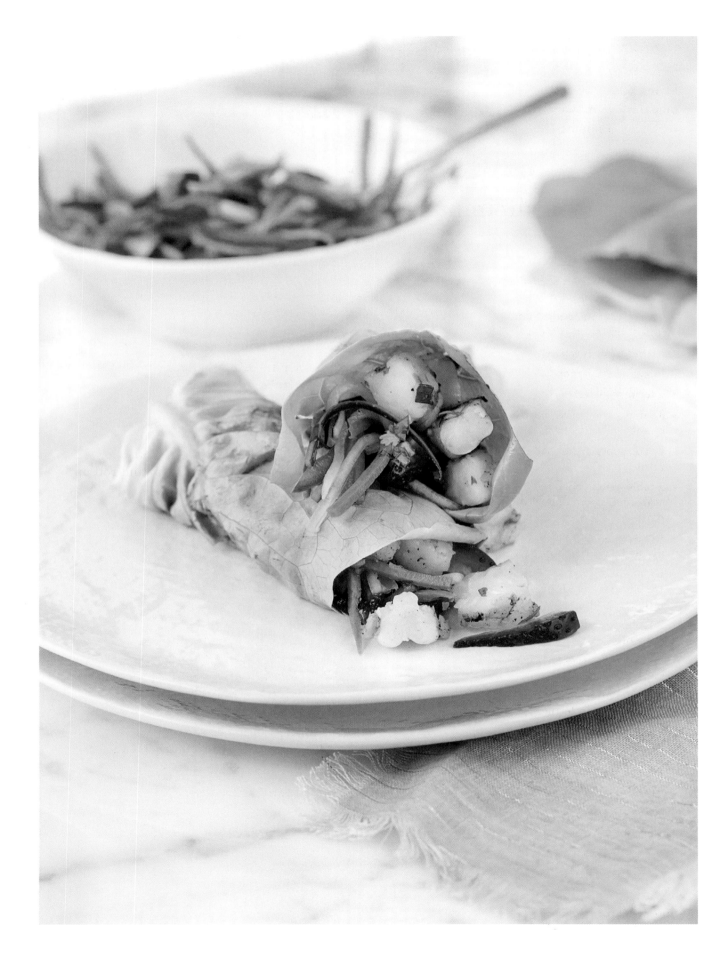

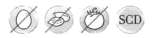

serves: 6

prep time: 10 minutes

cook time: 12 to 13 minutes

Wild salmon fillets are roasted and then topped with a creamy dill and garlic sauce for a light and nourishing meal that takes no time at all. A lemony side of Green Beans Almondine (page 212) complements this dish nicely.

# creamy dill salmon

## ingredients

FISH

- 6 (6-ounce) wild salmon fillets, skin-on, pin bones removed
- 1 tablespoon melted ghee or extra-virgin olive oil
- sea salt and cracked black pepper

SAUCE

- 2 tablespoons ghee or extra-virgin olive oil, divided
- 5 cloves garlic, crushed into a paste
- ½ cup dry white wine or Chicken Stock (page 242)
- 3 tablespoons full-fat coconut milk
- 2 teaspoons Dijon mustard
- 2 teaspoons fresh lemon juice
- ¼ cup chopped fresh dill
- ½ teaspoon sea salt
- ¼ teaspoon cracked black pepper

## method

1. Preheat the oven to 400°F. Line a rimmed baking sheet with parchment paper.

2. Rub the salmon fillets with the tablespoon of melted ghee, then season on both sides with salt and pepper. Place the fillets skin side down on the prepared baking sheet. Set aside while you begin the sauce.

3. Make the sauce: Melt 1 tablespoon of the ghee in a saucepan over medium-high heat. Sauté the garlic until fragrant and lightly browned, about 1 minute.

4. Pour in the wine and bring to a boil. Simmer for 5 minutes, until reduced by half.

5. Meanwhile, place the salmon in the oven and roast for 6 to 7 minutes, until the fillets flake slightly in the center.

6. Whisk the remaining 1 tablespoon of the ghee, coconut milk, Dijon mustard, lemon juice, dill, salt, and pepper into the sauce and simmer on low until the fish is ready.

7. Remove the skin from the salmon and serve hot with the sauce spooned over the top.

tidbits:

Purchase a whole-side wild salmon fillet and slice it crosswise into individual 6-ounce portions yourself to save a little on the price. For this recipe, look for a side of salmon that is about 2½ pounds.

Any leftover sauce will taste wonderful on other fish or chicken.

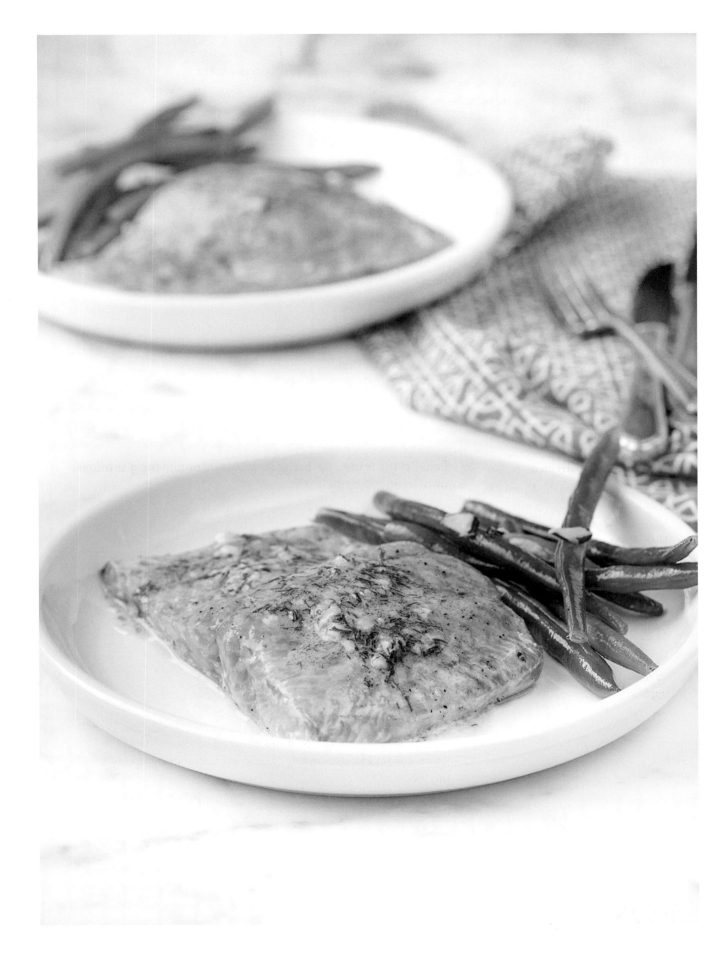

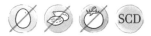

serves: 6
prep time: 15 minutes
cook time: 15 minutes

Buttery parsnips are turned into linguine noodles and serve as a brilliant vessel for this crab, asparagus, leek, and white wine sauce. Shrimp or leftover Roasted Chicken (page 118) can be substituted for the crab if desired.

# crab and asparagus linguine

## ingredients

- ¼ cup ghee, extra-virgin olive oil, or bacon fat
- ½ cup thinly sliced leeks, white and green parts
- 6 cloves garlic, crushed into a paste
- 12 ounces asparagus, trimmed and thinly sliced
- 2 pounds parsnips, peeled and spiral sliced or cut into noodles using a julienne peeler*
- ½ cup dry white wine, such as Sauvignon Blanc
- 1½ teaspoons sea salt
- 1½ pounds fresh crab meat, lump and claw
- ¼ cup chopped fresh parsley
- squeeze of fresh lemon juice

*Substitute celeriac spiral noodles for SCD.*

## method

1. Heat the ghee in a deep skillet over medium-high heat. Sauté the leeks and garlic until fragrant, about 2 minutes.

2. Add the asparagus and parsnip noodles and sauté for 5 minutes longer, until the asparagus is bright green and the noodles are crisp-tender.

3. Add the wine and stir to release any browned bits on the bottom of the pan. Reduce the heat to medium and simmer for 8 minutes to reduce the liquid by half.

4. Stir in the salt, crab meat, and parsley and cook for 2 minutes, until the crab is warm. Finish with a small squeeze of lemon juice right before serving.

make-ahead tip:
Save time by chopping all the vegetables and making the noodles the night before. This dish will come together in 20 minutes if you have everything prepared ahead of time!

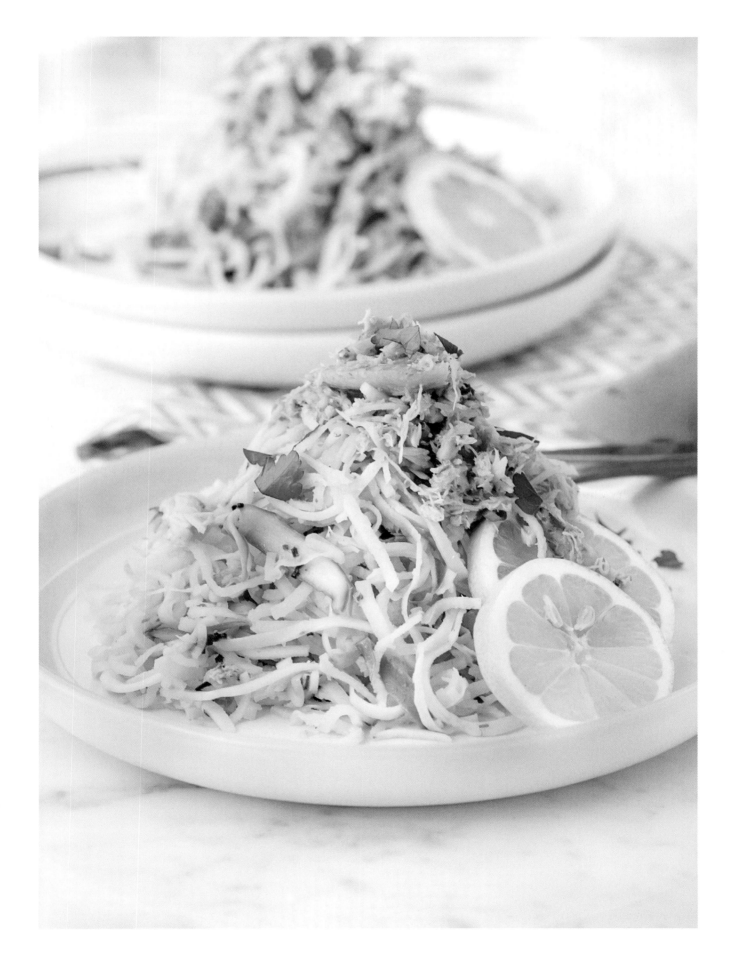

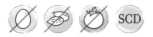

serves: 6

prep time: 10 minutes

cook time: 15 to 22 minutes

Mild cod fillets are poached in a leek-flavored broth and perched atop a savory garlic-sage-flavored puree of butternut squash and carrots.

# 30 minutes or less  poached cod with butternut squash and carrot puree

## ingredients

### PUREE

- 3 cups Chicken Stock (page 242)
- 1 small butternut squash (about 2 pounds), peeled and cubed (about 5 cups)
- 3 large carrots, peeled and cubed
- 3 cloves garlic, peeled
- 1½ teaspoons sea salt, divided
- 1 teaspoon chopped fresh sage
- 1 tablespoon ghee (optional)

### COD

- 6 (6-ounce) cod fillets, skinless
- 1 leek, washed and thinly sliced, white and green parts

## method

1. In a deep skillet with a lid, bring the Chicken Stock, squash, carrots, garlic, and 1 teaspoon of the salt to a boil. Reduce the heat to medium-low, cover, and cook for 10 to 15 minutes, until fork-tender.

2. With a slotted spoon, transfer the vegetables to a food processor with 2 tablespoons of the cooking liquid. (Leave the rest of the liquid in the skillet; do not discard.)

3. Poach the cod: Add the cod and leek to the liquid in the skillet, cover, and poach on medium-low heat for 5 to 7 minutes.

4. While the cod is poaching, make the puree: Add the sage, remaining ½ teaspoon of the salt, and ghee, if using, to the food processor and purée until smooth.

5. Remove the cod and leeks to a plate lined with paper towels to drain any excess liquid. Serve the fish on top of the puree.

make-ahead tip:

Preparing a butternut squash at home is easy to do and will save you money, but it takes a little time. Peel and cube it the night before to cut down your preparation time at dinnertime.

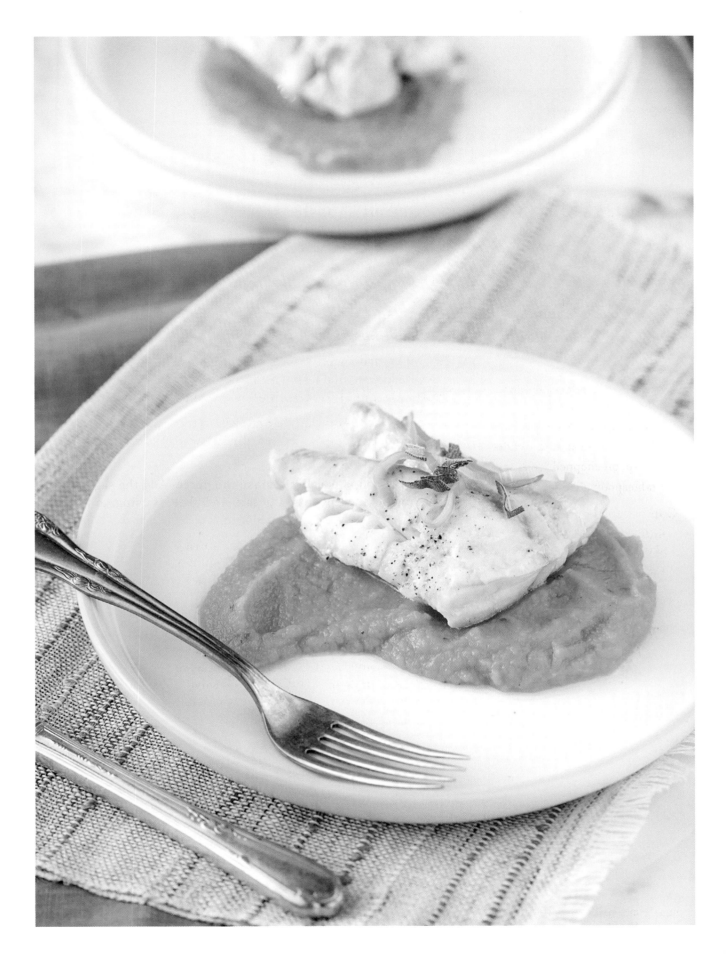

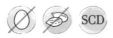

serves: 6

prep time: 10 minutes

cook time: 50 to 55 minutes

Juicy tomatoes roast with garlic, shrimp, and nutrient-rich herbs to create a light and fresh pasta dish. The best part? Cleanup is minimal with only two pans!

# roasted tomato and shrimp pasta

## ingredients

- 1 (3-pound) spaghetti squash
- 3 tablespoons plus 1 teaspoon melted ghee or extra-virgin olive oil, divided
- 1½ teaspoons sea salt, divided
- ½ teaspoon cracked black pepper, divided
- 2½ pounds Roma tomatoes, quartered
- 4 cloves garlic, minced
- 2 pounds medium wild-caught shrimp, peeled, deveined, and tails removed
- ½ cup chopped fresh parsley
- 2 cups chopped chard, spinach, or baby kale
- juice of 1 lemon

### tidbits:
If dairy is tolerated, a nice Parmesan cheese or feta tastes wonderful with this dish.

For a quick lunch, top any extra spaghetti squash with the Shortcut Spaghetti with Meat Sauce (page 168).

## method

1. Preheat the oven to 375°F.

2. Carefully cut the squash in half lengthwise. Scoop out and discard the seeds.

3. Rub 1 teaspoon of the ghee all over the skin of the squash and on the surface of the cut sides. Sprinkle the cut sides with ½ teaspoon of the salt and ¼ teaspoon of the pepper.

4. Place the halves cut side down on a rimmed baking sheet.

5. Place the tomatoes in a 9-by-12-inch baking dish and drizzle with the remaining 3 tablespoons of ghee, garlic, remaining 1 teaspoon of salt, and remaining ¼ teaspoon of pepper. Toss to combine.

6. Place both the squash and the tomato mixture in the oven, with the tomatoes on the higher rack.

7. Roast for 30 to 35 minutes, stirring the tomatoes once halfway through. The squash should be slightly soft to the touch.

8. Pull the squash out and set aside until cool enough to handle.

9. Add the shrimp, parsley, chard, and lemon juice to the tomato dish and stir to combine. Return the dish to the oven and continue roasting for 20 minutes, until the shrimp are pink and cooked through.

10. Use a fork to loosen the strings of noodles from the squash and transfer them to serving bowls. Top with the shrimp and tomato sauce.

### make-ahead tip:
Complete Steps 1 through 8 up to 3 days in advance and store the squash and tomato mixture in the refrigerator. Bring it to room temperature before adding the remaining ingredients and roasting.

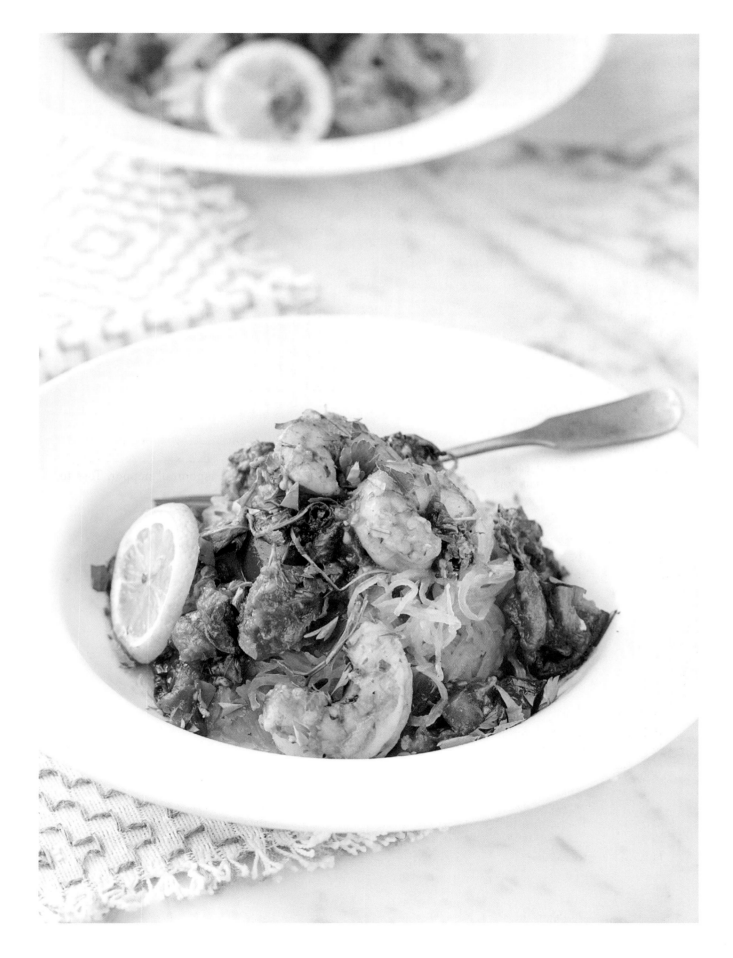

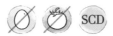

serves: 6

prep time: 10 minutes

cook time: 12 to 15 minutes

The delicate flavor of orange roughy is enhanced with an Italian Pesto Sauce and is sure to please even picky eaters. This versatile dish can be paired with Roasted Basil Eggplant (page 232) or with a side of zucchini noodles tossed in the leftover Pesto Sauce.

# pesto orange roughy

## ingredients

- 2 teaspoons melted ghee or extra-virgin olive oil
- 1½ pounds orange roughy fillets or other mild white fish
- sea salt and cracked black pepper
- ¼ cup Pesto Sauce (page 256)

## method

1. Preheat the oven to 400°F. Drizzle the ghee into a medium baking dish.

2. Season the fillets all over with salt and pepper and place them in the baking dish.

3. Spread the Pesto Sauce all over the top of the fish.

4. Bake for 12 to 15 minutes, until the fish flakes easily with a fork and is slightly firm to the touch.

make-ahead tip:

The Pesto Sauce can be prepared up to 3 days in advance and stored in an airtight container in the refrigerator. Orange roughy is easy to store in the freezer and thaws quickly, so keep some on hand for nights when dinner is rushed.

If preparing the Roasted Basil Eggplant (page 232) to serve with this dish, the eggplant can be roasted on the upper rack of the oven while the fish bakes on the center rack. Increase the oven temperature to 425°F after the fish is pulled from the oven and continue roasting for 7 to 10 minutes, until the eggplant is tender. Alternatively, roast the eggplant first and reheat right before serving.

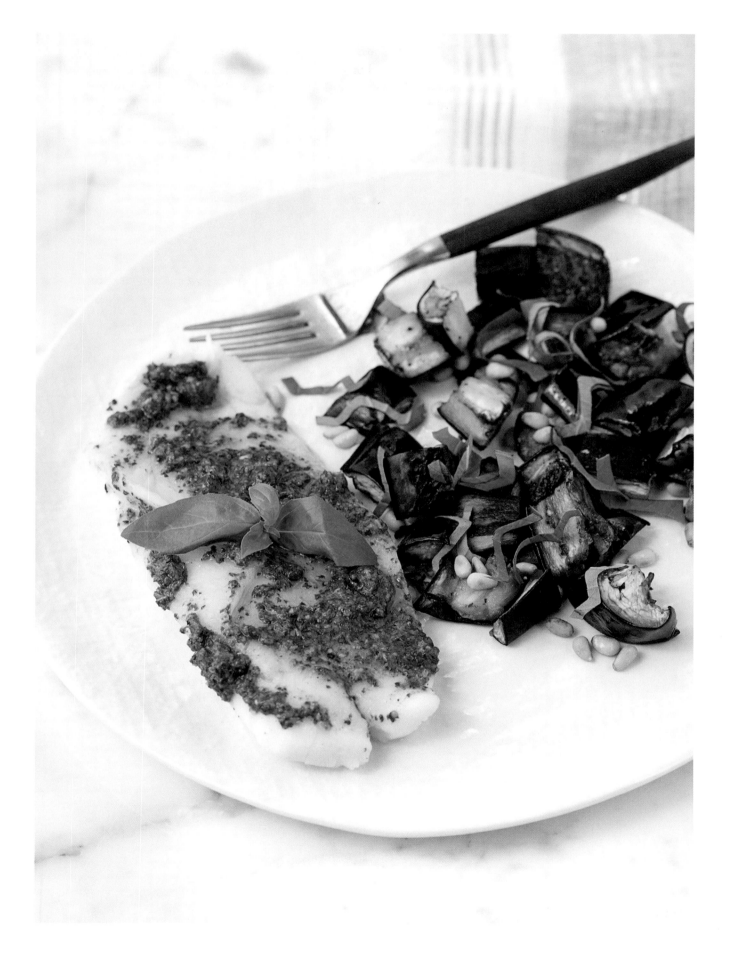

serves: 6

prep time: 12 minutes

cook time: 10 minutes

This fresh summertime meal is packed with flavor with the use of my smoky barbecue rub and delightful peach salsa to top the salmon. Serve with a simple green salad or my Smoky Roasted Sweet Potatoes (page 222).

# 30 minutes or less  barbecue salmon with grilled peach salsa

## ingredients

- 1 (2-pound) wild salmon fillet, skin-on
- ¼ cup Barbecue Dry Rub (page 244)

### SALSA

- 1 teaspoon melted ghee or coconut oil
- 2 large ripe peaches, pitted and halved
- 1 large avocado, pitted and diced
- 5 fresh basil leaves, chopped
- 2 tablespoons diced red onion
- 1 teaspoon fresh lime juice
- ¼ teaspoon sea salt

## method

1. Slice the salmon evenly into 6 fillets and spread the rub all over the top and sides.

2. Preheat a grill or grill pan to medium-high heat.

3. Sear the salmon fillets, skinless side down first. Close the grill lid and cook for 2 minutes on the first side. Do not move them until it is time to flip them over.

4. Using tongs in one hand and a metal spatula in the other, carefully turn the fish over so that the skin side is down, and reduce the heat to medium. For charcoal grills, finish cooking over indirect heat farthest from the coals.

5. Close the grill lid and finish cooking for another 3 to 5 minutes, depending on thickness of the fillets. The salmon will start to flake along the center of the fillet when done.

6. Rub the melted ghee on the peach halves and grill, cut side down, for 2 minutes.

7. Chop the grilled peaches and mix with the remaining salsa ingredients. Spoon the salsa over the salmon and serve.

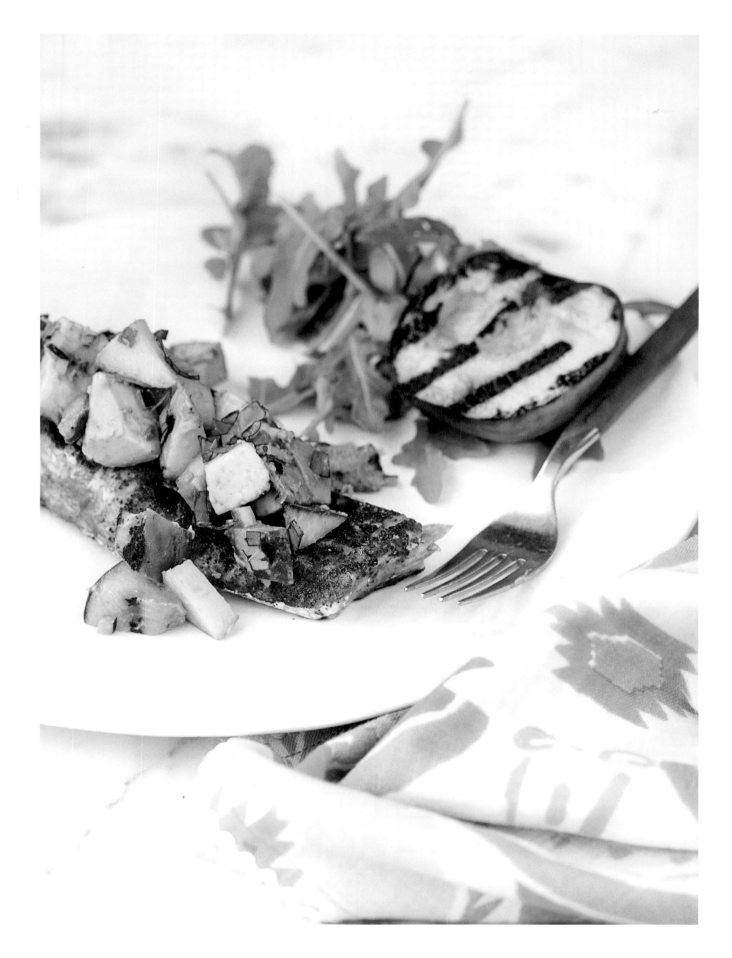

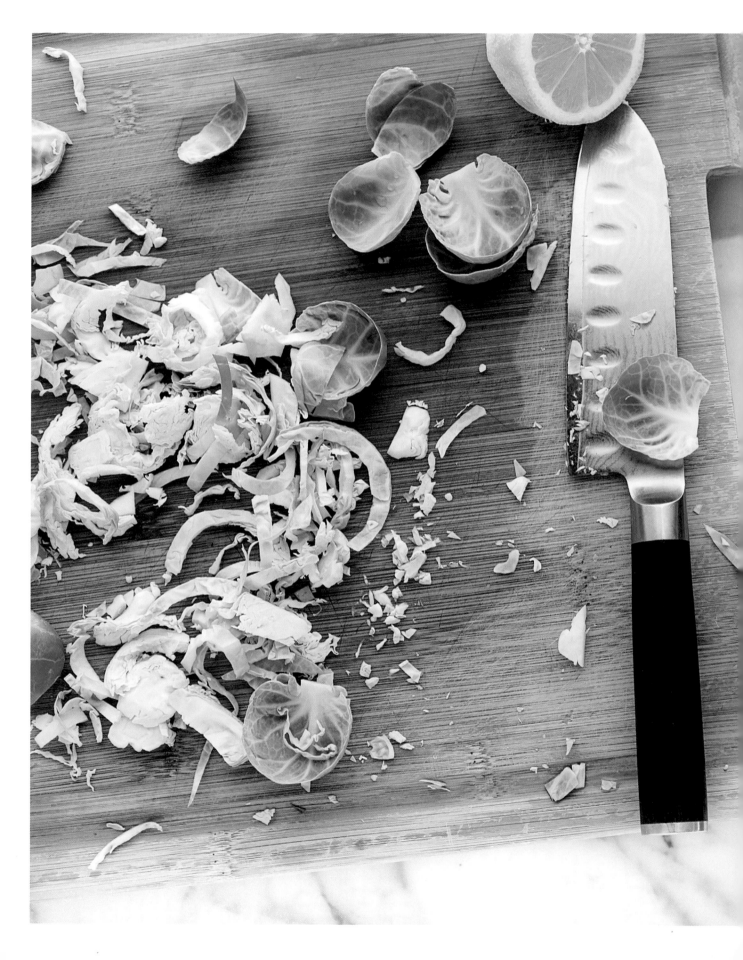

# sides

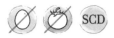

serves: 6

prep time: 10 minutes

cook time: 10 minutes

This dish is a wonderful addition to any meal. Green beans are in a gray area for Paleo because they are a legume and may be tougher to digest, but many people find that they can tolerate them and continue to enjoy them. Green beans are mostly pod and the beans are not fully ripe, but as always, listen to your own body.

## green beans almondine

### ingredients

- 1½ pounds green beans, trimmed
- ¼ cup sliced almonds
- 1½ tablespoons ghee or extra-virgin olive oil
- ¾ teaspoon fresh lemon juice
- ½ teaspoon sea salt
- ¼ teaspoon cracked black pepper

### method

1. Fill a large pot with 1 inch of water and arrange a steamer basket over the top.

2. Place the green beans in the steamer basket and bring the water to a boil. Cover and steam for 5 minutes, until the beans are bright green and crisp-tender.

3. Transfer the beans to a colander to drain. Discard the cooking water and wipe the pot dry. Return the pot to the stove.

4. Add the almonds to the pot and toast on medium heat for 5 minutes, until golden brown and aromatic, stirring frequently.

5. Add the ghee, lemon juice, salt, pepper, and beans to the pot. Toss to coat and transfer to a serving plate.

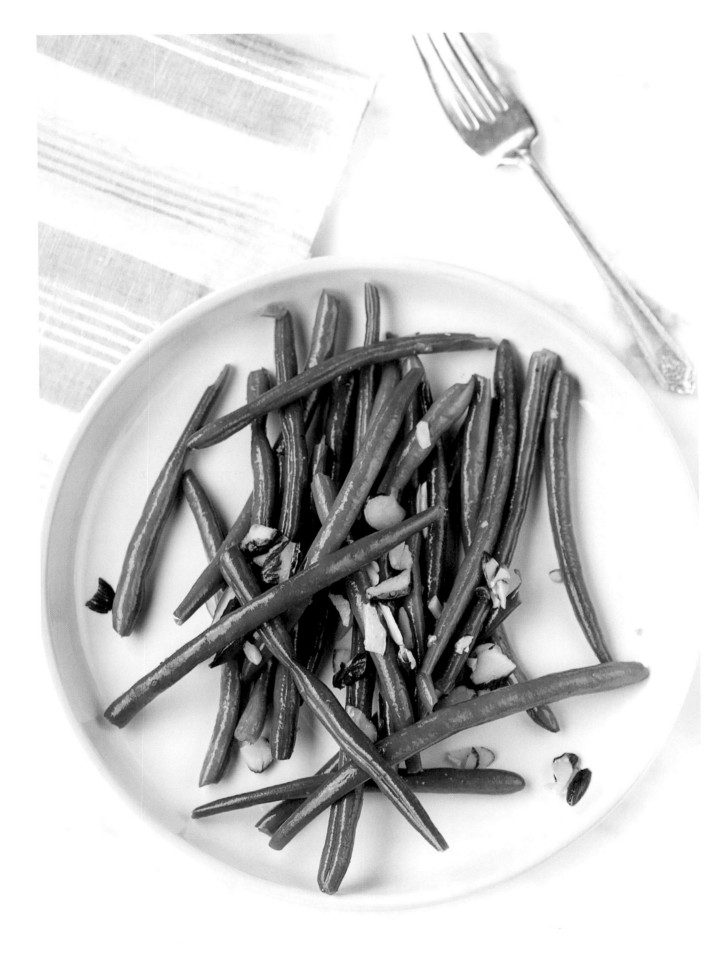

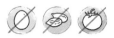

serves: 6

prep time: 10 minutes

cook time: 10 to 12 minutes

Mashed cauliflower is a fabulous alternative and favorite Paleo stand-in for mashed white potatoes, but my stomach cannot handle too many cruciferous vegetables. To create a low-starch alternative to both the potato and the cauliflower mash, I like to use a mix of parsnips and turnips, which makes a wonderfully creamy mash.

# creamy mashed root vegetables

## ingredients

- 1½ pounds parsnips, peeled and cubed
- 1 pound turnips, peeled and cubed
- ½ cup Chicken Stock (page 242)
- ¼ cup ghee
- ¾ teaspoon sea salt
- pinch of cracked black pepper
- chopped fresh parsley, for garnish

## method

1. Fill a pot with cold water and add the parsnips and turnips. Bring to a boil, then partially cover and cook for 10 to 12 minutes, until fork-tender.

2. Drain the vegetables and transfer them to a food processor.

3. Add the Chicken Stock, ghee, salt, and pepper and purée until smooth. Garnish with chopped parsley.

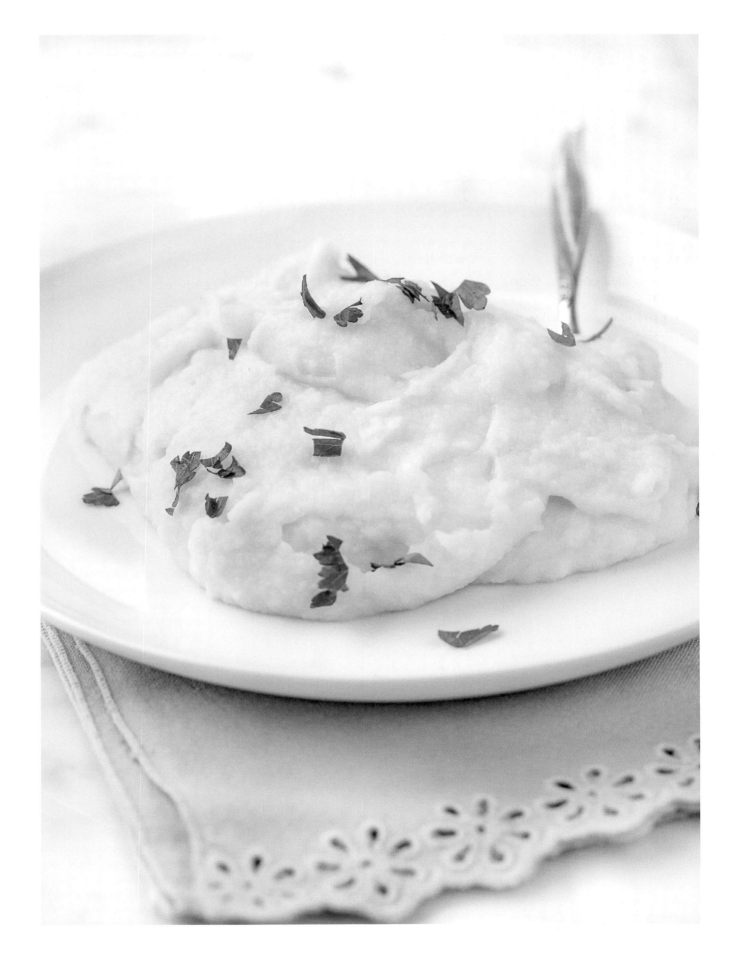

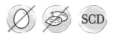

serves: 6

prep time: 20 minutes

cook time: 30 minutes

This Indian-style side dish is perfect to serve under my Chicken Tikka Masala (page 130). I've substituted cauliflower rice for the traditional white rice, and it has become a new favorite in our kitchen!

# vegetable biryani

## ingredients

- ½ cup Chicken Stock (page 242)
- 5 threads saffron
- 3 tablespoons ghee
- 1 cup peeled and diced carrots
- 1 cup diced parsnips*
- ½ yellow onion, diced
- ½ head cauliflower, cut into florets
- ¾ teaspoon sea salt
- 4 whole cloves
- 2 green cardamom pods
- ¾ teaspoon garam masala
- ½ teaspoon cayenne pepper
- ½ teaspoon ground ginger
- ¼ teaspoon ground turmeric
- ¼ cup frozen peas, thawed

*Substitute peeled and diced celeriac for SCD.*

## method

1. In a small saucepan, bring the Chicken Stock to a boil, then add the saffron. Cover and remove from the heat.

2. Melt the ghee in a large skillet over medium heat. Add the carrots, parsnips, and onion and sauté for 5 to 7 minutes.

3. "Rice" the cauliflower using a food processor with a grating attachment or a box grater. Pick out any large fragments that didn't get shredded and save for another use.

4. Add the cauliflower, salt, and all of the spices to the skillet and continue to sauté over medium heat for 5 minutes, until the cauliflower is crisp-tender.

5. Pour in the saffron broth and the peas, then cover and cook for 15 minutes, until the cauliflower is tender and the liquid has been absorbed.

make-ahead tip:

Chop the vegetables and rice the cauliflower up to 2 days in advance to save a few steps at mealtime. Reheat any leftovers in a dry skillet, uncovered, over medium-high heat for 5 to 7 minutes.

tidbits:

Saffron, cardamom pods, and garam masala are standard Indian spices, but they may be difficult to locate. They can be found at many health food stores and spice shops and on Amazon.

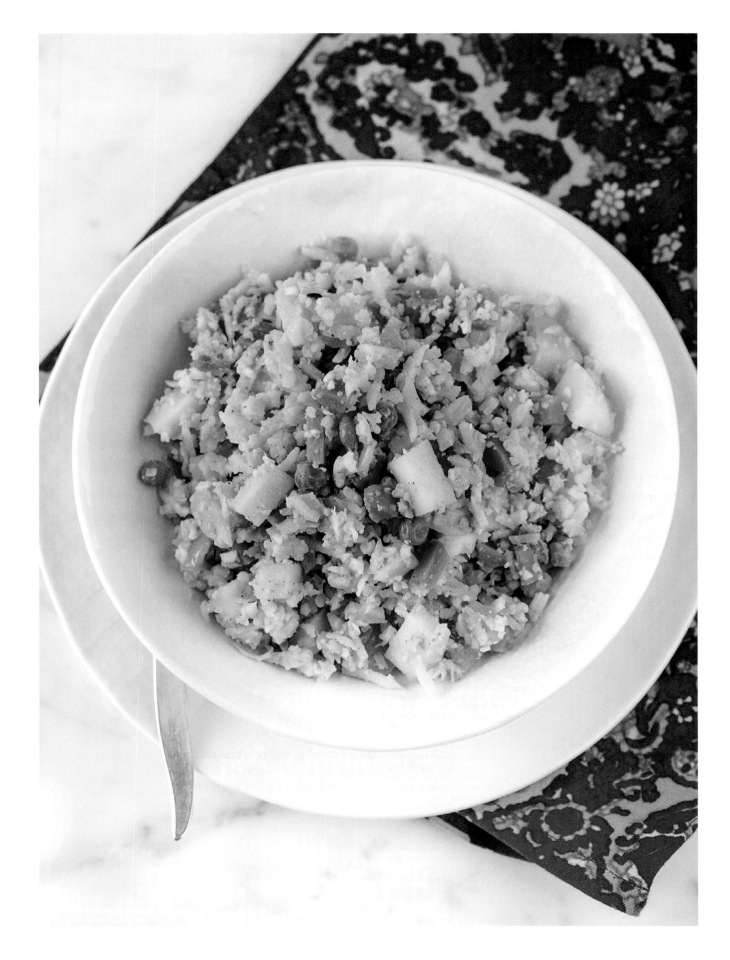

One head of cauliflower, three different flavor profiles!

serves: 6 to 8
prep time: 15 minutes
cook time: 20 to 25 minutes

# cauliflower rice three ways

## basic cauli-rice Ø 🥥 🍅 SCD

### ingredients

- 1 small head cauliflower, cut into florets
- 2 teaspoons ghee or extra-virgin olive oil
- 1 teaspoon cold-pressed sesame oil
- ½ cup diced yellow onion
- 1 clove garlic, minced
- ¼ cup water
- ¾ teaspoon sea salt

### method

1. "Rice" the cauliflower using a food processor with a grating attachment or a box grater. Pick out any large fragments that didn't get shredded and save for another use.

2. Melt the ghee and sesame oil in a large skillet over medium heat. Add the onion and garlic and sauté for 5 minutes, until the onion has softened.

3. Add the cauliflower to the pan and sauté for 5 minutes.

4. Add the water and salt and increase the heat to medium-high. Cook for 15 minutes, until the cauliflower is tender and the liquid has been absorbed.

## coconut, cilantro, & lime cauli-rice Ø 🥥 🍅 SCD

### ingredients

- 1 small head cauliflower, cut into florets
- 2 teaspoons coconut oil
- 1 tablespoon fresh lime juice
- 2 teaspoons honey
- ¼ cup chopped fresh cilantro
- ¼ cup full-fat coconut milk
- ¾ teaspoon sea salt

### method

1. "Rice" the cauliflower using a food processor with a grating attachment or a box grater. Pick out any large fragments that didn't get shredded and save for another use.

2. Melt the coconut oil in a large skillet over medium heat. Add the cauliflower to the pan and sauté for 5 minutes.

3. Add the remaining ingredients and cook for 15 minutes, until the cauliflower is tender and the liquid has been absorbed.

make-ahead tip:

The cauliflower can be riced up to 2 days in advance to save a few steps at mealtime.

To reheat cauli-rice, add the leftovers to a dry pan and heat, uncovered, over medium-high heat for 3 to 5 minutes, until warmed through.

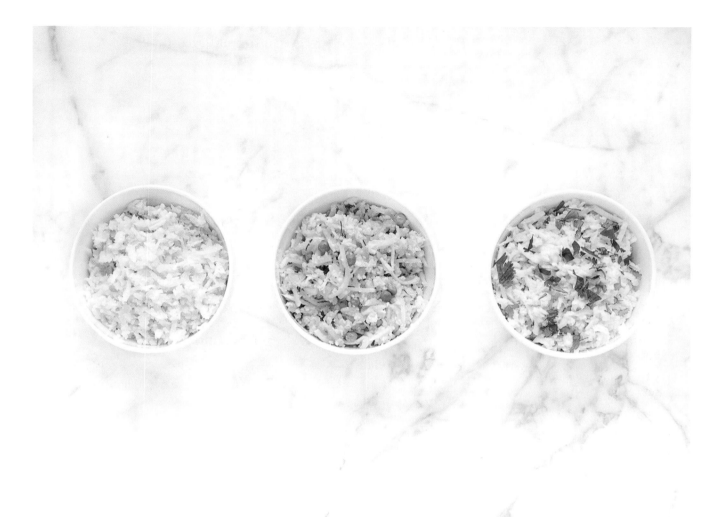

## saffron cauli-rice ⊘ ⌀ ⌀ SCD

### ingredients

- ¼ cup Chicken Stock (page 242)
- ½ teaspoon saffron threads
- 2 teaspoons ghee or extra-virgin olive oil
- ½ cup diced yellow onion
- 1 clove garlic, minced
- 1 teaspoon garam masala
- ¾ teaspoon sea salt
- 1 small head cauliflower, cut into florets
- ¼ cup peas

### method

1. In a small saucepan, bring the Chicken Stock to a boil, then add the saffron. Cover and remove from the heat.

2. Melt the ghee in a large skillet over medium heat. Add the onion, garlic, garam masala, and salt and sauté for 5 minutes, until the onion has softened.

3. "Rice" the cauliflower using a food processor with a grating attachment or a box grater. Pick out any large fragments that didn't get shredded and save for another use.

4. Add the cauliflower to the skillet and continue to sauté over medium heat for 5 minutes.

5. Pour in the saffron broth and the peas and increase the heat to medium-high. Cook for 15 minutes, until the cauliflower is tender and the liquid has been absorbed.

 SCD

serves: 6

prep time: 5 minutes plus
10 minutes marinating time
cook time: 6 minutes

Asparagus and scallions are seasoned in an Asian-style marinade and then grilled.

# 30 minutes or less grilled sesame asparagus and scallions

## ingredients

- 1 pound asparagus, trimmed
- 1 bunch scallions, trimmed

MARINADE

- 2 teaspoons cold-pressed sesame oil
- 2 teaspoons coconut aminos*
- 2 cloves garlic, minced
- ½ teaspoon peeled and minced fresh ginger
- ¾ teaspoon sea salt
- ¼ teaspoon cracked black pepper

* For SCD, omit the coconut aminos and increase the sea salt to 1 teaspoon.

## method

1. Toss the asparagus and scallions with the marinade ingredients in a shallow glass dish and marinate for 10 minutes.

2. Preheat a grill or grill pan to medium heat.

3. Lay the asparagus and scallions lengthwise on the grill so they do not fall through the grates and grill, covered, for 3 minutes.

4. Turn the vegetables over and grill for an additional 3 minutes, until tender and cooked through.

make-ahead tip:
You can prepare the vegetables the night before and marinate them covered in the refrigerator.

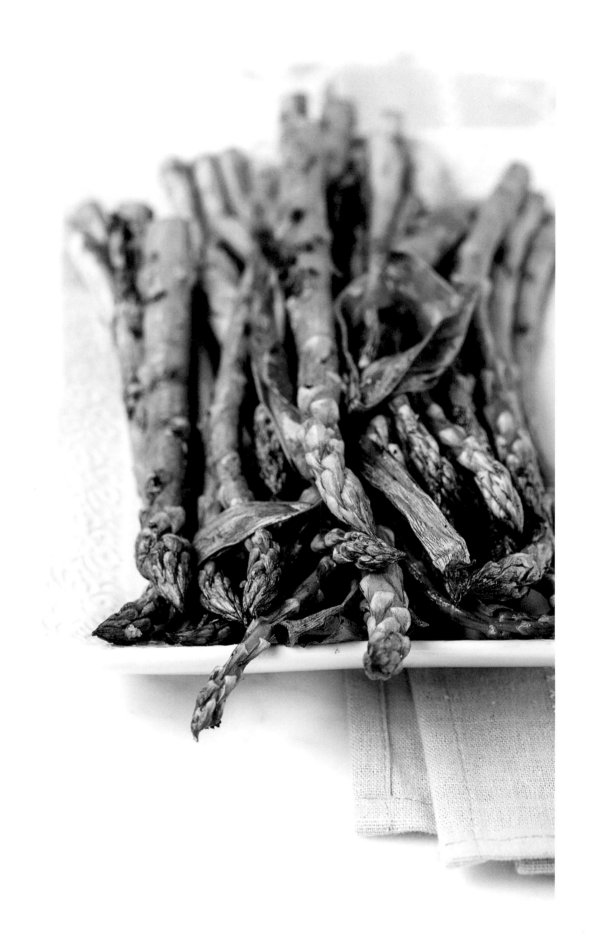

serves: 6
prep time: 10 minutes
cook time: 30 minutes

I could eat these sweet potatoes for breakfast, lunch, and dinner, and I'm known for picking at them right from the tray before they even hit the table.

# smoky roasted sweet potatoes

## ingredients

- 2 pounds sweet potatoes, scrubbed clean and diced
- 8 ounces bacon, chopped
- 1½ teaspoons chili powder
- ¾ teaspoon sea salt
- ½ teaspoon ground cinnamon
- ¼ teaspoon cayenne pepper

## method

1. Preheat the oven to 400°F.

2. In a large bowl, toss together all of the ingredients. Spread onto 2 rimmed baking sheets.

3. Place in the oven and roast for 15 minutes.

4. Toss to coat the potatoes in the rendered bacon fat. Continue roasting for 15 minutes, until the potatoes are crisp.

tidbits:
If there are any leftovers, serve with a fried egg over the top the next morning!

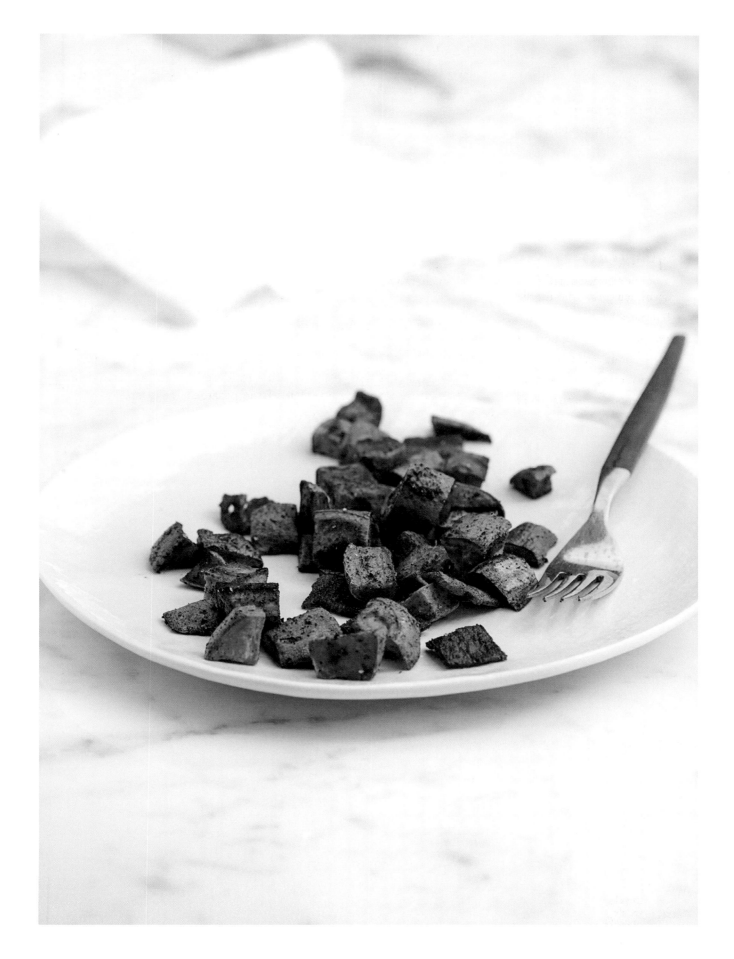

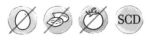

serves: 6

prep time: 15 minutes

cook time: 15 minutes

Shredding Brussels sprouts makes them melt in your mouth when roasted and also shortens their cooking time. This dish pairs well with Rosemary-Lemon Pork Chops (page 174) and adds a depth of flavor to fish and poultry dishes.

## 30 minutes or less lemon-roasted asparagus and brussels sprouts

### ingredients

- 12 ounces asparagus, trimmed and halved crosswise
- 1 pound Brussels sprouts, trimmed and shredded (see Tidbits)
- 1 tablespoon ghee or bacon fat, melted
- zest of 1 lemon, grated
- 2 tablespoons fresh lemon juice
- ¾ teaspoon sea salt
- ¼ teaspoon cracked black pepper
- 2 cloves garlic, minced

### method

1. Preheat the oven to 400°F.

2. In a large bowl, toss together the asparagus, Brussels sprouts, ghee, lemon zest and juice, salt, pepper, and garlic. Spread in a single layer on a rimmed baking sheet.

3. Roast for 10 minutes, stir, then continue roasting for another 5 minutes, until the vegetables are crisp-tender.

tidbits:

My favorite way to shred Brussels sprouts is in a food processor, but it can easily be done by hand using a knife and cutting into shreds.

If you live in an area where Brussels sprouts and asparagus cannot be found in the same season, artichoke hearts or mini artichokes are a wonderful substitute for the Brussels sprouts.

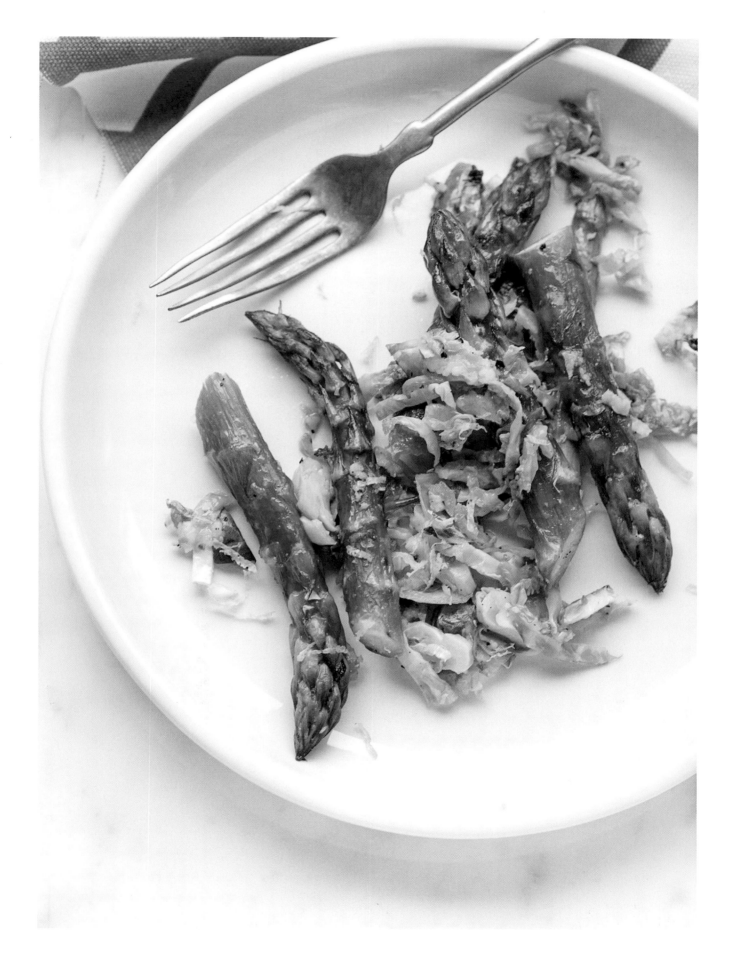

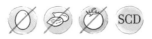

serves: 6

prep time: 5 minutes

cook time: 6 to 8 minutes

This savory and tangy sautéed spinach gets its flavors from vinegar and fruits. It pairs well with pork dishes or slow-roasted meats, particularly Slow Cooker Braised Pork Shoulder (page 184).

# catalan-style spinach

## ingredients

- 2 tablespoons extra-virgin olive oil or ghee
- 1 small apple, peeled, cored, and julienned
- 2 pounds baby spinach
- 3 tablespoons raisins
- 2 teaspoons red wine vinegar
- ¾ teaspoon sea salt
- cracked black pepper to taste

## method

1. Heat the olive oil in a sauté pan or Dutch oven over medium-high heat.

2. Add the apple and sauté for 3 to 5 minutes, until softened.

3. Add the spinach, raisins, vinegar, salt, and pepper and sauté until the spinach is wilted, about 3 minutes.

4. Serve immediately.

tidbits:
Spinach is large in volume until it cooks down. If your pot is not big enough, cook it in two batches and then add it all back together to reheat quickly prior to serving.

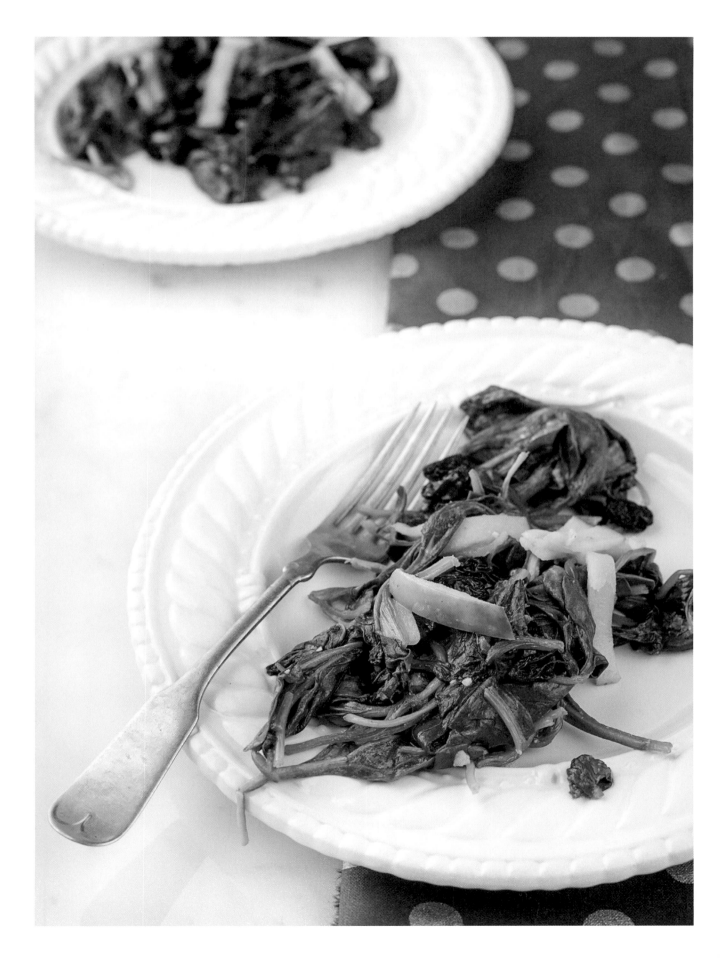

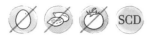

serves: 6 to 8

prep time: 15 minutes

cook time: 15 minutes

The anise essence of fennel is brought to the forefront when it's roasted, and it is especially complemented with notes of orange and balsamic vinegar in this recipe.

# thyme-roasted fennel and carrots

## ingredients

- 3 medium fennel bulbs, stalks discarded, bulbs cut into ½-inch-thick wedges
- 1 pound carrots, peeled and cut into 3-inch pieces or left whole if long and thin
- 6 cloves garlic, peeled
- 4 sprigs fresh thyme leaves
- 2 tablespoons fresh orange juice
- 1½ tablespoons balsamic vinegar
- 2 tablespoons melted ghee or coconut oil
- 1½ teaspoons sea salt
- ½ teaspoon cracked black pepper

## method

1. Preheat the oven to 425°F.

2. In a large bowl, toss together the fennel, carrots, garlic, thyme, orange juice, vinegar, ghee, salt, and pepper. Spread in a single layer in a roasting pan or on a rimmed baking sheet.

3. Roast until the fennel has caramelized slightly and the carrots have begun to wrinkle slightly, about 15 minutes.

make-ahead tip:
Toss all of the ingredients together and store, tightly wrapped, in the refrigerator for up to 2 days before roasting.

tidbits:
Make sure to purchase high-quality balsamic vinegar that does not contain additional sugar or additives.

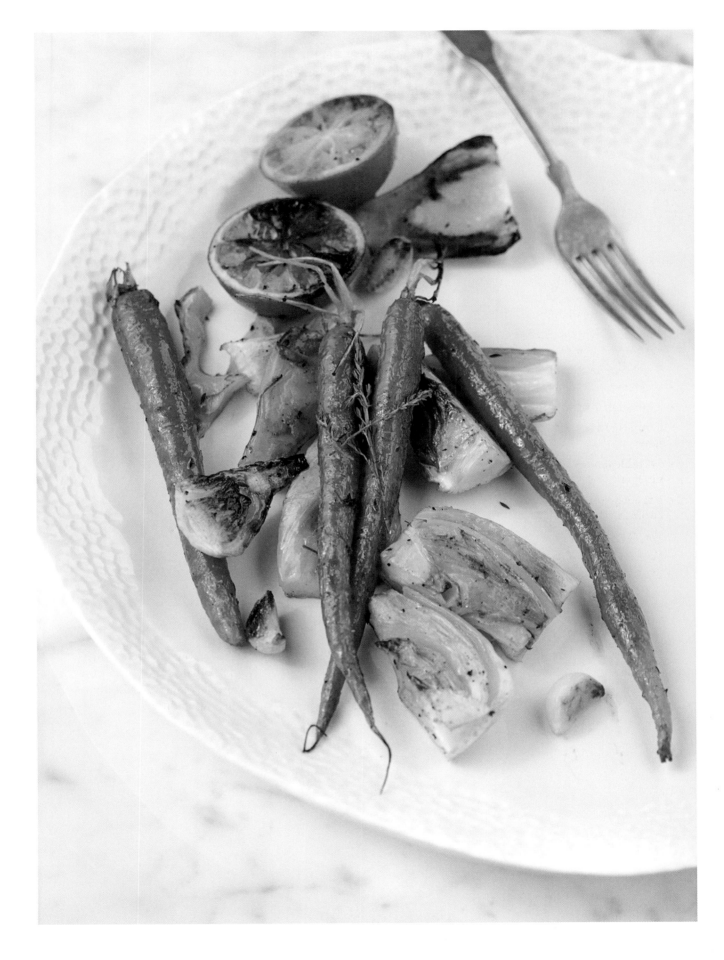

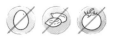

serves: 6 to 8

prep time: 15 minutes

cook time: 8 minutes

Crisp jicama stands in for the typical cabbage and a tangy dressing for the mayo to give this slaw a unique flavor and crunch. It is so refreshing on a warm summer day!

## 30 minutes or less | jicama apple bacon slaw

### ingredients

- 3 ounces bacon, chopped
- 3 cups peeled and shredded jicama
- 3 medium carrots, peeled and shredded
- 2 small apples, peeled and shredded
- 2 tablespoons fresh lime juice
- 2 tablespoons apple cider vinegar
- 1 teaspoon honey
- ½ teaspoon sea salt
- ¼ teaspoon cracked black pepper
- ¼ cup chopped fresh cilantro

### method

1. Cook the bacon in a skillet over medium heat until crispy, about 8 minutes. Drain on paper towels. Allow to cool to room temperature.

2. When the bacon has cooled, toss it and the rest of the ingredients together in a bowl. Refrigerate for 15 minutes before serving.

make-ahead tip:
The slaw can be stored in the refrigerator, tightly wrapped, for up to 3 days.

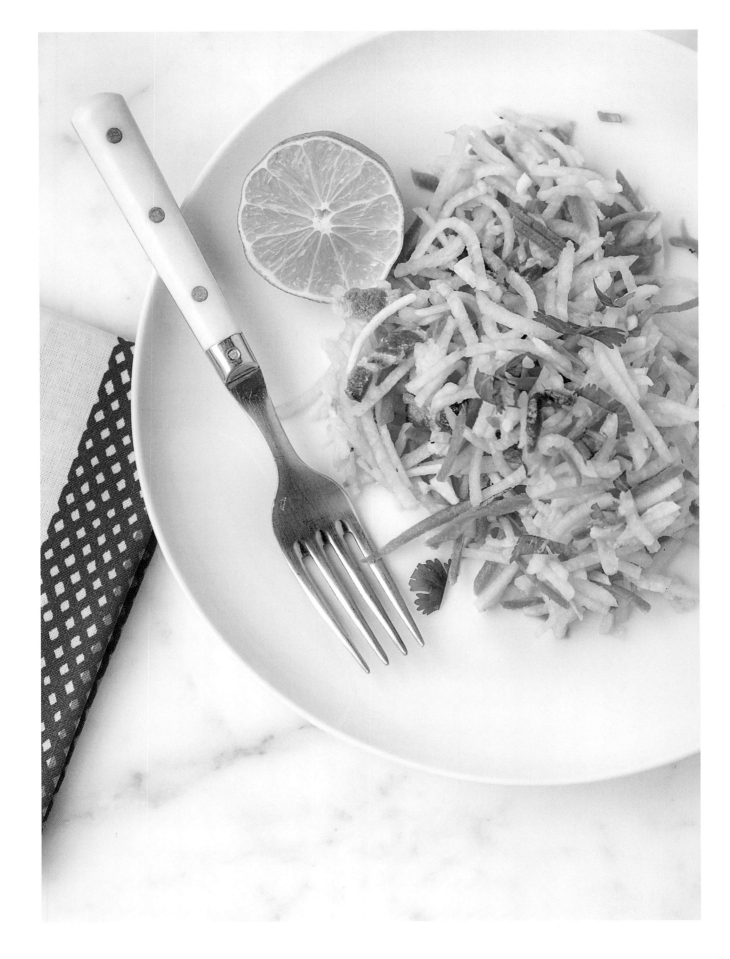

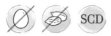

SCD

serves: 6

prep time: 15 minutes

cook time: 20 minutes

This dish goes really well with fish and poultry, or you can toss it with zucchini noodles and a little Pesto Sauce (page 256) for a quick vegetarian pasta dish.

# roasted basil eggplant

## ingredients

- 1½ pounds eggplant, cut into 1-inch cubes
- 3 tablespoons melted ghee, melted bacon fat, or extra-virgin olive oil
- 1 teaspoon white vinegar
- ¾ teaspoon sea salt
- ½ teaspoon cracked black pepper
- 3 tablespoons pine nuts*
- ¼ cup chopped fresh basil, for garnish

\* Omit for nut-free.

## method

1. Preheat the oven to 425°F.

2. In a large bowl, toss together the eggplant, ghee, vinegar, salt, and pepper. Spread in a single layer on a rimmed baking sheet or roasting pan.

3. Roast for 15 minutes, then add the pine nuts and toss to incorporate. Continue roasting for 5 minutes, until the eggplant is tender and lightly browned and the nuts are lightly toasted.

4. Top with basil and serve.

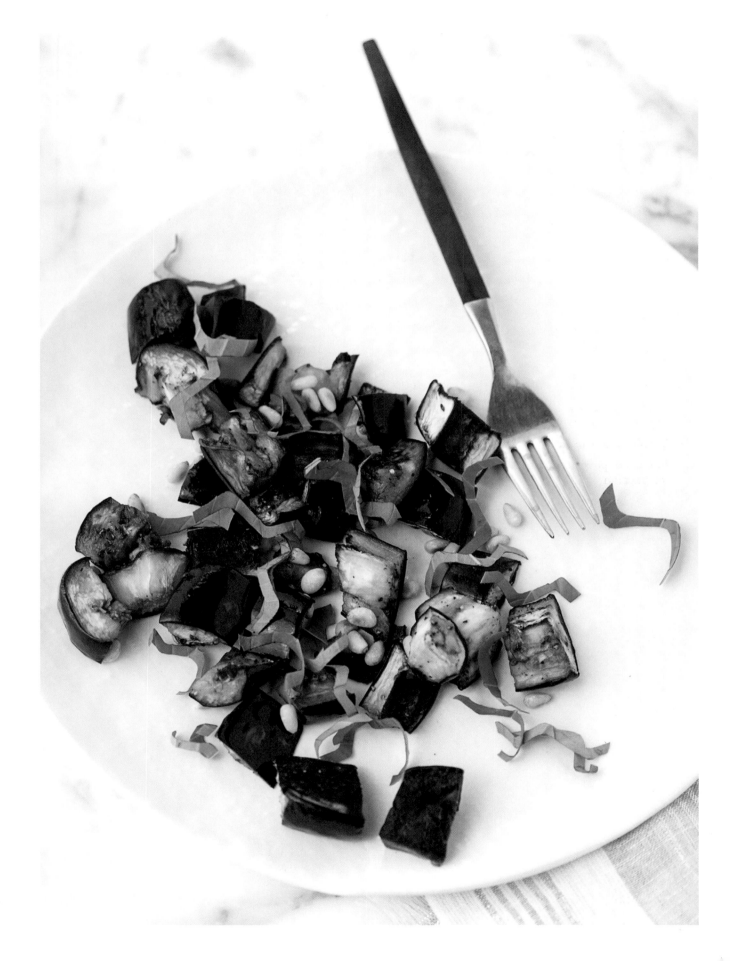

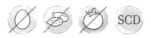

serves: 6
prep time: 20 minutes
cook time: 25 minutes

Tahini is a paste made from ground sesame seeds and is used in a lot of Mediterranean and Middle Eastern recipes. This Greek-inspired side dish quickly became one of my favorite recipes to accompany just about any protein, but it goes exceptionally well with my Mediterranean Braised Lamb (page 176). I could eat it on its own, it's that good!

# roasted squash and beets in tahini sauce

## ingredients

- 1 pound butternut squash, peeled and cut into 1-inch cubes
- 1 pound golden beets, peeled and cut into ½-inch wedges
- 2½ tablespoons melted ghee or cold-pressed sesame oil
- 2 tablespoons tahini
- 2 teaspoons fresh lemon juice
- 2 teaspoons chopped fresh oregano leaves
- 1 teaspoon chopped fresh rosemary
- ½ teaspoon sea salt
- ¼ teaspoon cracked black pepper
- 2 tablespoons shelled raw pistachios*

*Omit for nut-free.*

## method

1. Preheat the oven to 400°F.

2. In a large bowl, toss together all of the ingredients except the pistachios. Spread in a single layer on a rimmed baking sheet.

3. Roast for 25 minutes. Stir and rotate the pan halfway through.

4. Stir in the pistachios and serve.

make-ahead tip:
The vegetables can be peeled and cut the night before and stored in an airtight container in the refrigerator.

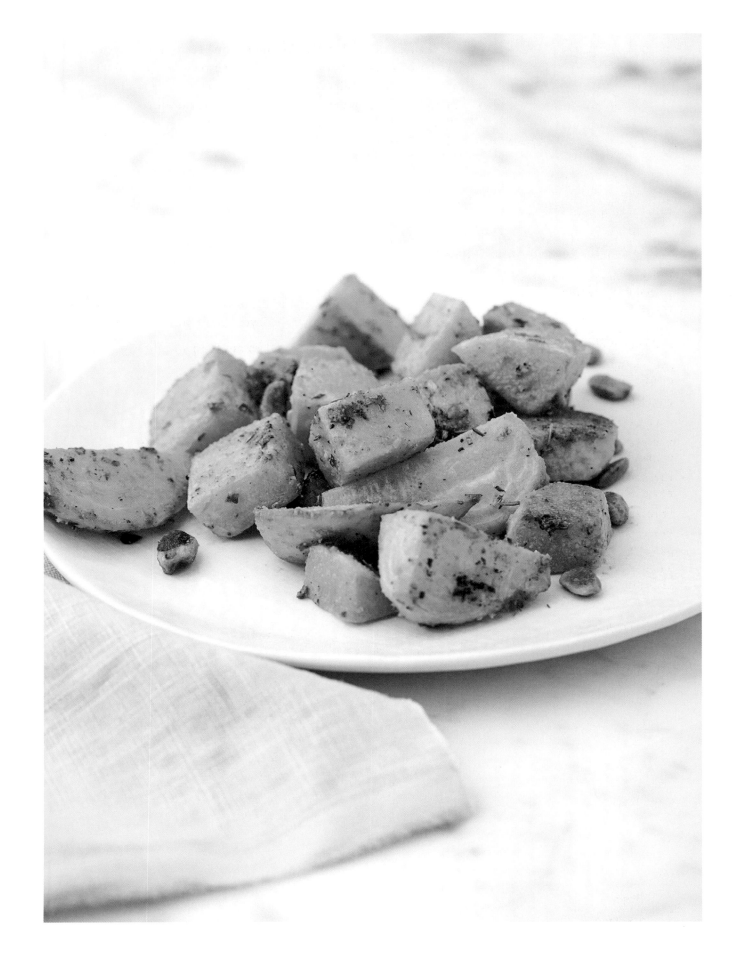

serves: 6 to 8

prep time: 10 minutes

cook time: 15 minutes

Summer squash is sautéed with garlic and cumin to create a side dish worthy of any Mexican meal.

# cumin-garlic summer squash

## ingredients

- 1 tablespoon ghee or olive oil, divided
- 2 cloves garlic, minced
- 3 medium zucchini, thinly sliced
- 3 medium yellow squash, thinly sliced
- 1 teaspoon ground cumin
- ½ teaspoon sea salt
- ¼ teaspoon cracked black pepper

## method

1. Heat 1½ teaspoons of the ghee in a skillet over medium-high heat.

2. Add the garlic and sauté for 2 minutes.

3. Add half of the zucchini and yellow squash and sauté for 5 minutes. Transfer to a plate.

4. Add the remaining 1½ teaspoons of ghee and vegetables to the skillet and sauté for 5 minutes. Return the first half of the vegetables to the pan and add the cumin, salt, and pepper. Toss to coat and cook for 2 minutes more.

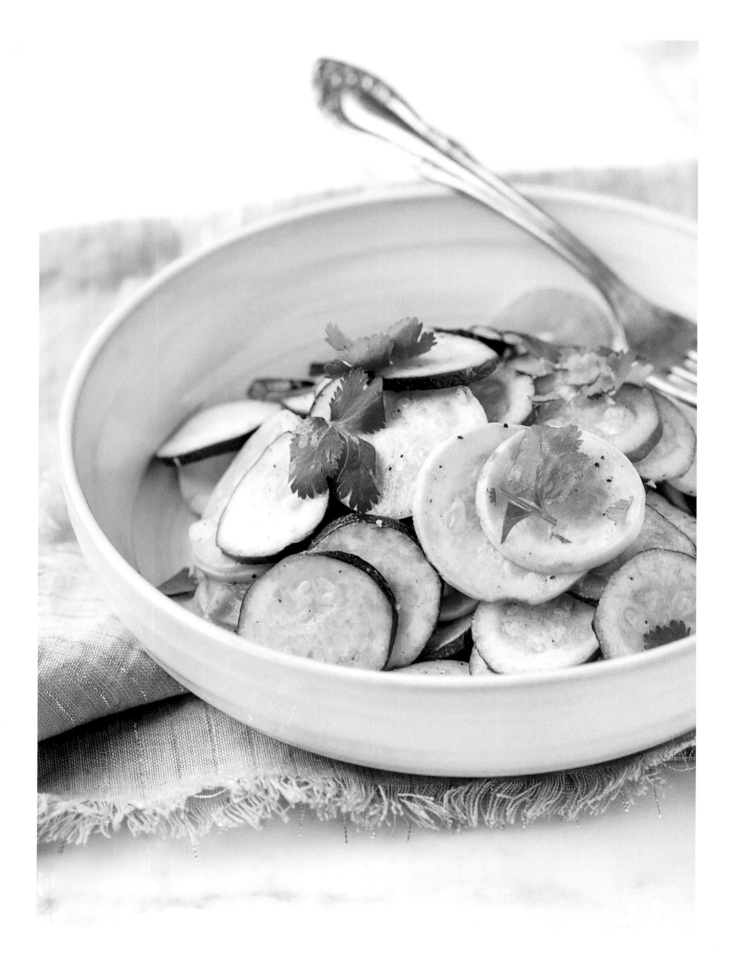

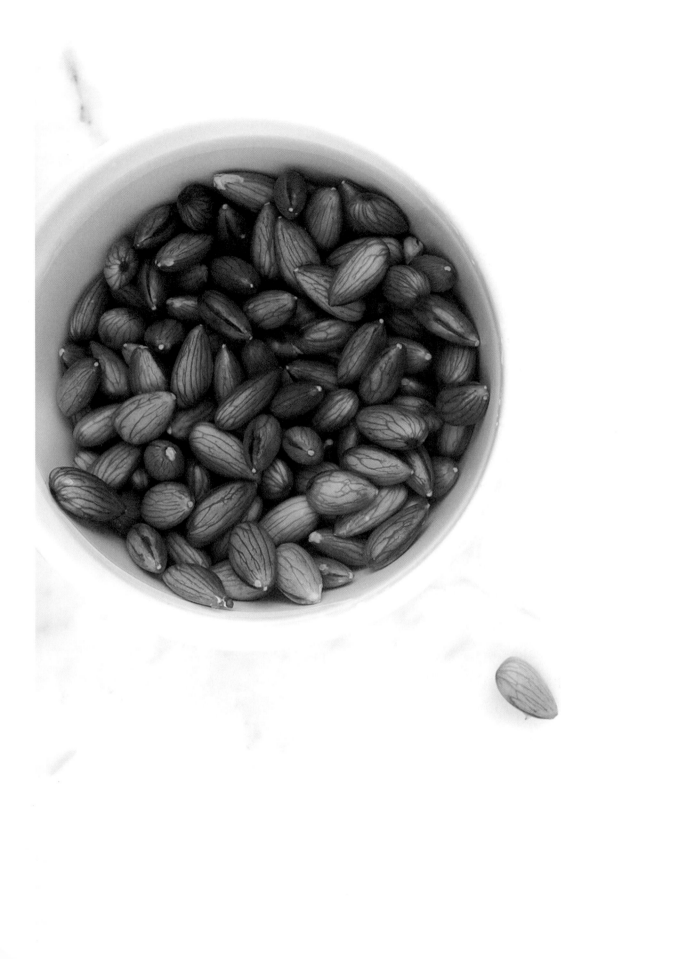

# basics

yield: 1 quart

prep time: 5 minutes, plus
10 hours to soak the almonds

Commercial almond milks are not only pricey, but also full of additives. All you need is a blender and some cheesecloth to create healthy dairy-free milk alternatives.

# almond milk

### ingredients

- 1 cup raw almonds
- 8 cups filtered water, divided
- ¼ teaspoon sea salt, divided
- 1 small date, pitted

### method

1. Place the almonds in a bowl with 4 cups of the filtered water and ⅛ teaspoon of the salt. Soak for 10 hours or overnight.

2. Drain the nuts and rinse well. Transfer them to a blender and fill with 4 cups of fresh filtered water. Add the date and the remaining ⅛ teaspoon of the salt and purée until smooth.

3. Strain the milk through a nut milk bag or a mesh sieve lined with 2 layers of cheesecloth. Squeeze the bag or use a spoon to press down on the nut pulp in the sieve and remove all of the liquid. Store the milk in the refrigerator for up to 5 days.

tidbits:

You can also make cashew, hazelnut, or brazil nut milk. Soak cashews for 4 hours. Hazelnuts and brazil nuts don't need to be soaked because they don't contain the enzyme inhibitors that prevent nuts from being digested properly—so you can make milk from those nuts at the drop of a hat.

There are many uses for leftover almond pulp, so be sure to save it and look online for ways to utilize it!

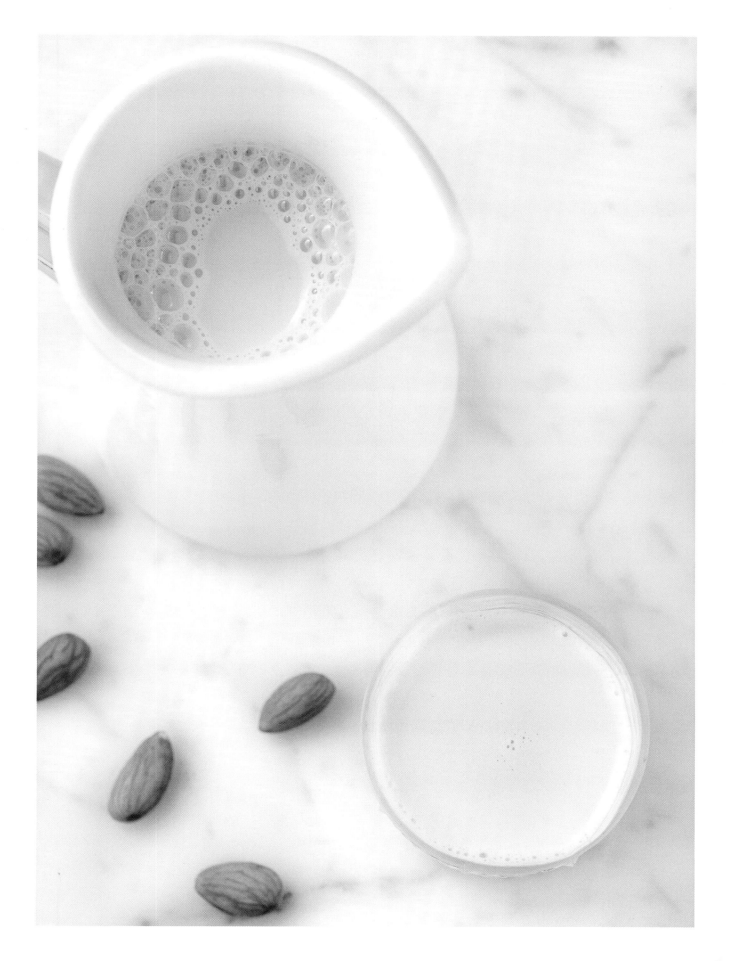

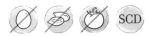

yield: 10 cups

prep time: 10 minutes

cook time: 12 to 24 hours

Homemade chicken stock is the secret to every good chef's flavorful soup, and it is simple and cost-efficient to make. It is packed full of minerals that are easily absorbed by our bodies, and the gelatin in the bones is a gut soother and healer. I like to make my chicken stock with meaty bone parts to provide an added depth of flavor.

# chicken stock

## ingredients

- 12 cups filtered water
- 1 to 2 pounds chicken bones and gizzards
- 1 tablespoon apple cider vinegar
- 1 yellow onion, peeled and quartered
- 3 large carrots, cut into large dice
- 4 cloves garlic, smashed
- 2 stalks celery with leaves
- 2 bay leaves
- 1 teaspoon sea salt
- ½ teaspoon cracked black pepper
- 1 bunch fresh parsley

## method

1. Place all of the ingredients except the parsley in a slow cooker and cook on low for 24 hours or on high for 12 hours. Turn off the slow cooker and skim the fat off the top. Stir in the parsley, cover, and let sit for 30 minutes.

2. Strain the broth through a fine-mesh sieve or cheesecloth. Store in the refrigerator or freezer for later use. Scoop off any solidified fat before using.

make-ahead tip:
Keep homemade stock in the refrigerator for up to 2 weeks or in the freezer for 6 months. Thaw overnight in the refrigerator or in a stockpot on low heat.

tidbits:
Break the chicken carcass or bones into parts if needed to fit into your slow cooker.

If you are drinking this stock on its own, more salt will need to be added. Otherwise, the recipes in this book call for the amount of salt needed based on using this homemade low-sodium stock. If you use store-bought stock to make the recipes in this book, be sure to buy low-sodium stock without sugars or additives and reduce the amount of salt called for in the recipes by half.

yield: 1½ cups

prep time: 5 minutes

Whether it's used on chicken, fish, or beef, this versatile smoky rub will give any dish a burst of flavor.

# barbecue dry rub

## ingredients

- ⅓ cup coconut crystals
- ¼ cup paprika
- ¼ cup chili powder
- 1 tablespoon garlic powder
- 1 tablespoon coarse sea salt
- 1 tablespoon dry mustard
- 2 teaspoons dried oregano leaves
- 2 teaspoons ground cumin
- ¾ teaspoon cracked black pepper
- ½ teaspoon cayenne pepper

## method

Mix all of the ingredients together in a small bowl. Store in an airtight container in the pantry for up to 3 months.

use it:
Barbecue Chicken (page 134)
Barbecue Tri-Tip with Grilled Watermelon Salad (page 170)
Barbecue Salmon with Grilled Peach Salsa (page 208)

yield: about ½ cup

prep time: 5 minutes

# taco seasoning

## ingredients

- 2½ tablespoons chili powder
- 1½ tablespoons sea salt
- 1½ tablespoons ground cumin
- 1 tablespoon ground dried oregano
- 2 teaspoons onion powder
- 2 teaspoons ground coriander
- 2 teaspoons paprika
- 1 to 3 teaspoons cayenne pepper
- ¼ teaspoon cracked black pepper

## method

Mix all of the ingredients together in a small bowl. Store in a jar in the pantry for up to 6 months.

tidbits:
I add only ½ teaspoon of cayenne pepper to the mix and then add more to the finished dish after I have served out my son Asher's portion.

use it:
Beef Tacos (page 146)
Mexican Chicken Soup (page 88)
Southwestern Frittata (page 50)

 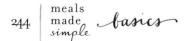

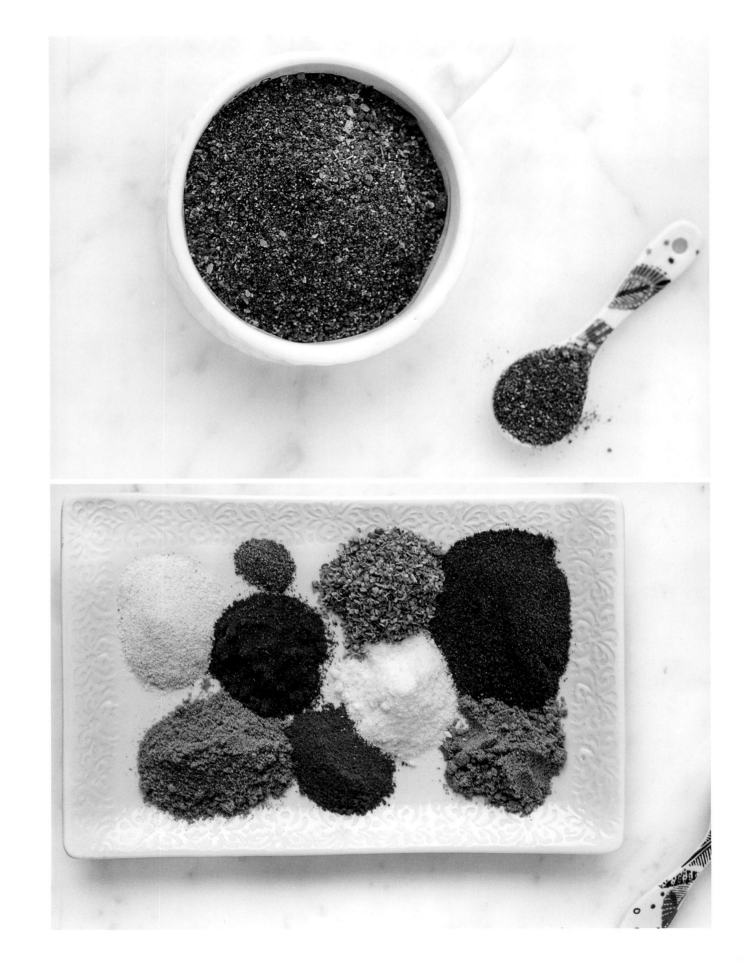

champagne vinaigrette                    herb ranch

greek                                    balsamic

# champagne vinaigrette Ø ⊘ ⊘ SCD

## ingredients

- 1½ tablespoons fresh lemon juice
- 2 teaspoons champagne vinegar
- 1 teaspoon Dijon mustard
- ¼ teaspoon sea salt
- pinch of cracked black pepper
- ¼ cup extra-virgin olive oil

## method

In a bowl, whisk together the lemon juice, vinegar, mustard, salt, and pepper in a bowl. Slowly whisk in the olive oil. Serve immediately or store, covered, in the refrigerator for up to 5 days. Shake before using to reincorporate the oil that may separate during refrigeration.

tidbits:

To make balsamic vinaigrette, swap the champagne vinegar for balsamic vinegar and add some chopped fresh herbs, such as thyme or basil.

# herb ranch dressing ⊘ ⊘ SCD

## ingredients

- 1 cup Mayonnaise (page 248)
- ½ cup full-fat coconut milk
- 2 cloves garlic, crushed into a paste
- 3 tablespoons chopped fresh parsley
- 2 tablespoons chopped fresh chives
- 2 tablespoons chopped fresh dill
- 1 tablespoon fresh lemon juice
- ½ teaspoon onion powder
- ½ teaspoon sea salt

## method

In a bowl, whisk together all of the ingredients. Refrigerate for up to 3 days.

# greek dressing Ø ⊘ ⊘ SCD

## ingredients

- ¼ cup fresh lemon juice
- 2 teaspoons red wine vinegar
- 2 cloves garlic, crushed into a paste
- 1 tablespoon chopped fresh oregano leaves
- ½ teaspoon Dijon mustard
- pinch of sea salt
- pinch of cracked black pepper
- ½ cup extra-virgin olive oil

## method

In a bowl, whisk together the lemon juice, vinegar, garlic, oregano, mustard, salt, and pepper.

Drizzle in the olive oil in a slow, steady stream while whisking continuously and vigorously, until it is all incorporated.

Serve immediately or store, covered, in the refrigerator for up to 5 days. Shake before using to reincorporate the oil that may separate during refrigeration.

yield: ¾ cup

prep time: 12 minutes

# mayonnaise

### ingredients

- 1 large egg yolk
- 1 teaspoon fresh lemon juice
- 1 teaspoon white vinegar
- ½ teaspoon sea salt
- ¼ teaspoon Dijon mustard
- ¾ cup macadamia nut oil

### method

1. Place the first 5 ingredients in a small blender or mini food processor and blend on low until combined.

2. With the blender on low, add the oil 1 drop at a time. When the mixture begins to thicken, add the remaining oil in a slow, steady stream with the blender still running, until all of the oil has been incorporated.

3. Cover and refrigerate, tightly covered, for up to 3 days.

tidbits:

Macadamia nut oil is used for its slightly sweet and mild flavor, but other oils, such as olive, avocado, or almond, may be substituted.

A small blender or mini food processor is essential for the method above; however, mayonnaise can also be made by hand. Place the first 5 ingredients in a medium bowl and whisk to combine. Add ¼ cup of the oil ½ teaspoon at a time, whisking vigorously. Gradually add the remaining ½ cup oil in a slow, steady stream, whisking constantly, until thick, about 5 to 7 minutes.

Alternatively, many find that using an immersion blender in a tall, slender container works well.

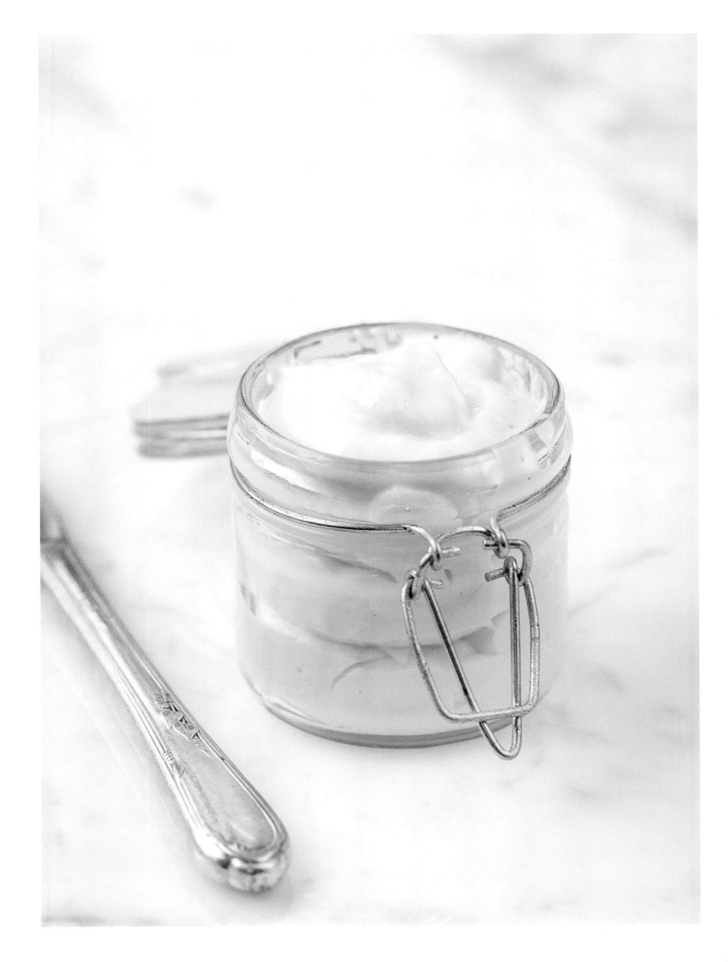

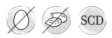

yield: 3 cups
prep time: 8 minutes
cook time: 30 to 40 minutes

# barbecue sauce

## ingredients

- 2 cups tomato puree
- ¾ cup honey
- ½ cup white vinegar
- ¼ cup tomato paste
- 2 tablespoons coconut crystals*
- 2 tablespoons coconut aminos*
- 2 teaspoons fish sauce
- 1½ teaspoons natural liquid smoke
- 1 teaspoon sea salt
- 1 teaspoon paprika
- 1 teaspoon chili powder
- 1 teaspoon Dijon mustard
- ½ teaspoon cayenne pepper
- ½ teaspoon minced garlic
- ½ teaspoon onion powder
- ½ teaspoon ground allspice
- ½ teaspoon cracked black pepper

* Omit for SCD.

## method

1. Place all of the ingredients in a saucepan over medium-high heat and whisk to combine.

2. Bring to a boil, then reduce the heat and simmer for 30 to 40 minutes, until the sauce has reduced by about half.

3. Let come to room temperature before storing in the refrigerator for later use. The sauce may be stored for up to 1 week.

make-ahead tip:
You can double this recipe and store half in the freezer for up to 6 months. Thaw in the refrigerator.

use it:
Barbecue Chicken Chopped Salad (page 108)

Barbecue Chicken (page 134)

Barbecue Beef Short Ribs (page 144)

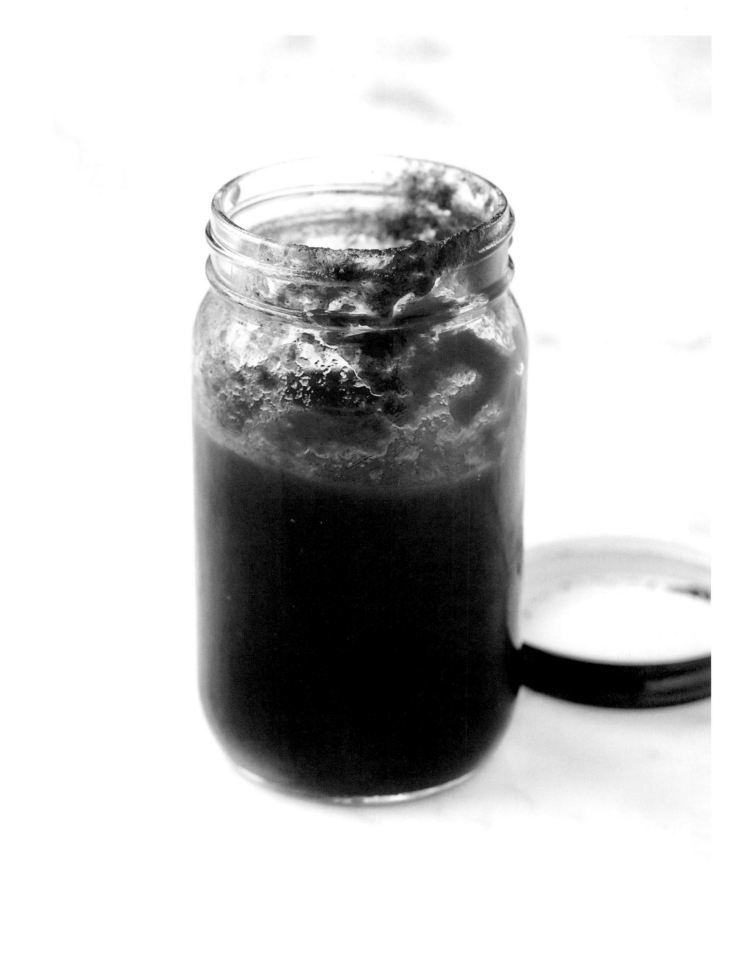

SCD

yield: ½ cup
prep time: 5 minutes
cook time: 4 minutes

## 30 minutes or less  hollandaise sauce

### ingredients

- 2 large egg yolks
- 3 tablespoons ghee, melted
- 2 teaspoons fresh lemon juice
- ¼ teaspoon sea salt
- 1 teaspoon water
- ⅛ teaspoon paprika

### method

1. Heat a medium saucepan filled halfway full with water over medium-high heat. Place a heatproof bowl over the saucepan to create a double boiler setup; make sure that the bottom of the bowl does not touch the water. Whisk the egg yolks vigorously in the bowl over the heat until pale in color and thickened slightly, about 2 minutes.

2. Slowly drizzle in the melted ghee, whisking continuously. Continue whisking until the sauce has thickened and doubled in volume. Remove from the heat and whisk in the lemon juice, salt, water, and paprika.

make-ahead tip:
While Hollandaise Sauce is best fresh, it can be gently reheated over a double boiler on low heat.

tidbits:
If the sauce is too thick, add a splash of water at a time until it reaches the desired consistency.

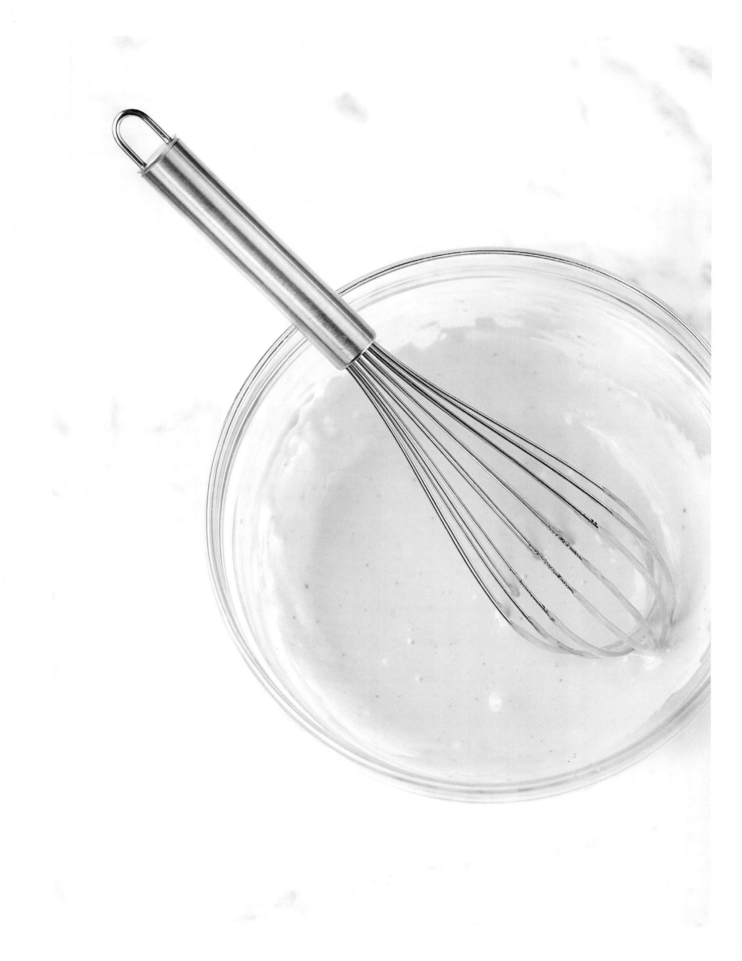

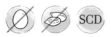

yield: 2 cups
prep time: 10 minutes
cook time: 45 minutes

# ketchup

### ingredients

- 1 tablespoon coconut oil
- ½ yellow onion, halved
- 1 clove garlic, crushed into a paste
- 3¼ cups tomato puree
- ½ cup honey
- ⅓ cup white vinegar
- 1 tablespoon tomato paste
- ½ teaspoon sea salt
- 8 whole cloves
- 10 whole allspice berries

### method

1. Heat the oil in a deep skillet or saucepan over medium heat. Add the onion and garlic and sauté for 5 minutes, until fragrant.

2. Add the remaining ingredients and bring to a boil. Reduce the heat to medium-low and simmer, uncovered, for 40 minutes, until the sauce has thickened and reduced by half.

3. Remove the onion, cloves, and allspice berries.

4. Let come to room temperature before storing in the refrigerator for later use.

make-ahead tip:
Double the recipe and store half in the freezer. Thaw in the refrigerator for a day before using.

Fresh Ketchup will keep, tightly wrapped, in the refrigerator for up to 1 week.

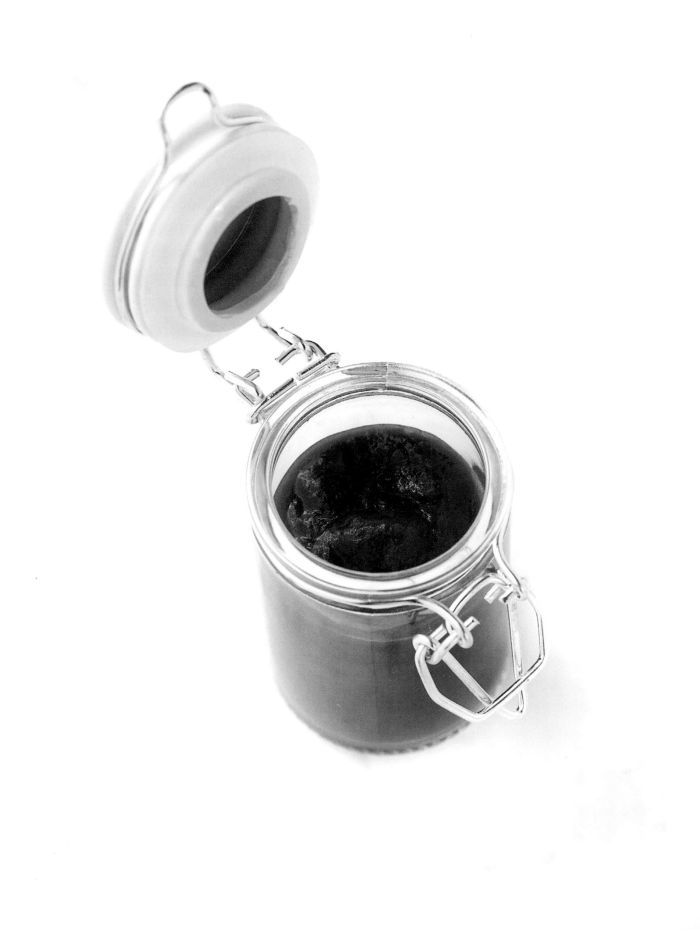

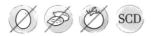

yield: 1 cup
prep time: 10 minutes
cook time: 5 minutes

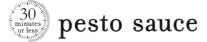 **pesto sauce**

### ingredients

- ⅓ cup pine nuts*
- 1½ cups packed basil leaves
- 3 cloves garlic
- 1½ teaspoons fresh lemon juice
- ½ teaspoon sea salt
- ⅓ cup extra-virgin olive oil

*For nut-free, substitute raw sunflower seed kernels or ¼ cup Parmesan cheese.*

### method

1. Lightly toast the pine nuts in a skillet over medium heat for 5 minutes, shaking the pan from time to time to make sure they don't burn.

2. Place all of the ingredients except the oil in a small food processor. Pulse a few times to chop the contents.

3. Slowly incorporate the oil while the food processor is running, until a paste has formed. Continue blending for 15 seconds until the sauce is smooth.

**make-ahead tip:**
Pesto Sauce can be prepared up to 3 days in advance and stored in an airtight container in the refrigerator. Add a thin layer of olive oil to the top before covering to keep the Pesto fresh. Stir to incorporate the oil before using.

**use it:**
Pesto-Stuffed Prosciutto Chicken (page 122)

Pesto Orange Roughy (page 206)

Pesto Pasta with Scallops (page 194)

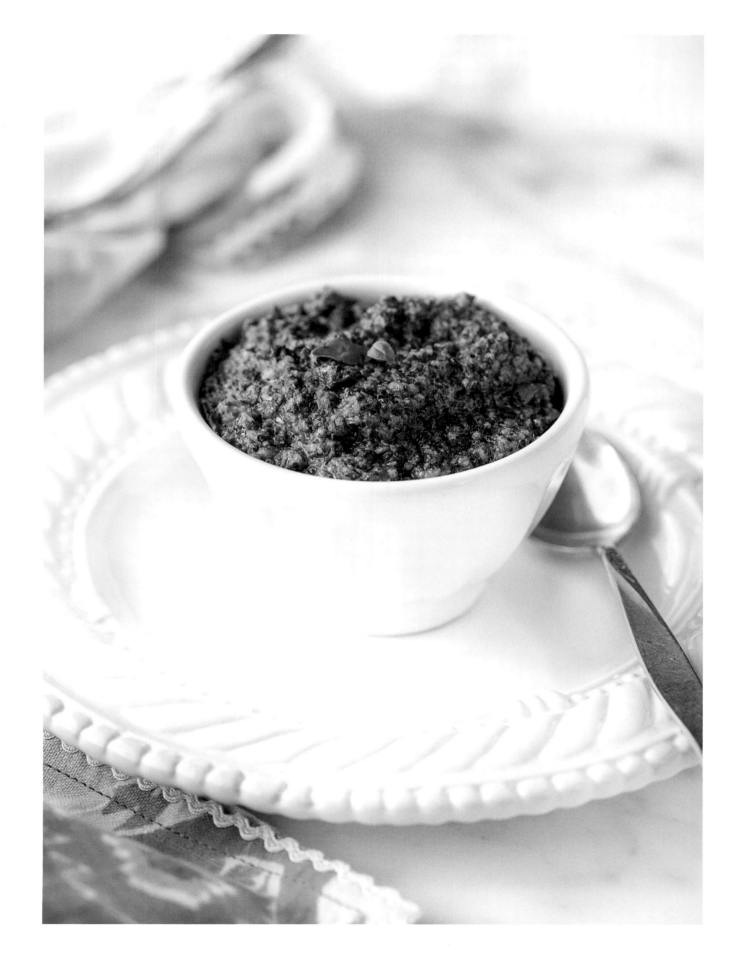

# mango-pineapple salsa

## ingredients

- ½ cup diced mango
- ½ cup diced pineapple
- ¼ cup diced avocado
- 2 tablespoons minced fresh cilantro
- 2 teaspoons fresh lime juice
- dash of sea salt
- 2 tablespoons minced jalapeño*
- 1 tablespoon minced red onion

## method

Mix together all of the ingredients. Serve immediately or store in the refrigerator for up to 2 days.

*Omit for nightshade-free.*

# roasted tomatillo salsa

## ingredients

- 2 pounds tomatillos, husked and rinsed
- 2 serrano peppers or 1 medium jalapeño
- ½ yellow onion
- 4 cloves garlic
- 1 teaspoon sea salt

## method

1. Preheat the oven to 425°F.

2. Bring a large pot of water to boil over high heat. Boil the tomatillos for 10 to 15 minutes, until the skins have shriveled slightly and the fruit has turned a dull army green. Drain and remove any stems.

3. Meanwhile, roast the serrano peppers, onion, and garlic on a rimmed baking sheet in the oven for 20 minutes.

4. Place the tomatillos, roasted vegetables, and salt in a food processor and blend until smooth. Seed the peppers prior to blending for a milder sauce. Serve immediately or store in the refrigerator for up to 5 days.

# guacamole

## ingredients

- 4 ripe avocados, pitted and diced
- ¼ cup minced red onion
- ½ jalapeño pepper, seeded and diced
- 2 cloves garlic, minced
- 1 tablespoon chopped fresh cilantro
- 2 tablespoons diced tomatoes
- juice of 1 lime
- ½ teaspoon sea salt
- pinch of cracked black pepper

## method

1. Place the avocados in a bowl and mash until mostly smooth. Alternatively, place in a food processor and pulse.

2. Add the remaining ingredients and stir to combine. If using a food processor, pulse 4 times to combine. Serve immediately.

 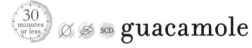

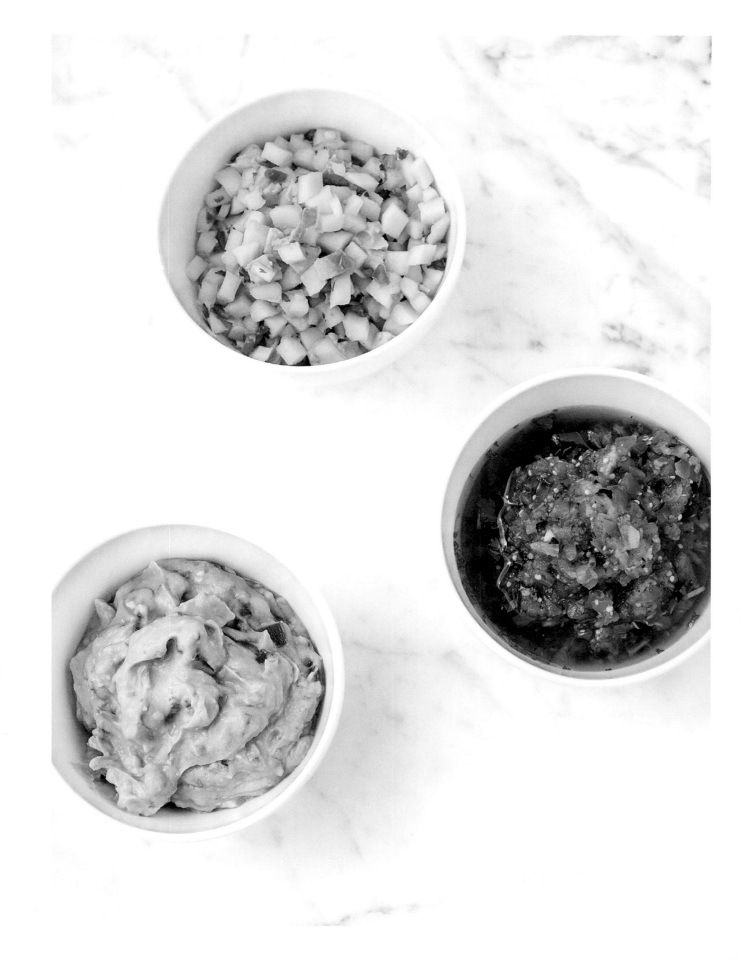

yield: 4 cups
prep time: 10 minutes

This multi-purpose flour mix can be made and stored in your pantry so you can whip together delicious baked goods like Freezer Waffles (page 66), Fluffy Pancakes (page 68), and Blueberry Muffins (page 72) in a flash.

# pancake mix

## ingredients

- 3 cups blanched almond flour
- 1 cup coconut flour
- 1 tablespoon baking soda
- 2 teaspoons cream of tartar
- ¾ teaspoon sea salt

## method

Whisk all of the ingredients together in a large bowl. Pour into an airtight container and store in the pantry for up to 1 month or in the refrigerator for up to 6 months. Fluff with a fork to break up any clumps before measuring and using for recipes.

tidbits:
Finely ground cashew flour or finely ground and sifted raw sunflower seed flour may be used in place of almond flour but will change the flavor and texture slightly.

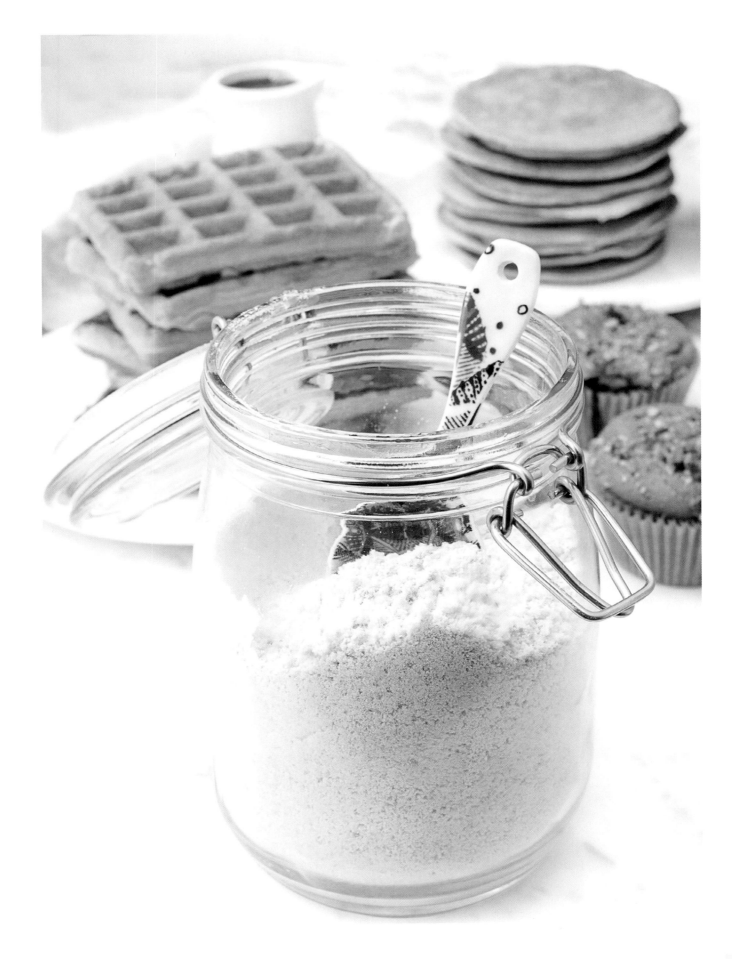

These wraps are great to have on hand when lettuce wraps are becoming mundane and something more substantial is in order. Use them for sandwiches, quesadillas, enchiladas, or simply as a crepe rolled with fruit and almond butter inside. I've discovered that the arrowroot powder in this recipe makes these wraps more pliable and also allows them to get crispier on the outside when used for quesadillas and paninis than the starch-free version from my first book, *Against All Grain*.

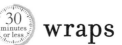

# wraps

## ingredients

- 6 large eggs, beaten
- 1 cup Almond Milk (page 240)*
- 6 tablespoons coconut flour, sifted
- ½ cup arrowroot powder
- 2 tablespoons melted ghee
- ½ teaspoon sea salt
- ghee or palm shortening, for the pan

*\* ½ cup coconut milk and ½ cup water may be substituted for nut-free.*

## method

1. Heat an 8-inch crêpe pan or well-seasoned griddle to medium-high heat.

2. Whisk together the eggs, Almond Milk, coconut flour, arrowroot powder, ghee, and salt. Let the batter sit for 10 minutes, then whisk again.

3. Melt a small amount of ghee in the pan and spread it all over.

4. Ladle ¼ cup of the batter onto the hot pan and quickly spread it into a paper-thin 8-inch circle with the back of the ladle or by turning the pan quickly with your wrist. Fill in any holes with a drop of batter. Cook for 45 seconds, until the sides start to lift, then gently flip the wrap. Cook for 30 seconds on the other side.

5. Move to a plate to cool and repeat the steps until all of the batter is used, greasing the pan between wraps when needed.

**use it:**
Breakfast Burritos (page 54)

Cuban Pork Panini (page 188)

California Chicken Wraps (page 128)

**make-ahead tip:**
The wraps will keep in the refrigerator for 5 days or the freezer for 6 months. Store with a piece of parchment paper between wraps and seal in a resealable bag. Thaw in the refrigerator for 2 hours prior to use.

**tidbits:**
A shallow, well-seasoned crêpe pan works best for this recipe, or use a large flat griddle to make multiple wraps at a time. Make sure to keep them very thin, and do not try to flip them until the sides start to lift.

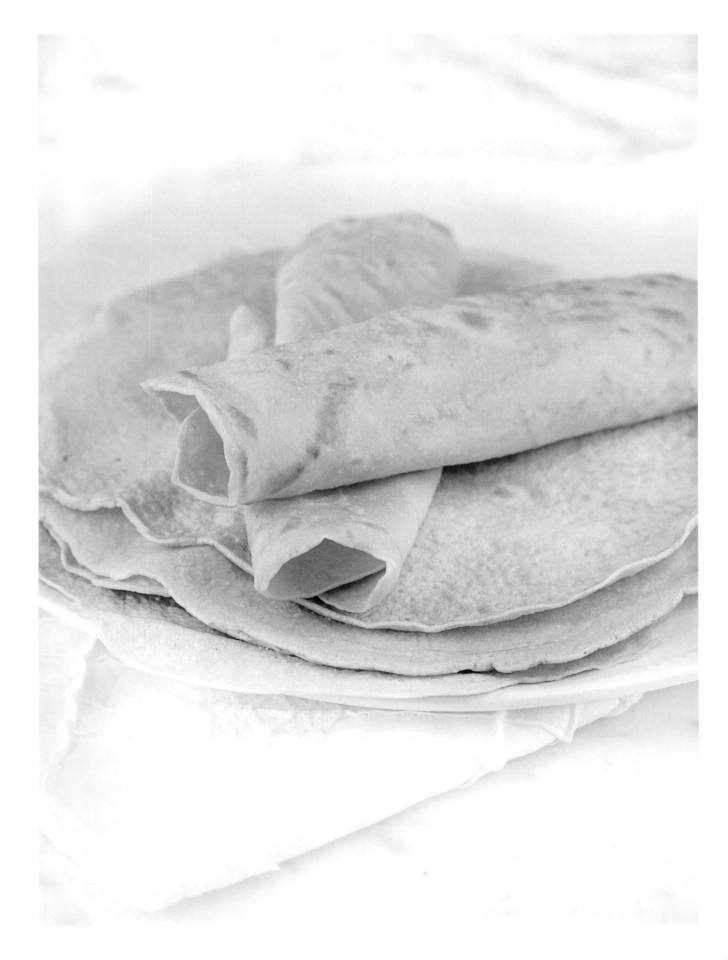

yield: 10 rolls

prep time: 10 minutes

cook time: 20 to 25 minutes

Make a batch of these rolls and keep them in the freezer to pull out for a quick lunch when a lettuce wrap just isn't cutting it! They work great for all types of sandwiches, burgers, and even breakfast sandwiches.

## 30 minutes or less | sandwich rolls

### ingredients

- ghee or coconut oil, for greasing the rings
- 8 large eggs
- ½ cup Almond Milk (page 240)
- 1 tablespoon plus 1 teaspoon apple cider vinegar
- 3 cups whole raw cashews (about 17½ ounces)
- ½ cup arrowroot powder*
- ¼ cup coconut flour
- 2 teaspoons baking soda
- 1 teaspoon sea salt

*For SCD, omit the arrowroot powder and increase the coconut flour to ½ cup.*

### method

1. Place a heatproof dish filled with 2 inches of water on the bottom rack of the oven. Preheat the oven to 325°F.

2. Lightly grease the inside of 10 (3¾-inch) English muffin rings with ghee and place them on a baking sheet lined with parchment paper.

3. Place all of the ingredients in a high-speed blender and process on low for 15 seconds. Scrape down the sides and process again on high for 15 to 30 seconds, until very smooth.

4. Fill each ring two-thirds full with batter. Bake for 20 to 25 minutes, until a toothpick inserted into the center comes out clean.

5. Allow the rolls to cool on the baking sheet for 15 minutes, then gently press them out of the rings from the bottom. Allow to cool on a wire rack before serving or storing.

**make-ahead tip:**
The rolls can be frozen for 6 months. Defrost the desired amount in the refrigerator overnight or place frozen rolls directly into a toaster.

**tidbits:**
Cleaned tuna cans with both ends cut off will work in place of the English muffin rings.

The steam bath created by the dish of water helps these rolls rise and stay moist.

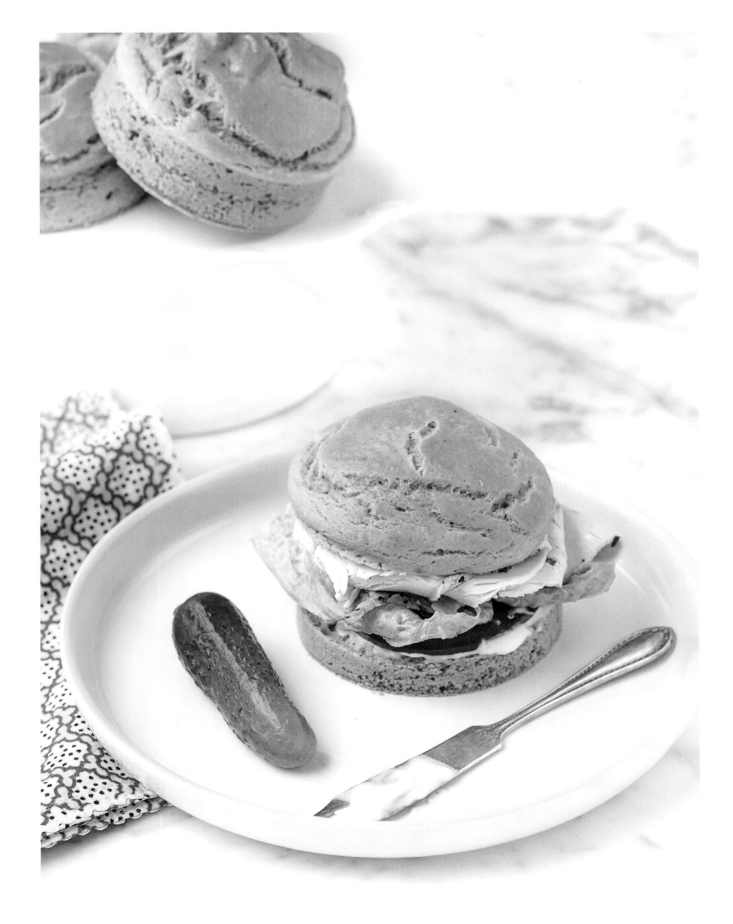

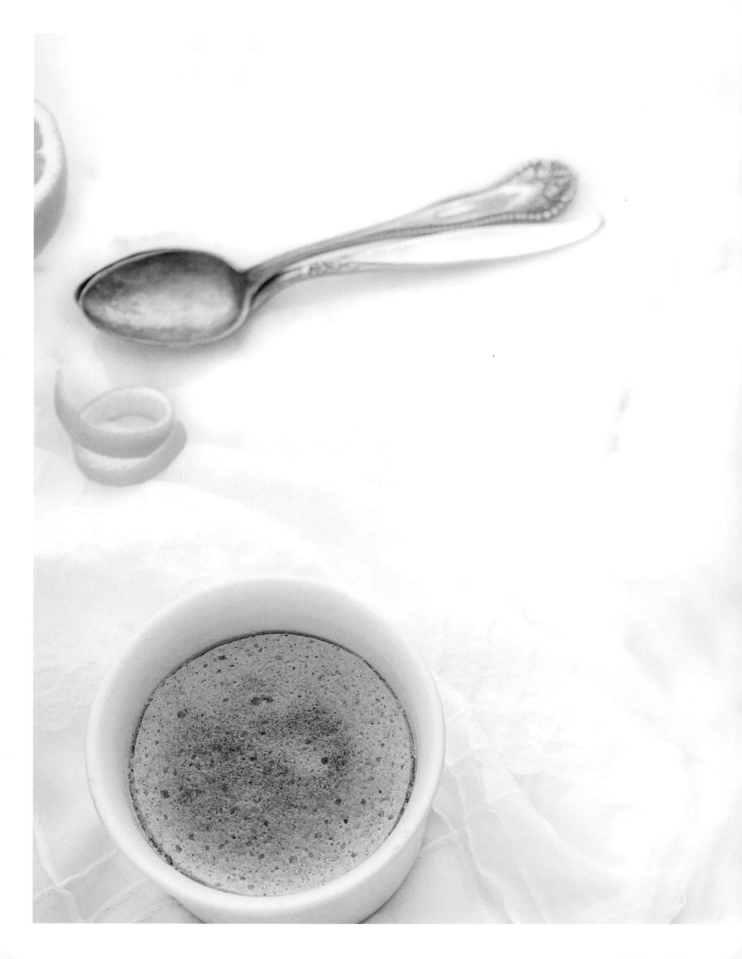

# simply sweets

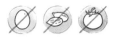

serves: 4 to 6

prep time: 5 minutes, plus
at least 6 hours refrigeration
time

This pudding is a breeze to throw together and is packed with omega-3 and fiber-rich chia seeds. I have always been sensitive to food textures and typically turn my nose up at chia desserts, but when you grind them in the blender you get a smooth pudding instead of the lumpy and crunchy texture that is often associated with chia recipes!

# 30 minutes or less  no-cook chocolate pudding

## ingredients

- 1 (13½-ounce) can full-fat coconut milk
- ½ cup hot water
- 4½ ounces pitted dates (about 18 small Deglet Noor)
- ½ cup raw cacao powder
- ¼ cup chia seeds
- 1 tablespoon melted coconut oil
- 2 teaspoons vanilla extract
- ¼ teaspoon sea salt
- dark chocolate shavings, unsweetened coconut flakes, or fresh berries, for garnish

## method

1. Place all of the ingredients in a high-speed blender. Blend until completely smooth, about 45 seconds.

2. Pour the pudding into serving bowls, cover, and refrigerate for at least 6 hours.

3. Garnish with dark chocolate shavings, unsweetened coconut flakes, or berries before serving.

tidbits:
Raw cacao powder is made from cold-pressed (as opposed to roasted) cacao beans and thus has more nutritional and health benefits than traditional cocoa powder. However, the two may be used interchangeably.

make-ahead tip:
The pudding may be made ahead and stored in the fridge for up to 3 days.

If a thin film forms on the top after chilling, remove it with a spoon before serving.

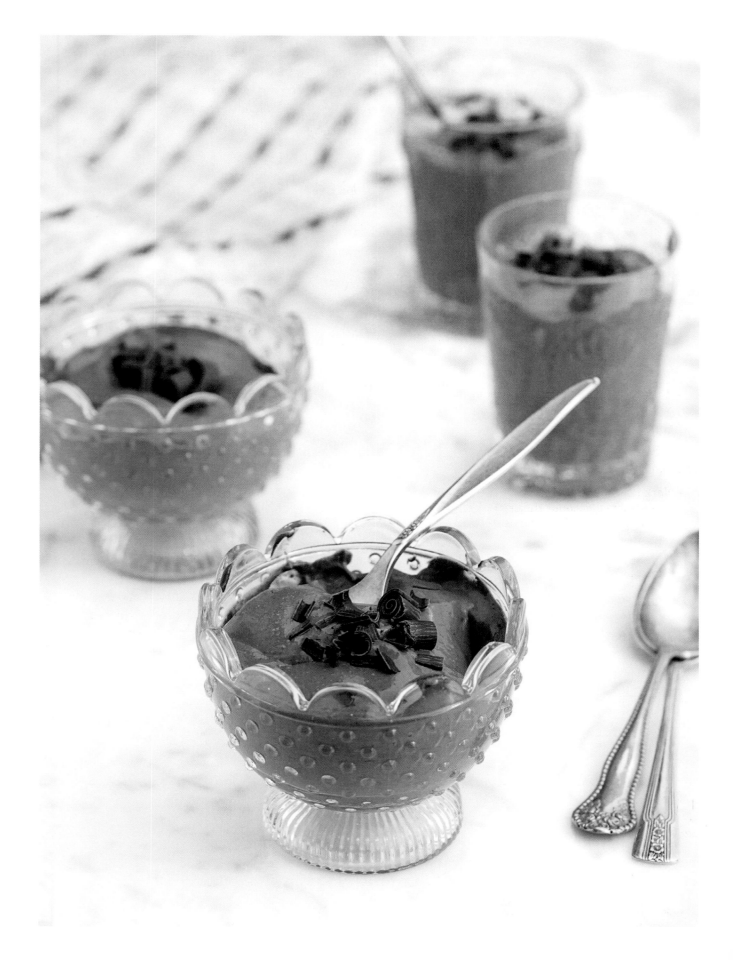

serves: 4

prep time: 15 minutes, plus at least 4 hours freezing time

This milkshake is a delightfully refreshing dessert that comes together quickly in a blender without the use of an ice cream machine.

# mint chocolate milkshake

## ingredients

- 1 (13½-ounce) can full-fat coconut milk
- 1 large avocado, pitted and diced
- 1 cup Almond Milk (page 240) or chilled coconut milk
- ¼ cup fresh mint leaves
- ¼ cup honey
- ¼ teaspoon peppermint extract
- dark chocolate chips or roasted cacao nibs

## method

1. Pour the coconut milk into a 12-cube ice tray and cover with plastic wrap. Place the diced avocado in a freezer-safe container and place it and the ice cube tray in the freezer. Freeze until hardened, about 4 hours or up to 2 days.

2. Remove the ice cube tray and avocado from the freezer and leave at room temperature for 15 minutes to defrost slightly.

3. Place the coconut milk cubes, avocado, and remaining ingredients in a blender. Blend on high until smooth.

4. Mix in the chocolate chips or cacao nibs and serve.

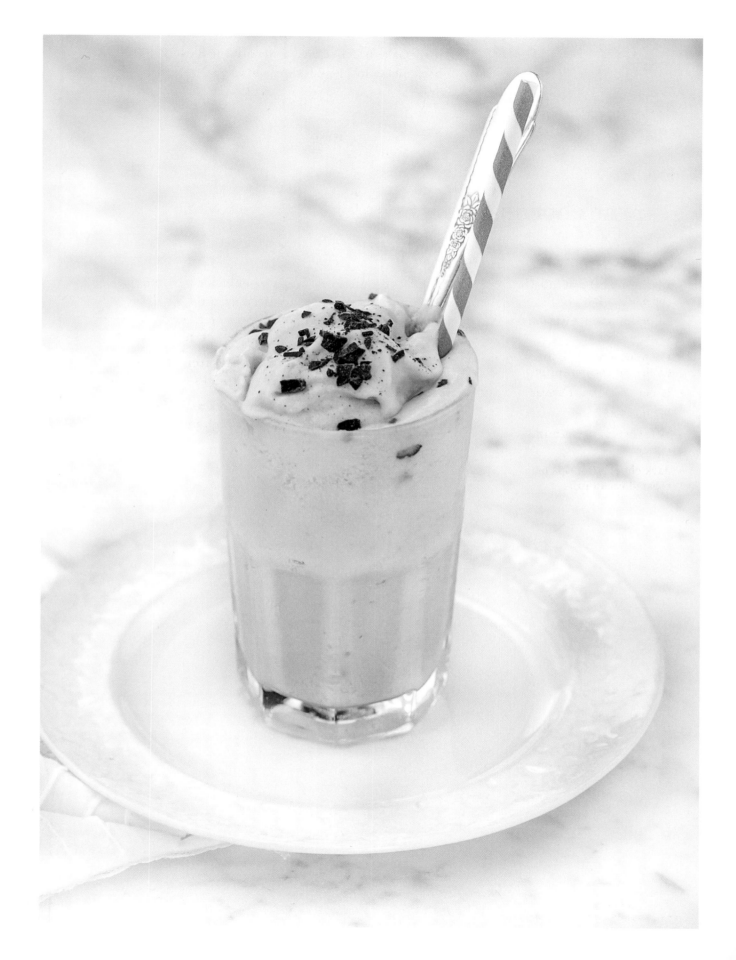

serves: 8

prep time: 35 minutes

cook time: 18 to 20 minutes

Strawberry shortcake is one of my favorite desserts and is the quintessential summertime treat. I love the fresh flavor of the strawberries and the simplicity of the biscuit and whipped cream.

# strawberry shortcake

## ingredients

- 1 batch Biscuits (page 56)
- 1½ pounds strawberries, stemmed and sliced
- 2 tablespoons coconut crystals or honey
- 2 teaspoons finely grated lemon zest
- Whipped Coconut Cream (recipe below)

## method

1. Make the Biscuits, following the recipe on page 56. Allow to cool completely on a wire rack.

2. While the Biscuits are baking, gently toss the strawberries, coconut crystals, and lemon zest together in a bowl. Refrigerate for 30 minutes to allow the juices to develop.

3. Slice the Biscuits in half and serve them with the strawberries and juices. Top with the Whipped Coconut Cream.

tidbits:
Try using fresh raspberries or peaches for a variation on this classic dessert!

make-ahead tip:
The biscuits can be made up to 3 days in advance and stored in the refrigerator to make this an even quicker dessert (just bring to room temperature before serving). The whipped coconut cream will keep in the refrigerator for 2 days. Whip it again right before serving.

# whipped coconut cream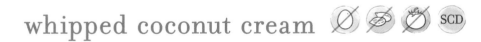

## ingredients

- 2 (13½-ounce) cans full-fat coconut milk, refrigerated for at least 24 hours
- 2 teaspoons honey (optional)

## method

1. Place a glass or metal bowl and beaters in the freezer to chill for 30 minutes.

2. Carefully remove the coconut milk from the fridge so as not to disturb the separation of the cream from the water that has taken place. Scoop off the cream that has risen to the top and place in the chilled bowl. Save the thinner coconut water for shakes or other uses.

3. Beat the cream on high until peaks form. If desired, drizzle in honey with the beaters running and mix until incorporated.

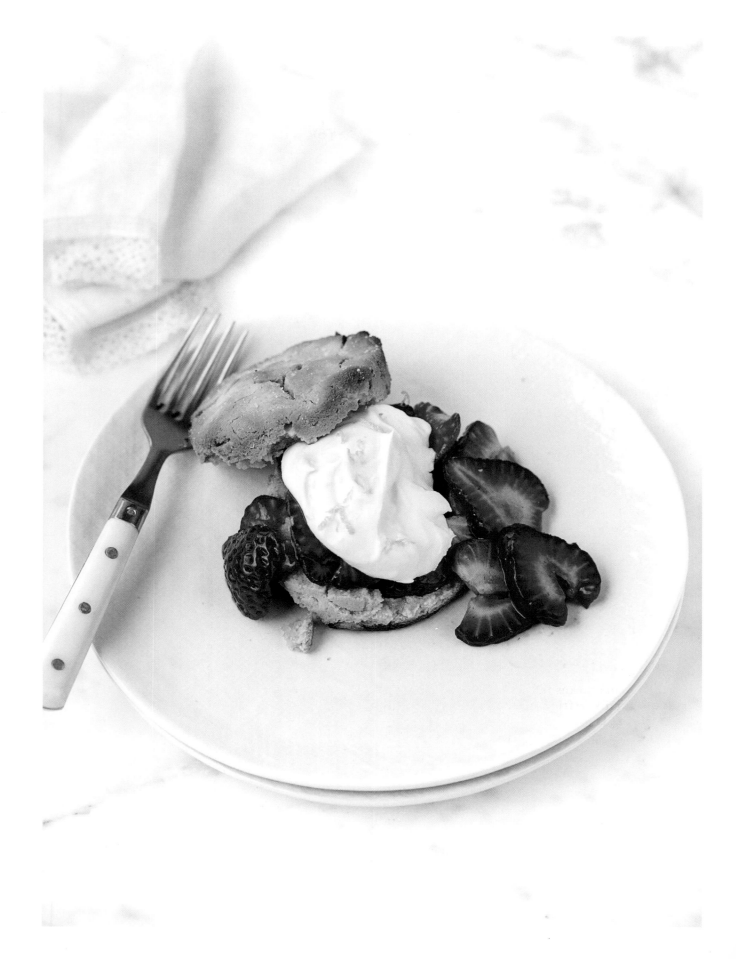

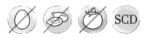

serves: 6

prep time: 10 minutes

cook time: 15 minutes

Stone fruits are roasted with vanilla and tarragon to release their juices into a sweet syrup, making for a delicious and simple dessert. With very little added sweetener, this also makes a great breakfast when topped with Nut-Free Granola (page 60).

## tarragon-vanilla stone fruits

*(30 minutes or less)*

### ingredients

- 2 yellow peaches, pitted and quartered
- 2 plums, pitted and quartered
- 2 nectarines, pitted and quartered
- 2 apricots, pitted and quartered
- 1 tablespoon coconut crystals or honey*
- 3 sprigs fresh tarragon
- 1 vanilla bean, split and seeds scraped
- 2 tablespoons melted coconut oil

FOR SERVING (OPTIONAL)

- dairy-free vanilla ice cream
- sliced almonds

* *Use honey for SCD.*

### method

1. Preheat the oven to 400°F.

2. In a large bowl, toss the fruits, coconut crystals, tarragon, vanilla bean seeds, and coconut oil together. Pour into a large baking dish.

3. Roast the fruit for 10 minutes, stir, and roast for an additional 5 minutes.

4. Serve with dairy-free ice cream and almonds, if desired.

make-ahead tip:

Complete Step 2 and store in the refrigerator for up to 1 day.

tidbits:

There are a lot of recipes for coconut or almond milk–based ice creams online and in cookbooks, including a few in my first book, *Against All Grain*, and my blog of the same name. Store-bought coconut milk–based ice cream can be substituted for homemade for convenience, if desired. Look for brands that are free of artificial sweeteners and carrageenan.

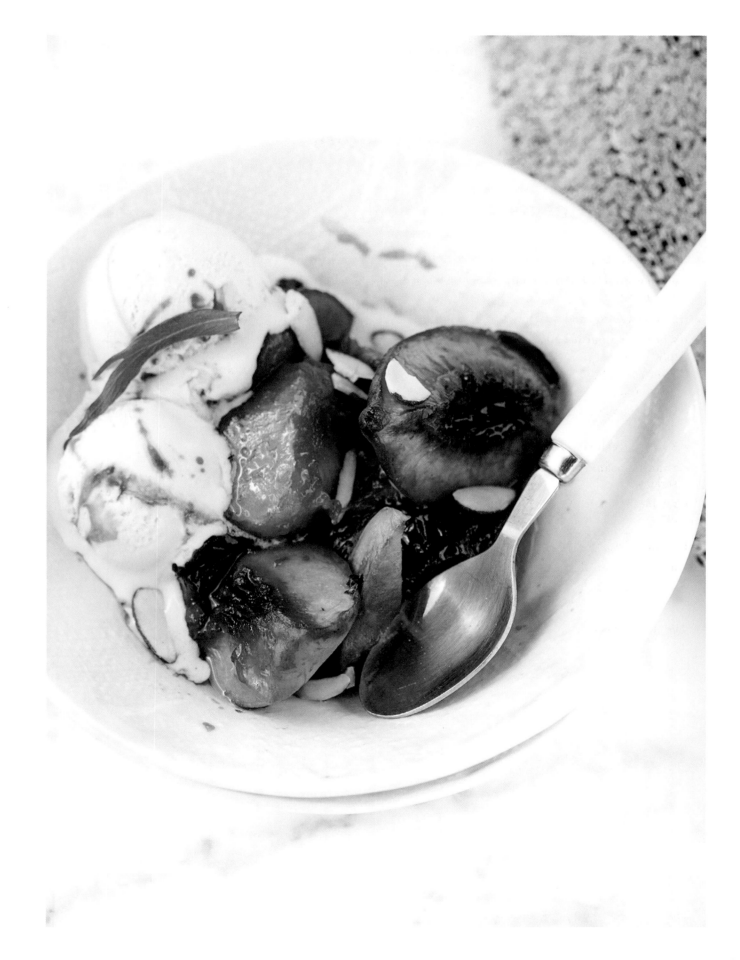

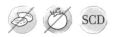

SCD

serves: 6
prep time: 20 minutes
cook time: 30 minutes

These cakes are so light and refreshing. Work your way through the fluffy cake on top to find a creamy lemon custard layer underneath.

# meyer lemon curd cakes

## ingredients

- coconut oil, for greasing the custard cups
- 3 large eggs, separated
- ½ cup honey
- zest of 1 Meyer lemon
- ½ cup fresh Meyer lemon juice
- ¼ cup full-fat coconut milk
- 1 vanilla bean, split and seeds scraped
- 1½ tablespoons coconut flour
- ¼ teaspoon sea salt

## method

1. Preheat the oven to 350°F. Fill a large roasting pan halfway full with boiling water. Lightly grease six 6-ounce custard cups with coconut oil and place them in the pan.

2. Whisk together the egg yolks, honey, lemon zest and juice, coconut milk, and vanilla bean seeds. Whisk in the coconut flour and salt until smooth. Let the batter sit for 10 minutes.

3. Meanwhile, beat the egg whites in the bowl of a stand mixer or with a handheld electric mixer until stiff peaks form.

4. Carefully fold the egg whites into the batter and continue folding until fully incorporated.

5. Divide the batter among the custard cups, then place the pan in the oven and bake for 30 minutes, rotating the pan once, until the tops are golden brown and the centers are set.

6. Remove the cups from the pan. Allow to cool completely before serving.

make-ahead tip:
The cakes can be made up to 3 days in advance and stored, covered, in the refrigerator.

tidbits:
These cakes taste wonderful with fresh berries on top.

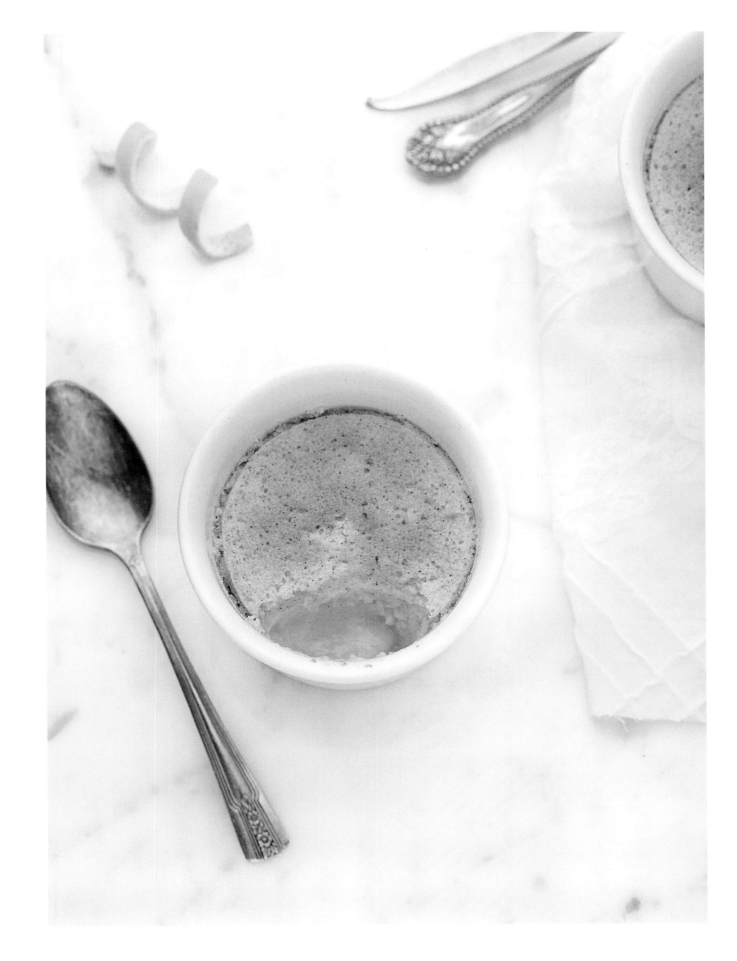

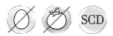

serves: 8

prep time: 20 minutes

cook time: 40 to 50 minutes

An old-fashioned classic gets a grain-free upgrade here, with rhubarb and strawberries baked in a crisp crust of nuts and coconut.

# strawberry-rhubarb crisp

## ingredients

- coconut oil, for greasing the pan
- 2 pounds strawberries, stemmed and halved
- 1 pound rhubarb, cut into 1-inch pieces
- ¼ cup coconut crystals or honey*
- ¼ cup fresh orange juice
- 2 tablespoons arrowroot powder*
- 1 teaspoon vanilla extract

TOPPING

- ½ cup blanched almond flour
- 1½ cups raw pecans
- 6 small dates, pitted
- 1 tablespoon coconut crystals or honey*
- 2 teaspoons ground cinnamon
- ¼ teaspoon sea salt
- 2 tablespoons solid ghee or coconut oil
- ¼ cup unsweetened shredded coconut

*For SCD, use honey and substitute coconut flour for the arrowroot powder.*

## method

1. Preheat the oven to 350°F. Lightly grease a 2- to 3-quart baking dish with coconut oil.

2. Place the strawberries, rhubarb, coconut crystals, orange juice, arrowroot powder, and vanilla in the baking dish and toss to combine.

3. Make the topping: Combine the almond flour, pecans, dates, coconut crystals, cinnamon, and salt in a food processor. Pulse until the mixture resembles small gravel.

4. Add the ghee and pulse until the mixture starts to clump slightly.

5. Stir in the shredded coconut, then spread the topping over the strawberry mixture.

6. Bake for 40 to 50 minutes, until the sides are bubbling and the topping is golden.

7. Allow the crisp to cool for 20 minutes before serving.

make-ahead tip:
The crisp topping can be made in advance and stored in the refrigerator, tightly wrapped, for up to 5 days.

tidbits:
When rhubarb is out of season, substitute an equal amount of peeled tart apples.

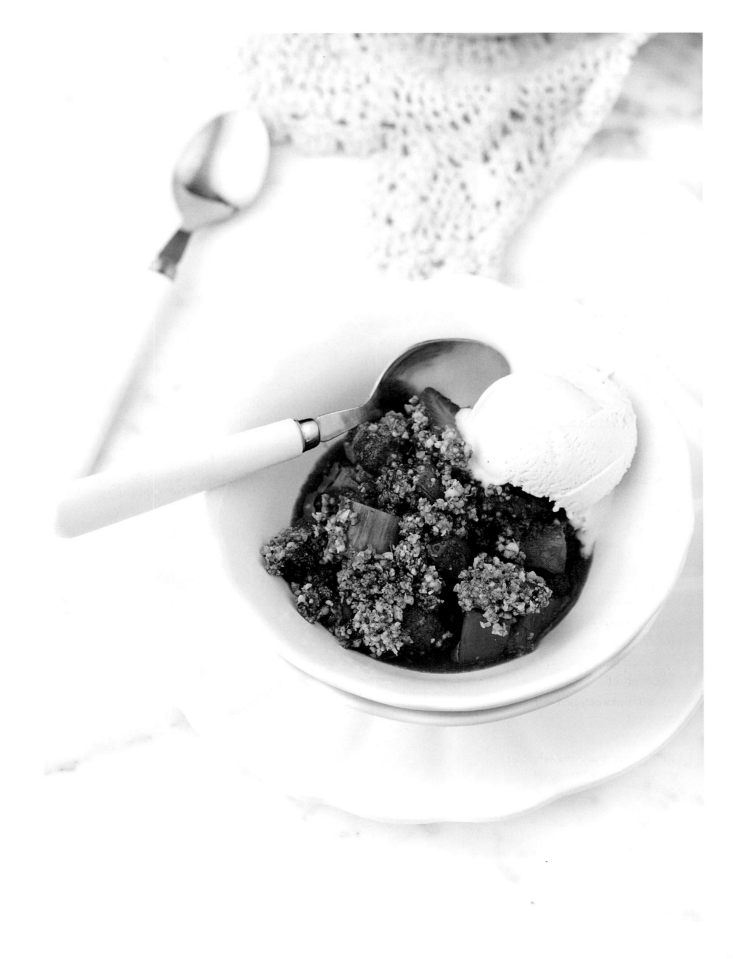

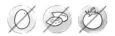

yield: 12 cookies

prep time: 10 minutes

cook time: 12 to 15 minutes

The Real Deal Chocolate Chip Cookies recipe from my book *Against All Grain* continues to be one of the most frequently made and loved, but I wanted to create a nut-free and coconut-free alternative with an egg-free option so that everyone with allergies could enjoy these classic cookies. This version has more of a crunch than the original but has the same gooey, chocolaty center characteristic of a good CCC!

# real deal chocolate chip cookies 2.0

## ingredients

- 1 large egg white or 1 flax-egg (see Tidbits)
- 2 tablespoons melted ghee, coconut oil, or palm shortening
- 1/3 cup coconut crystals
- 3 tablespoons honey
- 1/2 cup tahini
- 1/4 cup arrowroot powder
- 1 1/2 teaspoons vanilla extract
- 1/4 teaspoon sea salt
- 1/4 teaspoon baking soda
- 1/4 cup chopped dark chocolate
- 1/4 cup dairy- and soy-free chocolate chips

## method

1. Preheat the oven to 350°F and line a baking sheet with parchment paper.

2. In the bowl of a stand mixer or using an electric hand mixer, beat the egg white or flax-egg, ghee, coconut crystals, and honey on medium speed until smooth.

3. Add the tahini, arrowroot powder, vanilla, salt, and baking soda and beat on medium speed for 15 seconds, then on high for 15 seconds, until well incorporated. Stir in the chocolate chips.

4. Drop spoonfuls of dough onto the baking sheet, then gently spread the dough a bit with the back of the spoon. The dough can also be left as mounds for less crispy cookies.

5. Bake for 12 to 15 minutes, until golden brown. Allow to cool on a wire rack.

make-ahead tip:
Double (or triple!) the recipe and store the cookies in a sealed container in the freezer for up to 6 months. The cookies are every bit as good straight out of the freezer, or thaw at room temperature for 30 minutes.

tidbits:
This dough is more thin and runny than a traditional cookie dough, so do not be alarmed.

To make the flax-egg: Combine 1 tablespoon finely ground golden flaxseed with 3 tablespoons warm water. Allow the mixture to thicken for 15 minutes in the refrigerator before using. Note that the cookies in the photo were made with an egg white; the flax-egg version looks slightly different.

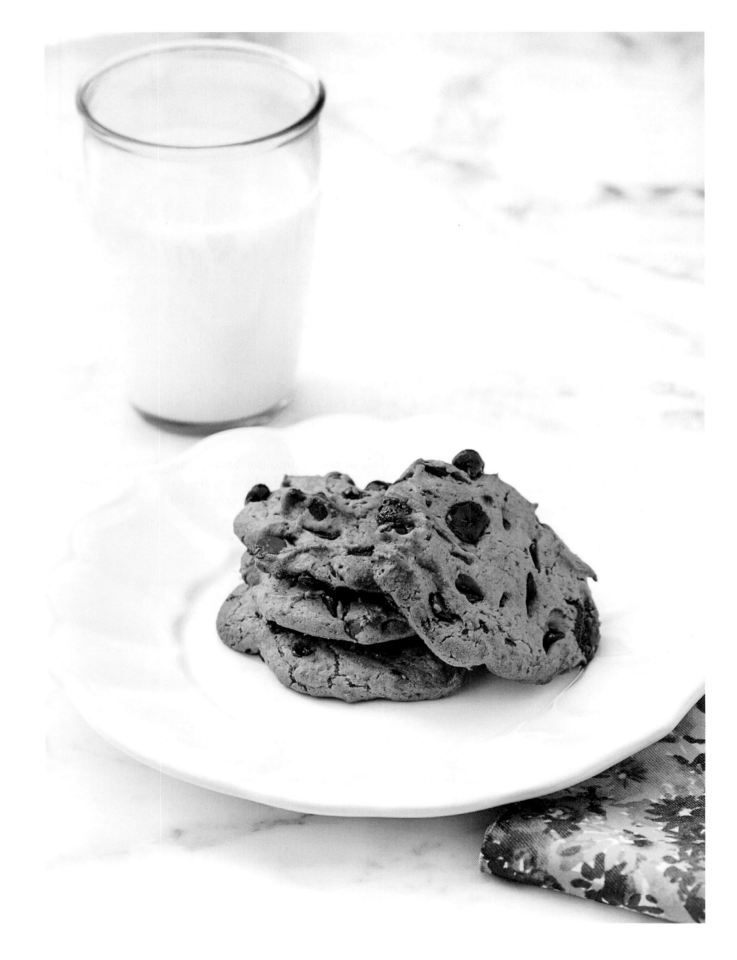

yield: 1 (8-by-11-inch) pan

prep time: 15 minutes

cook time: 35 to 40 minutes

There's a cake brownie, and there's a fudge brownie. I love both, and the nut-free cake brownies from my first book are one of my favorites, but these fudge brownies are so rich and chewy, they may take the cake.

# fudgy brownies

## ingredients

- ½ cup palm shortening or unsalted butter, plus extra for greasing the baking dish
- 8 ounces unsweetened chocolate, chopped
- 1 cup honey
- 1 teaspoon vanilla extract
- ¾ cup coconut crystals
- ½ cup blanched almond flour
- 1 tablespoon coconut flour
- 1 tablespoon arrowroot powder
- ¼ teaspoon sea salt
- ¼ teaspoon baking soda
- 4 large eggs

## method

1. Preheat the oven to 350°F. Lightly grease an 8-by-11-inch baking dish and place a piece of parchment paper in the bottom with flaps on the side for easy release.

2. Bring 1 inch of water in a saucepan to a boil. Reduce to a simmer and place a heatproof glass or metal bowl over the top to create a double boiler. Slowly melt the palm shortening and the chocolate together, stirring constantly. Stir in the honey and vanilla, then remove from heat and let cool.

3. In a food processor, grind the coconut crystals, almond flour, coconut flour, arrowroot powder, salt, and baking soda for 30 seconds.

4. Add the chocolate mixture and blend until smooth. Add 1 egg at a time, blending for 15 seconds between additions to fully combine.

5. Pour the batter into the prepared baking dish and bake for 35 to 40 minutes, until a toothpick comes out clean when inserted into the center. Allow to cool in the pan for 30 minutes, then release the sides with a knife and lift the brownies out of the pan with the parchment paper. Enjoy warm or let cool completely on a wire rack.

tidbits:

Using unsweetened chocolate ensures that it contains no refined sugar, soy, or dairy.

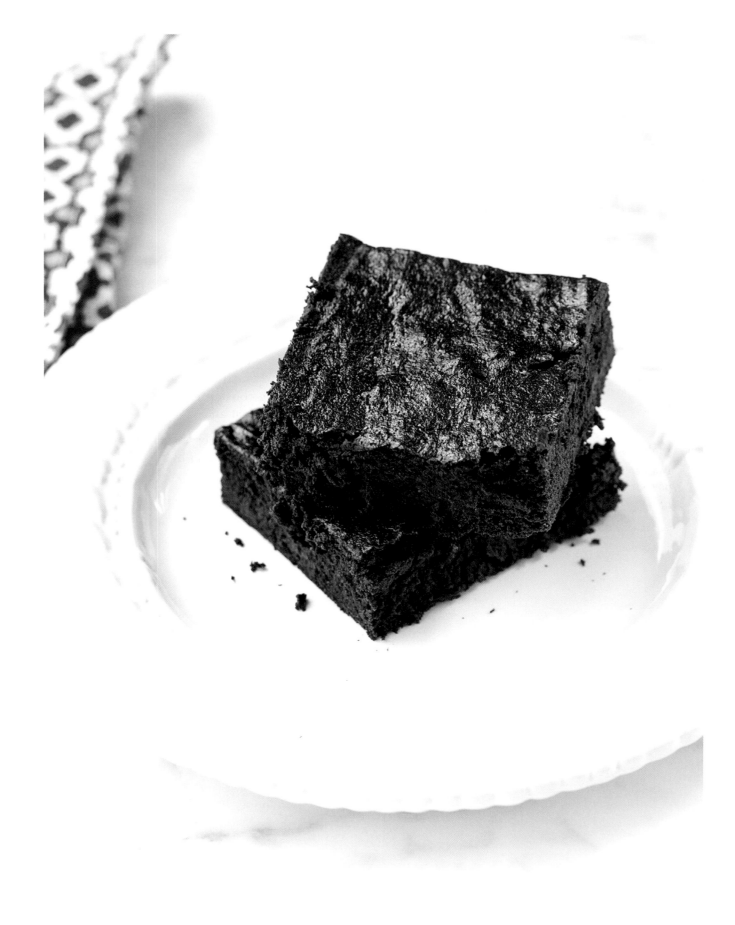

yield: 12 clusters

prep time: 12 minutes, plus
30 minutes refrigeration time

cook time: 8 minutes

I love a quick and easy dessert that doesn't require any baking. These clusters are so rich and dark that just one is satisfying enough!

# dark chocolate almond clusters

## ingredients

- 3½ ounces unsweetened chocolate, chopped
- 2½ teaspoons palm shortening or coconut oil
- 2 tablespoons grade B maple syrup or honey
- ½ teaspoon vanilla extract
- 2 cups almonds, raw or roasted and unsalted
- ¾ teaspoon coarse sea salt

## method

1. Bring 1 inch of water in a saucepan to a boil. Reduce to a simmer and place a heatproof glass or metal bowl over the top to create a double boiler. Slowly melt the chocolate and palm shortening together, stirring constantly. Stir in the maple syrup and vanilla, then remove from the heat and let cool for 10 minutes, until slightly thickened.

2. Line a baking sheet with parchment paper.

3. Stir the almonds into the chocolate, then spoon mounds onto the prepared baking sheet. Sprinkle with the salt. Place in the refrigerator to set for 30 minutes, until hardened. Store any leftover clusters in the refrigerator for up to 1 week.

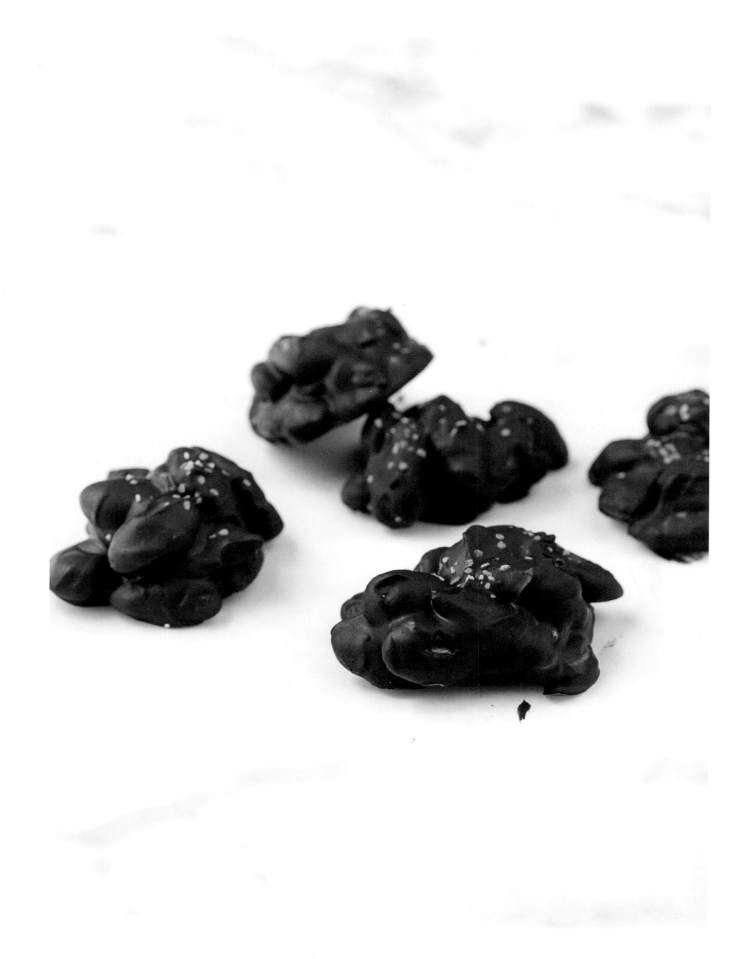

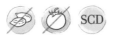

yield: 12 cupcakes

prep time: 15 minutes

cook time: 18 to 20 minutes

These perfectly moist and sweet cupcakes are packed with freshly grated carrots and just the right blend of spices. Eat them on their own, or spread the lemon-coconut frosting on top for an extra-special treat.

# carrot cake cupcakes

## ingredients

### CUPCAKES

- 4 large eggs, at room temperature
- ½ cup honey
- ¼ cup coconut oil, melted
- ½ teaspoon vanilla extract
- ½ cup coconut flour, sifted
- 1 teaspoon baking soda
- ¾ teaspoon ground cinnamon
- ½ teaspoon ground nutmeg
- ¼ teaspoon ground ginger
- ¼ teaspoon sea salt
- 1¼ cups grated carrots
- ¼ cup chopped raisins or chopped pecans (optional)

### FROSTING

- ¼ cup coconut butter
- 3 tablespoons honey
- 1 tablespoon coconut oil, softened
- 1 tablespoon full-fat coconut milk
- ½ teaspoon fresh lemon juice
- ¼ teaspoon apple cider vinegar

### FOR GARNISH:

- ¼ cup unsweetened shredded coconut

## method

1. Preheat the oven to 350°F and line a muffin tin with parchment paper liners.

2. Beat the eggs, honey, coconut oil, and vanilla in the bowl of a stand mixer on medium speed for 30 seconds, or use an electric hand mixer.

3. Add the coconut flour, baking soda, spices, and salt and beat again to combine fully. Fold in the carrots and, if desired, the raisins or pecans.

4. Bake the cupcakes for 18 to 20 minutes, until a toothpick inserted in the center comes out clean. Remove the cupcakes from the pan and allow to cool completely on a wire rack before serving or frosting.

5. For the frosting, combine all of the frosting ingredients in a small food processor or in the bowl of a stand mixer and beat until smooth. If the frosting is too thin, place in the refrigerator for 10 minutes, then beat again. Top with the shredded coconut.

tidbits:
Coconut butter is a spread made from the meat of the coconut and can also be found under the names coconut manna and creamed coconut.

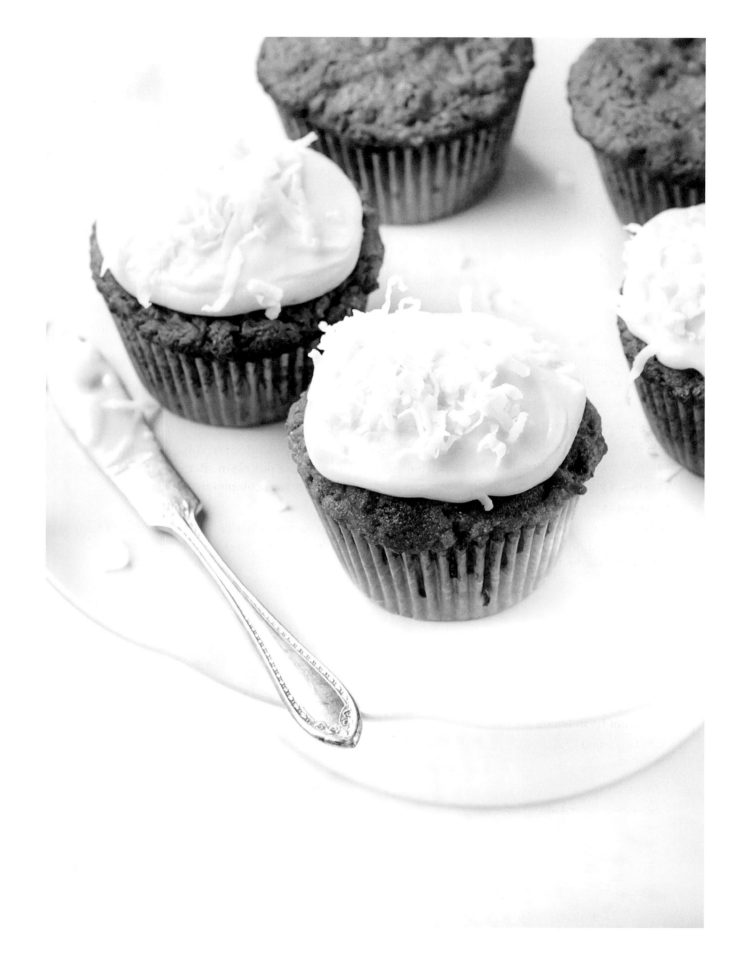

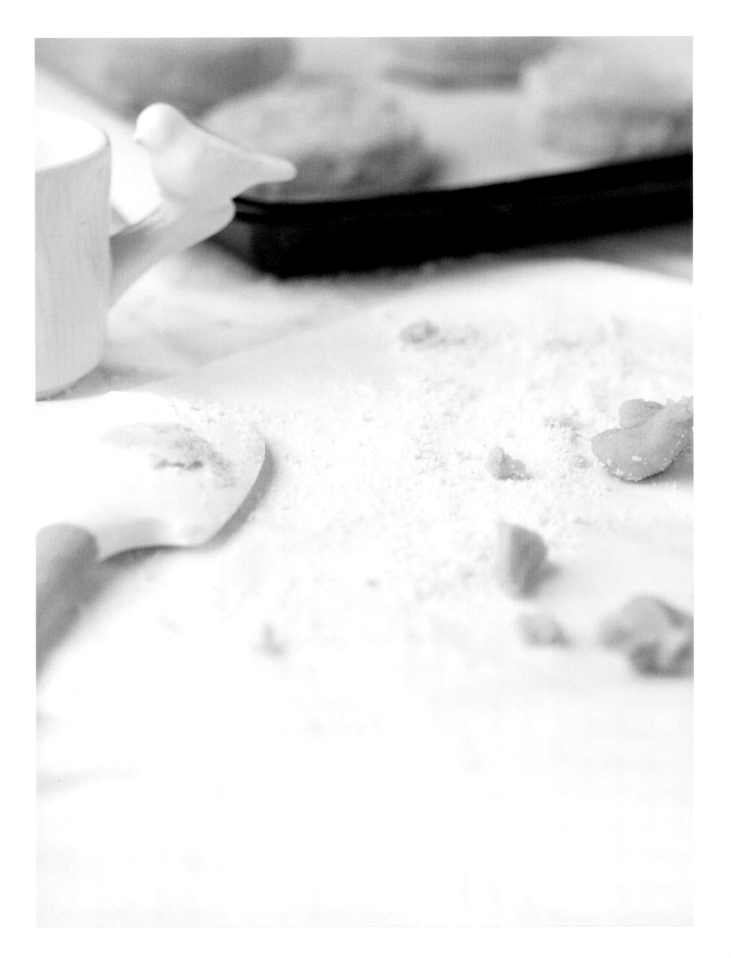

# acknowledgments

To my husband, Ryan, and my son, Asher—your endless support and love bless me beyond measure. I am so grateful to have you both, and you are what I live for daily. My greatest delight comes from making something with you both in mind and seeing you enjoy it at the table.

To our parents—you have rallied for Ryan and me more times than we can count, and we are so thankful for you. Thank you for playing with Asher while I worked, and for always being willing taste-testers and dishwashers.

To Eileen, Maddie, Sydney, and all of the Brooks ladies—thank you for your invaluable contributions to the team and for treating my mission to help heal people through food as your own. Thank you for all of the assistance you provide with the day-to-day tasks of running my life, website, social media sites, and books.

To Erich, Michele, and the Victory Belt team—you seamlessly saw my vision through and created a beautiful book that I am proud to call my own. Thank you for carrying me through to the finish line with this book.

To my fabulous recipe testers—thank you for all of your feedback, constructive criticism, and praise. Because of you, I feel confident releasing these recipes to the masses.

To my incredible community of friends, family, and faithful fans, both near and far— thank you for believing in me, cheering me on, and supporting me always. I create these recipes for you, and I am honored that you receive them so graciously.

And finally, to my sweet daughter, Aila—

You and I wrote this book together. I began it right when I found out
we were expecting you, and finished it during the hardest moments of
my life. For every word, photo, and chapter—you were with me.
You inspired every recipe.

There were times when you refused to allow me to enjoy a type of food
and times when you inspired something completely creative with your
little cravings. This book will forever serve as a celebration of you, a
constant reminder of the inextinguishable light that you provide and
the joy that you bring us. We cannot wait until the day when we can
see your sweet face again and hold you in our arms.

# snacking made simple

While I prefer to make everything homemade for quality and cost reasons, the reality is that I often run out of time like most of you do. I am always stumbling across new products, and the list of grain-free convenience foods is fortunately growing. These are my current favorite quick bites when I'm short on time and need something fast with ingredients I can trust. Most of these snacks, as well as the ingredient brands below, can be ordered in bulk online through my website at www.againstallgrain.com/shop or can be found in health food stores.

VEGGIE-GO'S
*organic all-fruit strips*

INKA
*plantain chips*

STEVE'S PALEO GOODS
*granola, granola bars, beef jerky, condiments*

PRIMAL PACS
*beef jerky*

MADE IN NATURE
*organic dried mango and other fruits*

SEA SNAX
*seaweed snacks*

BAREFOOT PROVISIONS
*paleo snacks and grocery items*

SIMPLE SQUARES
*organic nut and fruit snacks*

ALTER ECO
*dark chocolate*

PALEO TREATS
*macaroons and other treats*

# shopping resources

BOB'S RED MILL
*baking soda, arrowroot powder*

BIONATURAE
*organic tomato puree, tomato paste*

PURE INDIAN FOODS
*organic ghee, clarified butter*

NATURAL VALUE
*full-fat coconut milk (BPA- and guar gum–free)*

SPECTRUM
*organic palm shortening (label will say vegetable shortening)*

DIGESTIVE WELLNESS OR WELLBEE
*superfine blanched almond flour, cashew meal, SCD-legal snacks*

LET'S DO ORGANIC
*coconut flour, shredded coconut, coconut butter*

ARTISANA
*raw nut butters, organic coconut oil*

TROPICAL TRADITIONS
*coconut products, sustainable organic palm shortening, organic grocery items, grass-fed meats*

NAVITAS NATURALS
*organic raw cacao powder*

COCONUT SECRET RAW
*organic vegan coconut aminos, coconut palm sugar*

RED BOAT
*fish sauce*

PURE WRAPS
*coconut wraps*

TESSEMAE'S
*salad dressings and sauces*

US WELLNESS MEATS
*grass-fed and pastured meats*

KEVALA
*organic seed and nut butters*

NUTS.COM
*organic nuts, seeds, baking ingredients, and snacks*

EAT SEED
*organic seeds, seed butters, and seed flours*

# recipe nutritional information

Nutritional values are estimates only and were not verified by a lab or a doctor. The calculations were made using a nutritional calculator. Variations may occur due to product availability, food preparation, ingredient substitutions, origin and freshness of ingredients, etc.

ALMOND MILK
PER 1 CUP SERVING: 40 calories, 3 grams total fat, 0 grams saturated fat, 1 gram protein, 2 grams carbohydrates, 0 grams sugar, 1 gram dietary fiber

ASHER'S "GREEN" SMOOTHIE
PER SERVING: 204 calories, 10.1 grams total fat, 2.1 grams saturated fat, 3 grams protein, 27.8 grams carbohydrates, 11.2 grams sugar, 7.9 grams dietary fiber

AUTUMN BREAKFAST SKILLET
PER SERVING: 358 calories, 16.6 grams total fat, 4.1 grams saturated fat, 37.7 grams protein, 14 grams carbohydrates, 3.5 grams sugar, 2.6 grams dietary fiber

BACON MUSHROOM SCRAMBLE
PER SERVING: 377 calories, 29.1 grams total fat, 8.2 grams saturated fat, 24.2 grams protein, 6.2 grams carbohydrates, 1.7 grams sugar, 3.6 grams dietary fiber

BALSAMIC STEAK PIZZA
PER SERVING: 464 calories, 37.4 grams total fat, 20.6 grams saturated fat, 12.4 grams protein, 15.6 grams carbohydrates, 5.2 grams sugar, 5.7 grams dietary fiber

BANANA CHOCO MALT
PER SERVING: 576 calories, 44.7 grams total fat, 3.6 grams saturated fat, 20.8 grams protein, 33.6 grams carbohydrates, 13.2 grams sugar, 14.3grams dietary fiber

BARBECUE BEEF SHORT RIBS
PER SERVING: 691 calories, 51.4 grams total fat, 24.8 grams saturated fat, 51.2 grams protein, 7.1 grams carbohydrates, 5.6 grams sugar, 0.6 grams dietary fiber

BARBECUE CHICKEN
PER SERVING: 615 calories, 11.6 grams total fat, 3.3 grams saturated fat, 110.5 grams protein, 10.3 grams carbohydrates, 8.4 grams sugar, 1.2 grams dietary fiber

BARBECUE CHICKEN CHOPPED SALAD
PER SERVING: 367 calories, 26.6 grams total fat, 5.5 grams saturated fat, 17.2 grams protein, 19.3 grams carbohydrates, 8.6 grams sugar, 7.9 grams dietary fiber

BARBECUE SALMON WITH GRILLED PEACH SALSA
PER SERVING: 368 calories, 21 grams total fat, 4.1 grams saturated fat, 33.4 grams protein, 11.3 grams carbohydrates, 6.2 grams sugar, 3.9 grams dietary fiber

BARBECUE SAUCE
PER 1 TABLESPOON SERVING: 23.9 calories, 0.1 grams total fat, 0 grams saturated fat, 0.3 grams protein, 6.1 grams carbohydrates, 5.3 grams sugar, 0.3 grams dietary fiber

BARBECUE TRI-TIP WITH GRILLED WATERMELON SALAD
PER SERVING: 492 calories, 22.5 grams total fat, 8.3 grams saturated fat, 54.8 grams protein, 11.5 grams carbohydrates, 7.9 grams sugar, 1.6 grams dietary fiber

BASIC CAULI-RICE
PER SERVING: 27 calories, 1.7 grams total fat, 0.8 grams saturated fat, 0.7 grams protein, 2.6 grams carbohydrates, 1.1 grams sugar, 1 gram dietary fiber

BEEF STROGANOFF
PER SERVING: 251 calories, 16.9 grams total fat, 5.8 grams saturated fat, 13 grams protein, 14.3 grams carbohydrates, 5 grams sugar, 2.9 grams dietary fiber

BEEF TACOS
PER SERVING: 464 calories, 14.4 grams total fat, 5.3 grams saturated fat, 70.5 grams protein, 9.8 grams carbohydrates, 4.7 grams sugar, 2.2 grams dietary fiber

BISCUITS
PER BISCUIT (MAKES 8): 442 calories, 33.2 grams total fat, 7.8 grams saturated fat, 13.1 grams protein, 22.1 grams carbohydrates, 9.1 grams sugar, 7.1 grams dietary fiber

BLT SALAD
PER SERVING: 416 calories, 33.8 grams total fat, 9.5 grams saturated fat, 21.1 grams protein, 8.3 grams carbohydrates, 4.1 grams sugar, 2.2 grams dietary fiber

BLUEBERRY MUFFINS (WITH TOPPING)
PER SERVING: 359 calories, 28.6 grams total fat, 8.2 grams saturated fat, 7.9 grams protein, 20.6 grams carbohydrates, 12.8 grams sugar, 5 grams dietary fiber

BLUEBERRY MUFFINS (WITHOUT TOPPING)
PER SERVING: 235 calories, 15.7 grams total fat, 5.8 grams saturated fat, 5.7 grams protein, 16.9 grams carbohydrates, 10.5 grams sugar, 3.7 grams dietary fiber

BREAKFAST BURRITOS
PER SERVING: 368 calories, 28.5 grams total fat, 8.6 grams saturated fat, 18.1 grams protein, 17.2 grams carbohydrates, 2.5 grams sugar, 7.4 grams dietary fiber

BUFFALO CHICKEN SALAD
PER SERVING: 383 calories, 14.4 grams total fat, 1.7 grams saturated fat, 56.4 grams protein, 7.7 grams carbohydrates, 4.1 grams sugar, 2.5 grams dietary fiber

CALIFORNIA CHICKEN WRAPS
PER SERVING: 595 calories, 35.5 grams total fat, 9.2 grams saturated fat, 48.2 grams protein, 17.6 grams carbohydrates, 4 grams sugar, 5.2 grams dietary fiber

CARROT CAKE CUPCAKES
PER SERVING: 210 calories, 21.3 grams total fat, 10 grams saturated fat, 3.7 grams protein, 21.7 grams carbohydrates, 17.4 grams sugar, 3.1 grams dietary fiber

## CATALAN-STYLE SPINACH
PER SERVING: 102 calories, 5.3 grams total fat, 0.8 grams saturated fat, 5.4 grams protein, 12.5 grams carbohydrates, 5.9 grams sugar, 4.1 grams dietary fiber

## CHAMPAGNE VINAIGRETTE
PER 2-TABLESPOON SERVING: 123.3 calories, 14.1 grams total fat, 2.1 grams saturated fat, 0 grams protein, 0.3 grams carbohydrates, 0 grams sugar, 0 grams dietary fiber

## CHICKEN AND RICE CASSEROLE
PER SERVING: 301 calories, 18.6 grams total fat, 6.5 grams saturated fat, 20.3 grams protein, 16 grams carbohydrates, 3.4 grams sugar, 3.3 grams dietary fiber

## CHICKEN CURRY
PER SERVING: 568 calories, 31.5 grams total fat, 17 grams saturated fat, 54.5 grams protein, 17.8 grams carbohydrates, 6.4 grams sugar, 5 grams dietary fiber

## CHICKEN STOCK
PER 2-TABLESPOON SERVING: 10 calories, 0 grams total fat, 0 grams saturated fat, 2 grams protein, 0 grams carbohydrates, 0 grams sugar, 0 grams dietary fiber

## CHICKEN TIKKA MASALA
PER SERVING: 464 calories, 19.5 grams total fat, 4.9 grams saturated fat, 58.1 grams protein, 12.8 grams carbohydrates, 5 grams sugar, 2.3 grams dietary fiber

## CHICKEN VERDE
PER SERVING: 337 calories, 22.8 grams total fat, 7 grams saturated fat, 30.8 grams protein, 2.5 grams carbohydrates, 0 grams sugar, 0.7 grams dietary fiber

## CHICKEN WALDORF SALAD
PER SERVING: 416 calories, 20.9 grams total fat, 2.7 grams saturated fat, 31.3 grams protein, 30.3 grams carbohydrates, 15.3 grams sugar, 3.3 grams dietary fiber

## CHIPOTLE BARBACOA
PER SERVING: 357 calories, 16.5 grams total fat, 5 grams saturated fat, 45.8 grams protein, 7.8 grams carbohydrates, 3.3 grams sugar, 1.4 grams dietary fiber

## CHORIZO VEGGIE SCRAMBLE
PER SERVING: 320 calories, 22.3 grams total fat, 8.9 grams saturated fat, 19.9 grams protein, 7.5 grams carbohydrates, 6.3 grams sugar, 2.1 grams dietary fiber

## COCONUT, CILANTRO, & LIME CAULI- RICE
PER SERVING: 40 calories, 2.7 grams total fat, 2.4 grams saturated fat, 0.8 grams protein, 3.9 grams carbohydrates, 2.5 grams sugar, 0.9 grams dietary fiber

## CRAB AND ASPARAGUS LINGUINE
PER SERVING: 327 calories, 11.1 grams total fat, 5.4 grams saturated fat, 17.6 grams protein, 34.2 grams carbohydrates, 8.8 grams sugar, 8.9 grams dietary fiber

## CREAMY DILL SALMON
PER SERVING: 235 calories, 10.5 grams total fat, 2.6 grams saturated fat, 32.4 grams protein, 2.8 grams carbohydrates, 1.8 grams sugar, 2.1 grams dietary fiber

## CREAMY MASHED ROOT VEGETABLES
PER SERVING: 185 calories, 8.6 grams total fat, 5.4 grams saturated fat, 2.3 grams protein, 25.2 grams carbohydrates, 8.1 grams sugar, 6.5 grams dietary fiber

## CUBAN PORK PANINI
PER SERVING: 525 calories, 33.5 grams total fat, 8.2 grams saturated fat, 31.5 grams protein, 20.2 grams carbohydrates, 2.1 grams sugar, 5.2 grams dietary fiber

## CUCUMBER MELON MINT COOLER
PER SERVING: 73 calories, 0.2 grams total fat, 0 grams saturated fat, 1 gram protein, 19 grams carbohydrates, 12.4 grams sugar, 2.9 grams dietary fiber

## CUMIN-GARLIC SUMMER SQUASH
PER SERVING: 53 calories, 2.6 grams total fat, 1.4 grams saturated fat, 2.5 grams protein, 7.1 grams carbohydrates, 3.4 grams sugar, 2.2 grams dietary fiber

## DARK CHOCOLATE ALMOND CLUSTERS
PER COOKIE: 150 calories, 13.2 grams total fat, 4.1 grams saturated fat, 4.4 grams protein, 8.1 grams carbohydrates, 2.7 grams sugar, 3.4 grams dietary fiber

## ENCHILADA STUFFED PEPPERS
PER SERVING: 450 calories, 23.4 grams total fat, 9.8 grams saturated fat, 38.4 grams protein, 20.3 grams carbohydrates, 4.8 grams sugar, 4.2 grams dietary fiber

## FISH TACOS (WITHOUT TORTILLAS)
PER SERVING: 143 calories, 4.8 grams total fat, 1.1 grams saturated fat, 16.6 grams protein, 10.6 grams carbohydrates, 6.2 grams sugar, 2.8 grams dietary fiber

## FLUFFY PANCAKES
PER SERVING (2 PANCAKES): 165 calories, 11.9 grams total fat, 3.8 grams saturated fat, 4.2 grams protein, 8.5 grams carbohydrates, 2.7 grams sugar, 3.3 grams dietary fiber

## FREEZER WAFFLES
PER SERVING (2 WAFFLES): 201 calories, 14.4 grams total fat, 4.6 grams saturated fat, 7.3 grams protein, 8.7 grams carbohydrates, 2.9 grams sugar, 3.3 grams dietary fiber

## FUDGY BROWNIES
PER SERVING: 344 calories, 22.3 grams total fat, 12.2 grams saturated fat, 5.8 grams protein, 38.1 grams carbohydrates, 30.6 grams sugar, 3.9 grams dietary fiber

## GARLIC-HERB CHICKEN THIGHS
PER SERVING: 533 calories, 26.8 grams total fat, 7.2 grams saturated fat, 60.6 grams protein, 11.4 grams carbohydrates, 3.5 grams sugar, 4 grams dietary fiber

## GINGER CHICKEN AND BROCCOLI
PER SERVING: 437 calories, 24.7 grams total fat, 7.2 grams saturated fat, 46.1 grams protein, 6.9 grams carbohydrates, 1.3 grams sugar, 2 grams dietary fiber

## GREEK LAMB BURGERS WITH TZATZIKI SAUCE
PER SERVING: 439 calories, 22 grams total fat, 6.3 grams saturated fat, 50.8 grams protein, 6.4 grams carbohydrates, 4.5 grams sugar, 0.7 grams dietary fiber

## Greek Salad Dressing

PER 2-TABLESPOON SERVING: 113.8 calories, 12.7 grams total fat, 1.9 grams saturated fat, 0.2 grams protein, 3.2 grams carbohydrates, 0.3 grams sugar, 0.4 grams dietary fiber

## Greek Salad with Garlic-Oregano Lamb

PER SERVING: 206 calories, 14.8 grams total fat, 3.9 grams saturated fat, 9.4 grams protein, 12.8 grams carbohydrates, 5.9 grams sugar, 2.9 grams dietary fiber

## Green Beans Almondine

PER SERVING: 86 calories, 5.3 grams total fat, 2.2 grams saturated fat, 2.9 grams protein, 9 grams carbohydrates, 1.8 grams sugar, 4.4 grams dietary fiber

## Green Veggie Scramble

PER SERVING: 380 calories, 31.2 grams total fat, 10.7 grams saturated fat, 20.6 grams protein, 6.7 grams carbohydrates, 1.8 grams sugar, 4 grams dietary fiber

## Grilled Greek Summer Squash Salad

PER SERVING: 69 calories, 4.3 grams total fat, 0.6 grams saturated fat, 2.6 grams protein, 7.8 grams carbohydrates, 4.2 grams sugar, 2.6 grams dietary fiber

## Grilled Sesame Asparagus and Scallions

PER SERVING: 37 calories, 1.6 grams total fat, 0 grams saturated fat, 2 grams protein, 4.9 grams carbohydrates, 1.8 grams sugar, 2 grams dietary fiber

## Guacamole

PER ¼-CUP SERVING: 208 calories, 19.6 grams total fat, 4.1 grams saturated fat, 2 grams protein, 9.3 grams carbohydrates, 0.8 grams sugar, 6.8 grams dietary fiber

## Hawaiian Chicken Burgers

PER SERVING: 395 calories, 25.7 grams total fat, 4.8 grams saturated fat, 27.4 grams protein, 16.5 grams carbohydrates, 9.6 grams sugar, 2 grams dietary fiber

## Herb Ranch Dressing

PER 2-TABLESPOON SERVING: 154.1 calories, 16.4 grams total fat, 3.3 grams saturated fat, 0.6 grams protein, 3.3 grams carbohydrates, 1 gram sugar, 0.4 grams dietary fiber

## Island Breeze

PER SERVING: 142 calories, 0.3 grams total fat, 0 grams saturated fat, 1.8 grams protein, 35 grams carbohydrates, 24.2 grams sugar, 5.4 grams dietary fiber

## Italian Wedding Soup

PER SERVING: 230 calories, 9 grams total fat, 2.4 grams saturated fat, 30 grams protein, 6.5 grams carbohydrates, 1.7 grams sugar, 1.9 grams dietary fiber

## Jicama Apple Bacon Slaw

PER SERVING: 110 calories, 4.5 grams total fat, 1.5 grams saturated fat, 4.6 grams protein, 13.4 grams carbohydrates, 7.1 grams sugar, 3.8 grams dietary fiber

## Ketchup

PER 1-TABLESPOON SERVING: 37.7 calories, 0.7 grams total fat, 0.5 grams saturated fat, 0.6 grams protein, 8.6 grams carbohydrates, 5.7 grams sugar, 1.1 grams dietary fiber

## Lemon-Oregano Chicken Kabobs

PER SERVING: 166 calories, 7.1 grams total fat, 1.7 grams saturated fat, 26.4 grams protein, 1.5 grams carbohydrates, 0 grams sugar, 0 grams dietary fiber

## Lemon-Roasted Asparagus and Brussels Sprouts

PER SERVING: 66 calories, 2.5 grams total fat, 1.5 grams saturated fat, 3.9 grams protein, 9.6 grams carbohydrates, 2.8 grams sugar, 4.1 grams dietary fiber

## Maple-Dijon Pork Tenderloin

PER SERVING: 558 calories, 27.5 grams total fat, 7.1 grams saturated fat, 55 grams protein, 21.9 grams carbohydrates, 16.8 grams sugar, 2.4 grams dietary fiber

## Mayonnaise

PER 2-TABLESPOON SERVING: 255.83 calories, 28 grams total fat, 2.3 grams saturated fat, 0.5 grams protein, 4.2 grams carbohydrates, 1.2 grams sugar, 0.2 grams dietary fiber

## Meatloaf Meatballs

PER SERVING: 350 calories, 13.8 grams total fat, 4.7 grams saturated fat, 45.4 grams protein, 7.5 grams carbohydrates, 4.8 grams sugar, 1.7 grams dietary fiber

## Mediterranean Braised Lamb

PER SERVING: 499 calories, 24.6 grams total fat, 7.1 grams saturated fat, 64.1 grams protein, 2.4 grams carbohydrates, 0 grams sugar, 0.8 grams dietary fiber

## Mexican Burgers

PER SERVING: 381 calories, 15.5 grams total fat, 5 grams saturated fat, 54.1 grams protein, 5.4 grams carbohydrates, 1.7 grams sugar, 2.6 grams dietary fiber

## Mexican Chicken Soup

PER SERVING: 240 calories, 6.3 grams total fat, 1.2 grams saturated fat, 25.5 grams protein, 22.2 grams carbohydrates, 8.9 grams sugar, 6 grams dietary fiber

## Meyer Lemon Curd Cakes

PER SERVING: 154 calories, 4.7 grams total fat, 2.9 grams saturated fat, 3.9 grams protein, 25.1 grams carbohydrates, 23.8 grams sugar, 0.8 grams dietary fiber

## Minestrone Soup

PER SERVING: 440 calories, 8.5 grams total fat, 2 grams saturated fat, 72.1 grams protein, 17.3 grams carbohydrates, 6 grams sugar, 4.1 grams dietary fiber

## Mint Chocolate Milkshake

PER SERVING: 347 calories, 28.2 grams total fat, 18.3 grams saturated fat, 2.9 grams protein, 25.7 grams carbohydrates, 19.1 grams sugar, 4.1 grams dietary fiber

## No-Cook Chocolate Pudding

PER SERVING: 223 calories, 9.7 grams total fat, 6.8 grams saturated fat, 5.2 grams protein, 31.5 grams carbohydrates, 14 grams sugar, 8 grams dietary fiber

## Nut-Free Granola

PER 1-CUP SERVING: 786 calories, 47.2 grams total fat, 20.9 grams saturated fat, 17.1 grams protein, 82.4 grams carbohydrates, 65 grams sugar, 11.1 grams dietary fiber

## Overnight Breakfast Casserole
PER SERVING: 380 calories, 27.8 grams total fat, 10 grams saturated fat, 27.3 grams protein, 16.9 grams carbohydrates, 2.5 grams sugar, 2 grams dietary fiber

## Pancake Mix
PER 1/3-CUP SERVING: 222.7 calories, 14.6 grams total fat, 2.3 grams saturated fat, 8 grams protein, 11.6 grams carbohydrates, 0.7 grams sugar, 6.3 grams dietary fiber

## Pepperoni Pizza Pasta
PER SERVING: 373 calories, 25.1 grams total fat, 8.1 grams saturated fat, 21.3 grams protein, 18.4 grams carbohydrates, 7.9 grams sugar, 5 grams dietary fiber

## Peruvian-Style Chicken
PER SERVING: 580 calories, 19.2 grams total fat, 5 grams saturated fat, 67.9 grams protein, 30.5 grams carbohydrates, 3.2 grams sugar, 5.6 grams dietary fiber

## Pesto Orange Roughy
PER SERVING: 138 calories, 6.2 grams total fat, 1.4 grams saturated fat, 20.5 grams protein, 0.4 grams carbohydrates, 0 grams sugar, 0 grams dietary fiber

## Pesto Pasta with Scallops
PER SERVING: 328 calories, 14.1 grams total fat, 2.6 grams saturated fat, 17.5 grams protein, 34.4 grams carbohydrates, 6.4 grams sugar, 5 grams dietary fiber

## Pesto Sauce
PER 1-TABLESPOON SERVING: 54.1 calories, 5.9 grams total fat, 0.7 grams saturated fat, 0.4 grams protein, 0.6 grams carbohydrates, 0.1 grams sugar, 0.1 grams dietary fiber

## Pesto-Stuffed Prosciutto Chicken
PER SERVING: 455 calories, 22.8 grams total fat, 4.9 grams saturated fat, 62.6 grams protein, 4 grams carbohydrates, 1.1 grams sugar, 1.1 grams dietary fiber

## Pineapple Beef Kabobs
PER SERVING: 323 calories, 9.2 grams total fat, 3 grams saturated fat, 37 grams protein, 23.4 grams carbohydrates, 15.4 grams sugar, 4 grams dietary fiber

## Poached Cod with Butternut Squash and Carrot Puree
PER SERVING: 269 calories, 4 grams total fat, 1.4 grams saturated fat, 31 grams protein, 21.2 grams carbohydrates, 4.9 grams sugar, 3.6 grams dietary fiber

## Pork Ragu
PER SERVING: 324 calories, 8 grams total fat, 2.6 grams saturated fat, 20.5 grams protein, 47.9 grams carbohydrates, 9.8 grams sugar, 8 grams dietary fiber

## Pork Stir-Fry
PER SERVING: 241 calories, 8 grams total fat, 2.8 grams saturated fat, 30.3 grams protein, 11.7 grams carbohydrates, 0.6 grams sugar, 3 grams dietary fiber

## Pumpkin Bread
PER 1-CUP SERVING: 246 calories, 14.9 grams total fat, 5.3 grams saturated fat, 4.6 grams protein, 26.4 grams carbohydrates, 14.7 grams sugar, 2.7 grams dietary fiber

## Quiche with Bacon, Zucchini, and Chard
PER SERVING: 307 calories, 22.4 grams total fat, 8.3 grams saturated fat, 22 grams protein, 4.2 grams carbohydrates, 2 grams sugar, 0.9 grams dietary fiber

## Real Deal Chocolate Chip Cookies 2.0
PER COOKIE: 122 calories, 7.5 grams total fat, 2.1 grams saturated fat, 2 grams protein, 12.3 grams carbohydrates, 7.6 grams sugar, 0.9 grams dietary fiber

## Roasted Basil Eggplant
PER SERVING: 95 calories, 7.5 grams total fat, 2.9 grams saturated fat, 1.8 grams protein, 7.1 grams carbohydrates, 2.8 grams sugar, 4.1 grams dietary fiber

## Roasted Beet and Bacon Salad
PER SERVING: 218 calories, 18.5 grams total fat, 3.4 grams saturated fat, 6.9 grams protein, 6.6 grams carbohydrates, 3.4 grams sugar, 2.1 grams dietary fiber

## Roasted Chicken and Vegetable Soup
PER SERVING: 210 calories, 7.3 grams total fat, 5.2 grams saturated fat, 20.4 grams protein, 15.7 grams carbohydrates, 4.8 grams sugar, 3.5 grams dietary fiber

## Roasted Chicken, Butternut, and Apple Salad
PER SERVING: 276 calories, 13 grams total fat, 2.4 grams saturated fat, 26 grams protein, 14.7 grams carbohydrates, 8 grams sugar, 5 grams dietary fiber

## Roasted Chickens with Thyme Gravy
PER SERVING: 305 calories, 19.6 grams total fat, 6.2 grams saturated fat, 20.3 grams protein, 8.9 grams carbohydrates, 3.1 grams sugar, 2.5 grams dietary fiber

## Roasted Squash and Beets in Tahini Sauce
PER SERVING: 162 calories, 9.2 grams total fat, 3.8 grams saturated fat, 3.5 grams protein, 18.8 grams carbohydrates, 8.1 grams sugar, 3.9 grams dietary fiber

## Roasted Tomatillo Salsa
PER 1/4-CUP SERVING: 17 calories, 0 grams total fat, 0.5 grams saturated fat, 0.5 grams protein, 3.1 grams carbohydrates, 0.2 grams sugar, 1 gram dietary fiber

## Roasted Tomato and Shrimp Pasta
PER SERVING: 217 calories, 5.3 grams total fat, 1.8 grams saturated fat, 21.8 grams protein, 25.5 grams carbohydrates, 5.3 grams sugar, 3 grams dietary fiber

## Ropa Vieja
PER SERVING: 372 calories, 17.1 grams total fat, 7.3 grams saturated fat, 43 grams protein, 9 grams carbohydrates, 4.9 grams sugar, 2.6 grams dietary fiber

## Rosemary-Lemon Pork Chops
PER SERVING: 188 calories, 13.1 grams total fat, 5.9 grams saturated fat, 16.1 grams protein, 0.7 grams carbohydrates, 0 grams sugar, 0 grams dietary fiber

## Saffron Cauli-Rice
PER SERVING: 25 calories, 1.1 grams total fat, 0.7 grams saturated fat, 1 gram protein, 3.3 grams carbohydrates, 1.4 grams sugar, 1.2 grams dietary fiber

## SANDWICH ROLLS

PER ROLL (MAKES 10): 227 calories, 13.9 grams total fat, 3.2 grams saturated fat, 9.5 grams protein, 14.5 grams carbohydrates, 0.5 grams sugar, 1.8 grams dietary fiber

## SAUSAGE AND PEPPERS ARRABBIATA

PER SERVING: 453 calories, 11.8 grams total fat, 3.6 grams saturated fat, 26.5 grams protein, 57.2 grams carbohydrates, 5.1 grams sugar, 9.9 grams dietary fiber

## SAUSAGE BREAKFAST SANDWICHES

PER SERVING: 213 calories, 10.5 grams total fat, 3.9 grams saturated fat, 22.5 grams protein, 7 grams carbohydrates, 6.4 grams sugar, 0 grams dietary fiber

## SHIRRED EGGS WITH HAM

PER SERVING: 211 calories, 15 grams total fat, 6.9 grams saturated fat, 16.5 grams protein, 2.3 grams carbohydrates, 0.6 grams sugar, 0.6 grams dietary fiber

## SLOW COOKER BRAISED PORK SHOULDER

PER SERVING: 629 calories, 44.5 grams total fat, 15.1 grams saturated fat, 47.3 grams protein, 7.1 grams carbohydrates, 3.1 grams sugar, 1.6 grams dietary fiber

## SMOKED SALMON AND SWEET POTATO SCRAMBLE

PER SERVING: 485 calories, 35.4 grams total fat, 16.8 grams saturated fat, 25.1 grams protein, 17.5 grams carbohydrates, 1.5 grams sugar, 2.4 grams dietary fiber

## SMOKY ROASTED SWEET POTATOES

PER SERVING: 386 calories, 16.2 grams total fat, 5.3 grams saturated fat, 16.4 grams protein, 43.2 grams carbohydrates, 0.8 grams sugar, 6.5 grams dietary fiber

## SOUTHWESTERN FRITTATA

PER SERVING: 211 calories, 10 grams total fat, 3.3 grams saturated fat, 23.4 grams protein, 6.3 grams carbohydrates, 1.1 grams sugar, 1.3 grams dietary fiber

## SPA SALAD

PER SERVING: 322 calories, 22.5 grams total fat, 3.1 grams saturated fat, 9.9 grams protein, 24.6 grams carbohydrates, 8 grams sugar, 9.9 grams dietary fiber

## SPAGHETTI SAUCE

PER SERVING: 425 calories, 11.7 grams total fat, 3.9 grams saturated fat, 46.6 grams protein, 1.8 grams carbohydrates, 15.6 grams sugar, 3.6 grams dietary fiber

## STRAWBERRY SHORTCAKE

PER SERVING: 446 calories, 30.2 grams total fat, 6.2 grams saturated fat, 13.6 grams protein, 30.4 grams carbohydrates, 14.6 grams sugar, 13.4 grams dietary fiber

## STRAWBERRY-RHUBARB CRISP

PER SERVING: 267 calories, 17 grams total fat, 10.2 grams saturated fat, 4.4 grams protein, 2 grams carbohydrates, 15.9 grams sugar, 14.4 grams dietary fiber

## SUMMER SHRIMP ROLLS

PER SERVING: 177 calories, 8.4 grams total fat, 1.1 grams saturated fat, 19 grams protein, 8.6 grams carbohydrates, 4.5 grams sugar, 3.1 grams dietary fiber

## TARRAGON-VANILLA STONE FRUITS

PER SERVING: 74 calories, 3.8 grams total fat, 3 grams saturated fat, 0.9 grams protein, 10.5 grams carbohydrates, 8.3 grams sugar, 1.8 grams dietary fiber

## THAI BEEF STEW

PER SERVING: 552 calories, 29.6 grams total fat, 18.2 grams saturated fat, 54.4 grams protein, 14.7 grams carbohydrates, 5.6 grams sugar, 3.1 grams dietary fiber

## THYME-ROASTED FENNEL AND CARROTS

PER SERVING: 90 calories, 3.8 grams total fat, 3 grams saturated fat, 1.9 grams protein, 14.1 grams carbohydrates, 3.1 grams sugar, 5 grams dietary fiber

## VEGETABLE BIRYANI

PER SERVING: 199 calories, 8.6 grams total fat, 4.1 grams saturated fat, 5.3 grams protein, 33.1 grams carbohydrates, 3 grams sugar, 12.1 grams dietary fiber

## WARM TACO SALAD WITH CREAMY AVOCADO-CILANTRO VINAIGRETTE

PER SERVING: 295 calories, 10.8 grams total fat, 4.1 grams saturated fat, 6.8 grams protein, 10.9 grams carbohydrates, 4.75 grams sugar, 2.9 grams dietary fiber

## WHITE PORK CHILI

PER SERVING: 258 calories, 13.4 grams total fat, 3.7 grams saturated fat, 6.8 grams protein, 25.3 grams carbohydrates, 4.7 grams sugar, 5.3 grams dietary fiber

## WRAPS

PER WRAP (MAKES 12): 101 calories, 5.4 grams total fat, 2.6 grams saturated fat, 4 grams protein, 7.7 grams carbohydrates, 0 grams sugar, 1.3 grams dietary fiber

# recipe dietary restriction guide

| | Page # | Egg-Free | Nut-Free | Nightshade-Free | SCD |
|---|---|---|---|---|---|
| southwestern frittata | 50 | ✓ | ✓ | | ✓ |
| autumn breakfast skillet | 52 | ✓ | ✓ | ✓ | ✓ |
| breakfast burritos | 54 | | ✓ | | |
| biscuits | 56 | | | ✓ | ✓ |
| quiche with bacon, zucchini, and chard | 58 | | ✓ | | |
| nut-free granola | 60 | ✓ | ✓ | ✓ | |
| overnight breakfast casserole | 62 | | ✓ | | |
| pumpkin bread | 64 | | ✓ | ✓ | |
| freezer waffles | 66 | | ✓ | | |
| fluffy pancakes | 68 | | ✓ | | |
| shirred eggs with ham | 70 | | ✓ | ✓ | ✓ |
| blueberry muffins | 72 | | ✓ | | |
| sausage breakfast sandwiches | 74 | | ✓ | ✓ | ✓ |
| banana choco-malt | 76 | ✓ | | | |
| cucumber melon mint cooler | 76 | ✓ | ✓ | ✓ | ✓ |
| asher's "green" smoothie | 76 | ✓ | ✓ | ✓ | ✓ |
| island breeze | 76 | ✓ | ✓ | ✓ | ✓ |
| chorizo veggie scramble | 78 | | ✓ | | ✓ |
| smoked salmon and sweet potato scramble | 78 | | ✓ | ✓ | |
| green veggie scramble | 79 | | ✓ | ✓ | ✓ |
| bacon mushroom scramble | 79 | | ✓ | ✓ | ✓ |
| italian wedding soup | 82 | | ✓ | | ✓ |
| minestrone soup | 84 | ✓ | ✓ | | ✓ |
| roasted chicken and vegetable soup | 86 | ✓ | ✓ | ✓ | ✓ |
| mexican chicken soup | 88 | ✓ | ✓ | | ✓ |
| white pork chili | 90 | ✓ | | | |
| roasted beet and bacon salad | 92 | ✓ | ✓ | ✓ | ✓ |
| spa salad | 94 | ✓ | ✓ | ✓ | ✓ |
| buffalo chicken salad | 96 | | ✓ | | ✓ |
| roasted chicken, butternut, and apple salad | 98 | ✓ | ✓ | ✓ | ✓ |
| chicken waldorf salad | 100 | | ✓ | ✓ | ✓ |
| warm taco salad with creamy avocado-cilantro vinaigrette | 102 | ✓ | ✓ | | ✓ |
| BLT salad | 104 | | ✓ | | ✓ |
| grilled greek summer squash salad | 106 | ✓ | ✓ | | ✓ |
| barbecue chicken chopped salad | 108 | | ✓ | | ✓ |
| greek salad with garlic-oregano lamb | 110 | | ✓ | | ✓ |
| tuna salad | 112 | | ✓ | ✓ | ✓ |
| peruvian-style chicken | 116 | ✓ | ✓ | | ✓ |
| roasted chickens with thyme gravy | 118 | ✓ | ✓ | | ✓ |
| garlic-herb chicken thighs | 120 | ✓ | ✓ | ✓ | ✓ |
| pesto-stuffed prosciutto chicken | 122 | ✓ | | ✓ | ✓ |
| hawaiian chicken burgers | 124 | ✓ | ✓ | | ✓ |
| ginger chicken and broccoli | 126 | | ✓ | ✓ | |
| california chicken wraps | 128 | | ✓ | ✓ | ✓ |
| chicken tikka masala | 130 | ✓ | | | |
| chicken curry | 132 | ✓ | ✓ | ✓ | ✓ |
| barbecue chicken | 134 | ✓ | ✓ | | |
| chicken verde | 136 | ✓ | | | ✓ |
| lemon-oregano chicken kabobs | 138 | ✓ | ✓ | ✓ | ✓ |
| chicken and rice casserole | 140 | ✓ | | ✓ | ✓ |
| barbecue beef short ribs | 144 | ✓ | | | ✓ |
| beef tacos | 146 | ✓ | ✓ | | ✓ |
| meatloaf meatballs | 148 | | ✓ | | |
| beef stroganoff | 150 | ✓ | | ✓ | ✓ |
| enchilada stuffed peppers | 152 | ✓ | | | ✓ |
| chipotle barbacoa | 154 | ✓ | ✓ | | ✓ |
| sausage and peppers arrabbiata | 156 | ✓ | ✓ | | ✓ |
| ropa vieja | 158 | ✓ | ✓ | | ✓ |
| slow cooker thai beef stew | 160 | ✓ | ✓ | | ✓ |
| pineapple beef kabobs | 162 | ✓ | ✓ | | ✓ |
| mexican burgers | 164 | ✓ | ✓ | | ✓ |
| pepperoni pizza pasta | 166 | ✓ | ✓ | | ✓ |
| shortcut spaghetti with meat sauce | 168 | ✓ | ✓ | | ✓ |
| barbecue tri-tip with grilled watermelon salad | 170 | ✓ | ✓ | | |

breakfast

soups and hearty salads

poultry

beef, pork, and lamb

# recipe dietary restriction guide

| | Page # | Egg-Free | Nut-Free | Nightshade-Free | SCD |
|---|---|---|---|---|---|
| **beef, pork, and lamb** | | | | | |
| balsamic steak pizza | 172 | | ✓ | | |
| rosemary-lemon pork chops | 174 | ✓ | ✓ | ✓ | ✓ |
| mediterranean braised lamb | 176 | ✓ | ✓ | ✓ | ✓ |
| greek lamb burgers with tzatziki sauce | 178 | ✓ | ✓ | ✓ | ✓ |
| maple-dijon pork tenderloin | 180 | ✓ | ✓ | ✓ | ✓ |
| pork stir-fry | 182 | ✓ | ✓ | ✓ | ✓ |
| slow cooker braised pork shoulder | 184 | ✓ | ✓ | ✓ | ✓ |
| pork ragu | 186 | ✓ | ✓ | ✓ | ✓ |
| cuban pork panini | 188 | ✓ | ✓ | ✓ | |
| **seafood** | | | | | |
| fish tacos | 192 | ✓ | ✓ | ✓ | ✓ |
| pesto pasta with scallops | 194 | ✓ | ✓ | ✓ | ✓ |
| summer shrimp rolls | 196 | ✓ | ✓ | ✓ | ✓ |
| creamy dill salmon | 198 | ✓ | ✓ | ✓ | ✓ |
| crab and asparagus linguine | 200 | ✓ | ✓ | ✓ | ✓ |
| poached cod with butternut squash and carrot puree | 202 | ✓ | ✓ | ✓ | ✓ |
| roasted tomato and shrimp pasta | 204 | ✓ | ✓ | | |
| pesto orange roughy | 206 | ✓ | | ✓ | |
| barbecue salmon with grilled peach salsa | 208 | ✓ | | ✓ | |
| **sides** | | | | | |
| green beans almondine | 212 | ✓ | | ✓ | ✓ |
| creamy mashed root vegetables | 214 | ✓ | ✓ | ✓ | |
| vegetable biryani | 216 | ✓ | ✓ | | ✓ |
| basic cauli-rice | 218 | ✓ | ✓ | ✓ | ✓ |
| coconut, cilantro, & lime cauli-rice | 218 | ✓ | ✓ | ✓ | ✓ |
| saffron cauli-rice | 218 | ✓ | ✓ | ✓ | ✓ |
| grilled sesame asparagus and scallions | 220 | ✓ | ✓ | | ✓ |
| smoky roasted sweet potatoes | 222 | ✓ | ✓ | | |
| lemon-roasted asparagus and brussels sprouts | 224 | ✓ | ✓ | ✓ | ✓ |
| catalan-style spinach | 226 | ✓ | ✓ | | |
| thyme-roasted fennel and carrots | 228 | ✓ | ✓ | ✓ | ✓ |
| jicama apple bacon slaw | 230 | ✓ | ✓ | ✓ | |
| roasted basil eggplant | 232 | ✓ | ✓ | | ✓ |
| roasted squash and beets in tahini sauce | 234 | ✓ | ✓ | | ✓ |
| cumin-garlic summer squash | 236 | ✓ | ✓ | ✓ | |
| **basics** | | | | | |
| almond milk | 240 | ✓ | | ✓ | ✓ |
| chicken stock | 242 | ✓ | ✓ | ✓ | ✓ |
| barbecue dry rub | 244 | ✓ | ✓ | | |
| taco seasoning | 244 | ✓ | ✓ | | |
| champagne vinaigrette | 247 | ✓ | ✓ | ✓ | ✓ |
| herb ranch dressing | 247 | | ✓ | ✓ | ✓ |
| greek dressing | 247 | ✓ | ✓ | ✓ | ✓ |
| mayonnaise | 248 | | | ✓ | ✓ |
| barbecue sauce | 250 | ✓ | ✓ | | ✓ |
| hollandaise sauce | 252 | | ✓ | | ✓ |
| ketchup | 254 | ✓ | ✓ | | ✓ |
| pesto sauce | 256 | ✓ | ✓ | ✓ | ✓ |
| mango-pineapple salsa | 258 | ✓ | ✓ | ✓ | ✓ |
| roasted tomatillo salsa | 258 | ✓ | ✓ | | |
| guacamole | 258 | ✓ | ✓ | | |
| pancake mix | 260 | ✓ | | ✓ | |
| wraps | 262 | | ✓ | ✓ | |
| sandwich rolls | 264 | | | ✓ | ✓ |
| **simply sweets** | | | | | |
| no-cook chocolate pudding | 268 | ✓ | ✓ | ✓ | |
| mint chocolate milkshake | 270 | ✓ | | ✓ | |
| strawberry shortcake | 272 | | | ✓ | ✓ |
| whipped coconut cream | 272 | ✓ | ✓ | ✓ | ✓ |
| tarragon-vanilla stone fruits | 274 | ✓ | ✓ | ✓ | ✓ |
| meyer lemon curd cakes | 276 | | ✓ | ✓ | ✓ |
| strawberry-rhubarb crisp | 278 | ✓ | | ✓ | ✓ |
| real deal chocolate chip cookies 2.0 | 280 | ✓ | ✓ | | ✓ |
| fudgy brownies | 282 | | | ✓ | |
| dark chocolate almond clusters | 284 | ✓ | | ✓ | |
| carrot cake cupcakes | 286 | | ✓ | ✓ | ✓ |

# 30-minute, one-pot, and slow cooker recipes

*breakfast*

*soups and hearty salads*

*poultry*

*beef, pork, and lamb*

# 30-minute, one-pot, and slow cooker recipes

# week 1 meal plan shopping list

- ☐ apple, 1 small
- ☐ arrowroot powder, ½ cup
- ☐ avocados, 2
- ☐ baby spinach, 2 pounds
- ☐ bacon, 1½ pounds
- ☐ beef stew meat, 3 pounds
- ☐ broccoli, 1 pound
- ☐ Brussels sprouts, 1 pound
- ☐ butternut squash, 1 (4 pounds)
- ☐ carrots, 2 pounds
- ☐ cauliflower, 1 small head
- ☐ cherry tomatoes, ¾ pound
- ☐ chicken breasts, boneless, skinless, 2 pounds
- ☐ chicken thighs, bone-in, skin-on, 4 pounds
- ☐ cilantro, fresh, ½ small bunch
- ☐ coconut flour, 6 tablespoons

- ☐ coconut milk, full-fat, 2 (13½-ounce) cans
- ☐ coconut oil, 3 tablespoons
- ☐ Dijon mustard, 3 tablespoons
- ☐ dry red wine, ¾ cup
- ☐ eggs, 6 large
- ☐ extra-virgin olive oil, 2 tablespoons (sub ghee)
- ☐ fennel bulb, 1 small
- ☐ fennel seeds, 1½ teaspoons
- ☐ fish sauce, 2 tablespoons
- ☐ garlic, 1 large head
- ☐ ghee, about ½ cup (sub bacon fat or palm shortening)
- ☐ ginger, fresh, ½ ounce
- ☐ honey, 2 tablespoons
- ☐ jicama, ¼ pound
- ☐ lime, 1 medium

- ☐ onions, yellow, 1 medium plus 2 small
- ☐ pancetta, 6 ounces
- ☐ parsley, fresh, ½ ounce
- ☐ pork shoulder roast, boneless, 1 (5 pounds)
- ☐ raisins, 3 tablespoons
- ☐ red wine vinegar, 2 teaspoons
- ☐ romaine lettuce, 3 heads
- ☐ sage, fresh, 2 or 3 sprigs
- ☐ sea salt
- ☐ Thai red curry paste, 4 ounces
- ☐ tomato paste, 4 ounces
- ☐ tomato puree, 8 ounces
- ☐ sea salt and cracked black pepper

## additional items you might need

### If making Almond Milk

- ☐ almonds, raw, 5 ounces
- ☐ date, 1 small

### If making Mayonnaise

- ☐ Dijon mustard, ¼ teaspoon
- ☐ egg, 1 large
- ☐ lemon, ¼ small
- ☐ macadamia nut oil, ¾ cup
- ☐ white vinegar, 1 teaspoon

### If making Herb Ranch Dressing

- ☐ chives, fresh, ½ small bunch
- ☐ coconut milk, full-fat, ½ cup
- ☐ dill, fresh, 2 or 3 sprigs
- ☐ garlic, 2 cloves
- ☐ lemon, ½ small
- ☐ onion powder, ½ teaspoon
- ☐ parsley, fresh, 6 sprigs

### If making Chicken Stock

- ☐ apple cider vinegar, 1 tablespoon
- ☐ bay leaves, 2
- ☐ carrots, 3 large (about ¾ pound)
- ☐ celery, with leaves, 2 stalks
- ☐ chicken bones and gizzards, 1 to 2 pounds
- ☐ garlic, 4 cloves
- ☐ onion, yellow, 1
- ☐ parsley, fresh, 1 bunch

# week 2 meal plan shopping list

- [ ] almonds, sliced, ¼ cup (about 1 ounce)
- [ ] apple cider vinegar, 1 tablespoon
- [ ] apples, Fuji, 2
- [ ] baby spinach, 8 ounces
- [ ] bay leaf, 1
- [ ] bell pepper, red, 1
- [ ] bell pepper, yellow, 1
- [ ] butter lettuce, 1 head
- [ ] butternut squash, 1 (2½ to 3 pounds)
- [ ] carrots, 2 pounds
- [ ] cauliflower, 2 small heads or 1 large head
- [ ] celery, 2 stalks
- [ ] chicken, boneless breasts or thighs, 2½ pounds
- [ ] cilantro, ½ bunch (about 1 ounce)
- [ ] coconut flour, 1½ tablespoons
- [ ] coconut milk, full-fat, 8 ounces
- [ ] coconut oil, 2 tablespoons
- [ ] cumin, ground, 2 teaspoons
- [ ] Dijon mustard, 2 teaspoons
- [ ] dill, fresh, ½ ounce
- [ ] dry white wine, ½ cup (sub Chicken Stock)
- [ ] eggs, 3 large
- [ ] escarole, 1 head
- [ ] flank steak, 2 pounds
- [ ] garlic, 2 large heads
- [ ] ghee, scant 1 cup (sub coconut oil or extra-virgin olive oil)
- [ ] green beans, 1½ pounds
- [ ] ground beef, 3 pounds
- [ ] honey, ⅔ cup (8 ounces)
- [ ] jalapeños, 2
- [ ] lemon, 1
- [ ] lime, 1 large
- [ ] Meyer lemons, 2
- [ ] onions, yellow, 6 medium (about 1¼ pounds)
- [ ] oregano leaves, dried, 2 teaspoons
- [ ] parsley, dried, 2½ teaspoons
- [ ] pimento-stuffed green olives, ¼ cup (about 2 ounces)
- [ ] prosciutto or bacon, 4 ounces
- [ ] roasting chickens, 2 (4 pounds each)

- [ ] rosemary, dried, 1½ teaspoons
- [ ] salmon, wild, skin-on, 6 (6-ounce) fillets
- [ ] sea salt, coarse, 1 tablespoon plus 1½ teaspoons
- [ ] sweet potato, 1 small
- [ ] thyme, fresh, 8 sprigs
- [ ] thyme leaves, dried, 1½ teaspoons
- [ ] tomatoes, diced, 1 (18-ounce) jar
- [ ] tomato puree, 16 ounces
- [ ] vanilla bean, 1

## additional items you might need

For Chicken Stock. If making stock for all recipes in Week 2, you'll need a double batch.

- [ ] apple cider vinegar, 1 tablespoon
- [ ] bay leaves, 2
- [ ] carrots, 3 large (about ¾ pound)
- [ ] celery with leaves, 2 stalks
- [ ] chicken bones and gizzards, 1 to 2 pounds
- [ ] garlic, 4 cloves
- [ ] onion, yellow, 1
- [ ] parsley, fresh, 1 bunch

### If making Champagne Vinaigrette

- [ ] champagne vinegar, 2 teaspoons
- [ ] Dijon mustard, 1 teaspoon
- [ ] lemon, 1 small
- [ ] olive oil, extra-virgin, ¼ cup

### If making Taco Seasoning

- [ ] cayenne pepper, 1 to 3 teaspoons
- [ ] chili powder, 2½ tablespoons
- [ ] coriander, ground, 2 teaspoons
- [ ] cumin, ground, 1 tablespoon plus 1½ teaspoons
- [ ] onion powder, 2 teaspoons
- [ ] oregano, dried ground, 1 tablespoon
- [ ] paprika, 2 teaspoons

### Serving suggestions for Beef Tacos

- [ ] avocado
- [ ] cilantro, fresh
- [ ] Guacamole
- [ ] lime quarters
- [ ] onion, red
- [ ] lettuce leaves, romaine, butter, or iceberg, large
- [ ] tomatoes

### If making Guacamole for Beef Tacos

- [ ] avocados, 4 ripe
- [ ] black pepper, cracked, pinch of
- [ ] cilantro, fresh, 2 sprigs
- [ ] garlic, 2 cloves
- [ ] jalapeño pepper, ½
- [ ] lime, 1
- [ ] onion, red, ½ small
- [ ] tomato, ½ small

### If making Pan-Fried Plantains

- [ ] coconut oil
- [ ] lime juice, fresh
- [ ] plantains, 2 very ripe

# week 3 meal plan shopping list

- ☐ apple cider vinegar, ¼ cup (2 ounces)
- ☐ apricots, 2
- ☐ arrowroot powder, 2 teaspoons
- ☐ baby greens, 6 ounces
- ☐ bell pepper, red, 1
- ☐ butternut squash, 1 pound
- ☐ cashew butter, raw, ½ cup (4½ ounces)
- ☐ chard, 1 small bunch (¾ to 1 pound) (sub spinach or baby kale)
- ☐ chicken legs, bone-in, skin-on, 6 (about 1½ pounds)
- ☐ coconut crystals or honey, 1 tablespoon
- ☐ coconut oil, 2 tablespoons
- ☐ coriander, ground, 1 teaspoon
- ☐ cumin, ground, 1 tablespoon plus 1 teaspoon
- ☐ Dijon mustard, 3 tablespoons
- ☐ English cucumber, 1
- ☐ garlic, 2 large heads
- ☐ ghee, ⅓ cup (sub bacon fat, coconut oil, cold-pressed

- sesame oil, or olive oil, depending on recipe)
- ☐ golden beets, 1 pound
- ☐ green olives, pitted, ¼ cup (about 2 ounces)
- ☐ hard cider or dry white wine, 1 cup (8 ounces)
- ☐ Kalamata olives, pitted, ¼ cup (about 2 ounces)
- ☐ lamb shoulder roast, trimmed and tied, 1 (5 pounds)
- ☐ lemons, 3
- ☐ lime, 1
- ☐ maple syrup, grade B, ⅓ cup (2¾ ounces) (sub honey)
- ☐ nectarines, 2
- ☐ olive oil, extra-virgin, ¾ cup (6 ounces)
- ☐ onion, red, ½
- ☐ onion, yellow, ½ medium
- ☐ oregano leaves, dried, 2 teaspoons
- ☐ oregano leaves, fresh, ¾ ounce (sub 3 tablespoons dried)
- ☐ parsley, fresh, ½ ounce
- ☐ peaches, 2

- ☐ pears, 2
- ☐ pepperoncini
- ☐ pistachios, raw, shelled, 2 tablespoons (½ ounce)
- ☐ plums, 2
- ☐ poblano peppers, 2
- ☐ pork tenderloins, 2 (1½ to 2 pounds each)
- ☐ prosciutto, 4 ounces
- ☐ Roma tomatoes, 2¾ pounds
- ☐ romaine lettuce, 2 heads
- ☐ rosemary, fresh, 1 sprig
- ☐ spaghetti squash, 1 (3 pounds)
- ☐ tahini, 2 tablespoons
- ☐ tarragon, fresh, 8 sprigs
- ☐ vanilla bean, 1
- ☐ white sweet potatoes, 2 medium (about ¾ pound)
- ☐ shrimp, wild-caught, medium, 2 pounds
- ☐ zucchini, 2 medium (about ¾ pound)

## additional items you might need

If making Roasted Tomatillo Salsa

- ☐ garlic, 4 cloves
- ☐ onion, yellow, ½
- ☐ serrano peppers, 2, or 1 medium jalapeño
- ☐ tomatillos, 2 pounds

If using toppings for Tarragon-Vanilla Stone Fruit

- ☐ dairy-free vanilla ice cream
- ☐ sliced almonds

If making Greek Dressing

- ☐ Dijon mustard, ½ teaspoon
- ☐ garlic, 2 cloves
- ☐ lemons, 2
- ☐ olive oil, extra-virgin, ½ cup (4 ounces)
- ☐ oregano, fresh, 2 sprigs
- ☐ red wine vinegar, 2 teaspoons

If making Chicken Broth

- ☐ apple cider vinegar, 1 tablespoon
- ☐ bay leaves, 2
- ☐ carrots, 3 large (about ¾ pound)
- ☐ celery with leaves, 2 stalks
- ☐ chicken bones and gizzards, 1 to 2 pounds
- ☐ garlic, 4 cloves
- ☐ onion, yellow, 1
- ☐ parsley, fresh, 1 bunch

# week 4 meal plan shopping list

- ☐ allspice, ground, ¼ teaspoon
- ☐ asparagus, ¾ pound
- ☐ bacon, ½ pound
- ☐ basil, fresh, ¼ ounce
- ☐ beef, ground, 3 pounds
- ☐ bell pepper, red, 1
- ☐ bell pepper, yellow, 1
- ☐ broccoli, 3 heads
- ☐ carrots, 5 large (about 1¼ pounds)
- ☐ cashew pieces, raw, ½ cup (about 3 ounces)
- ☐ cauliflower, 2 small heads
- ☐ cayenne pepper, ¼ teaspoon
- ☐ chicken breasts or thighs, boneless, skinless, 3 pounds
- ☐ chicken breasts, boneless, skinless, 2 pounds
- ☐ chicken thighs, boneless, skinless, 3 pounds
- ☐ chili powder, 1½ teaspoons
- ☐ cilantro, fresh, ¼ ounce plus more for optional garnish
- ☐ cinnamon, ground, ½ teaspoon
- ☐ coconut aminos, 8½ ounces
- ☐ coconut milk, full-fat, 2 cups (about 1¼ [13½-ounce] cans)

- ☐ coconut oil, expeller-pressed, 3 tablespoons (sub ghee)
- ☐ coriander, ground, 1¾ teaspoons
- ☐ crab meat, fresh, lump and claw, 1½ pounds
- ☐ cremini mushrooms, 8 ounces
- ☐ crushed red pepper, 1¼ teaspoons
- ☐ cumin, ground, 1 tablespoon plus 1 teaspoon
- ☐ dry white wine, such as Sauvignon Blanc, 8 ounces
- ☐ eggs, 2 large
- ☐ fish sauce, 1½ teaspoons
- ☐ garlic, 3 heads
- ☐ ghee, ⅓ cup (sub extra-virgin olive oil or bacon fat, depending on recipe)
- ☐ ginger, fresh, 1½ to 2 ounces
- ☐ Italian seasoning, 1½ teaspoons
- ☐ leek, 1 small
- ☐ lemon, 1
- ☐ nutmeg, ground, ¾ teaspoon
- ☐ onion, red, ½
- ☐ onions, yellow, 3 medium
- ☐ parsley, fresh, 1 bunch

- ☐ parsnips, 2 pounds
- ☐ peas, frozen, ½ cup (about 2½ ounces)
- ☐ Roma tomatoes, 2
- ☐ romaine lettuce, 1 head
- ☐ salsa of choice, ½ cup (4 ounces)
- ☐ scallions, 6
- ☐ sesame oil, cold-pressed, 2 teaspoons
- ☐ sesame oil, toasted (or dark), 2 tablespoons
- ☐ spicy Italian sausage, 2 pounds
- ☐ sweet potatoes, 5 pounds
- ☐ tomatoes, diced, 1 (18-ounce) jar
- ☐ turmeric, ground, 2½ teaspoons
- ☐ yellow squash, 2 medium (about ¾ pound)
- ☐ zucchini, 2 medium (about ¾ pound)

## additional items you might need

### If making Greek Dressing

- ☐ Dijon mustard, ½ teaspoon
- ☐ garlic, 2 cloves
- ☐ lemons, 2 large
- ☐ olive oil, extra-virgin, ½ cup (4 ounces)
- ☐ oregano leaves, fresh, 1 to 2 sprigs
- ☐ red wine vinegar, 2 teaspoons

### If making Guacamole

- ☐ avocados, 4 ripe
- ☐ cilantro, fresh, 2 sprigs
- ☐ garlic, 2 cloves
- ☐ jalapeño pepper, ½
- ☐ lime, 1
- ☐ onion, red, ½ small
- ☐ tomatoes, ½ small

# week 5 meal plan shopping list

- ☐ allspice, ground, ½ teaspoon
- ☐ almonds, sliced, ¼ cup (about 1 ounce)
- ☐ apple cider vinegar, 2 tablespoons
- ☐ apples, 2 small
- ☐ avocados, 2 ripe
- ☐ bacon, 3 ounces
- ☐ basil, fresh, 1½ ounces
- ☐ beef stew meat, 3 pounds
- ☐ broccoli, 1 head
- ☐ Brussels sprouts, 1 pound
- ☐ carrots, 2 pounds
- ☐ cauliflower, 1 small head
- ☐ cayenne pepper, 1 teaspoon
- ☐ chicken breasts, boneless, skinless, ¾ pound*
- ☐ chicken parts, bone-in, skin-on, 5 pounds
- ☐ chicken thighs, bone-in, skin-on, 4 pounds
- ☐ chili powder, ¼ cup plus 1 teaspoon
- ☐ cilantro, fresh, scant 1 ounce
- ☐ coconut aminos, 2 tablespoons
- ☐ coconut crystals, ½ cup (3½ ounces)
- ☐ coconut milk, full-fat, 2 (13½-ounce) cans

- ☐ coconut oil, 3 tablespoons
- ☐ cumin, ground, 2 teaspoons
- ☐ Dijon mustard, 1 tablespoon
- ☐ dill, fresh, ¼ ounce
- ☐ dry mustard, 1 tablespoon
- ☐ eggplant, 1½ pounds
- ☐ fish sauce, 2 tablespoons plus 2 teaspoons
- ☐ garlic, 1 head plus 1 clove
- ☐ garlic powder, 1 tablespoon
- ☐ ghee, scant 1 cup (sub bacon fat or extra-virgin olive oil, depending on the recipe)
- ☐ ginger, fresh, ½ ounce
- ☐ green beans, 1½ pounds
- ☐ honey, ¾ cup plus 1 tablespoon (6½ ounces)
- ☐ jicama, 1 pound
- ☐ lemon, 1
- ☐ limes, 2
- ☐ liquid smoke, natural, 1½ teaspoons
- ☐ olive oil, extra-virgin, ⅓ cup (2¾ ounces)
- ☐ onion powder, ½ teaspoon
- ☐ onion, yellow, 1 medium
- ☐ orange roughy fillets or other mild white fish, 1½ pounds

- ☐ oregano leaves, dried, 2 teaspoons
- ☐ paprika, ¼ cup plus 1 teaspoon
- ☐ parsley, fresh, 3 sprigs
- ☐ pine nuts, ½ cup (2½ ounces)
- ☐ romaine lettuce, 2 heads
- ☐ sage, fresh, 1 sprig
- ☐ scallion, 1
- ☐ sea salt, coarse, 1 tablespoon
- ☐ Thai red curry paste, 4 ounces
- ☐ tomato paste, 5 ounces
- ☐ tomato puree, 16 ounces
- ☐ tomatoes, 2 medium
- ☐ white vinegar, ½ cup plus 1 teaspoon
- ☐ salmon, wild, skin-on, 6 (6-ounce) fillets

\* Needed only if you do not have the equivalent of 2 cups leftover diced cooked chicken on hand.

## additional items you might need

If making Herb Ranch Dressing
- ☐ chives, fresh, ¼ bunch
- ☐ coconut milk, full-fat, ½ cup (4 ounces)
- ☐ dill, fresh, 1 or 2 sprigs
- ☐ garlic, 2 cloves
- ☐ lemon, ½
- ☐ onion powder, ½ teaspoon
- ☐ parsley, fresh, ¼ ounce

If making Chicken Stock
- ☐ apple cider vinegar, 1 tablespoon
- ☐ bay leaves, 2
- ☐ carrots, 3 large (about ¾ pound)
- ☐ celery with leaves, 2 stalks
- ☐ chicken bones and gizzards, 1 to 2 pounds
- ☐ garlic, 4 cloves
- ☐ onion, yellow, 1
- ☐ parsley, fresh, 1 bunch

If making Mayonnaise
- ☐ Dijon mustard, ¼ teaspoon
- ☐ egg, 1 large
- ☐ lemon, ¼
- ☐ macadamia nut oil, ¾ cup (12 ounces)
- ☐ white vinegar, 1 teaspoon

# week 6 meal plan shopping list

- ☐ apple cider vinegar, 2 tablespoons plus ¼ teaspoon
- ☐ beef stock, low-sodium, 8 ounces*
- ☐ beef, ground, 1½ pounds
- ☐ bell peppers, red, 2
- ☐ butternut squash, 1 small (about 2 pounds)
- ☐ carrots, 5 large (about 1¼ pounds)
- ☐ cashew pieces, raw, scant ¾ cup (3 ounces)
- ☐ cashews, raw, ½ cup (about 2½ ounces)
- ☐ cauliflower, 2 small heads
- ☐ cayenne pepper, ¼ teaspoon
- ☐ chicken breast halves, boneless, skinless, 6 (about 3 pounds)
- ☐ chicken thighs, boneless, skinless, 2½ pounds
- ☐ chuck, ground, 2 pounds
- ☐ cilantro, fresh, ¼ ounce
- ☐ coconut aminos, ½ cup (4 ounces)
- ☐ coconut flour, 2 tablespoons (sub almond meal, ½ cup)
- ☐ cod, skinless, 6 (6-ounce) fillets

- ☐ cremini mushrooms, 8 ounces
- ☐ crushed red pepper, ¼ teaspoon
- ☐ Dijon mustard, 1 tablespoon plus 1 teaspoon
- ☐ dry sherry, ½ cup (4 ounces)
- ☐ eggs, 2 large
- ☐ garam masala, 2 tablespoons plus 2½ teaspoons
- ☐ garlic, 1 large head
- ☐ ghee, up to ⅔ cup (sub extra-virgin olive oil)
- ☐ ginger, fresh, ½ to ¾ ounce
- ☐ ginger, ground, 1 teaspoon
- ☐ honey, ¼ cup (3¼ ounces)
- ☐ leek, 1
- ☐ lemon, 1 large
- ☐ olive oil, extra-virgin, 1 teaspoon (sub ghee or coconut oil)
- ☐ onion, red, 1 large
- ☐ onion, yellow, 2 medium
- ☐ oregano, dried, ground, 1 teaspoon
- ☐ paprika, ½ teaspoon
- ☐ parsley, fresh, ½ ounce
- ☐ parsnips, 1½ pounds
- ☐ peas, ¼ cup (about 1¼ ounces)

- ☐ pineapple juice, unsweetened, ⅓ cup (2⅔ ounces)
- ☐ pineapple, 1 small (about 1½ pounds)
- ☐ pork, ground, lean, ½ pound
- ☐ prosciutto, thinly sliced, 12 slices
- ☐ saffron threads, ½ teaspoon
- ☐ sage, fresh, 1 sprig
- ☐ scallion, 1
- ☐ sesame oil, cold-pressed, 1 tablespoon
- ☐ shallot, 1
- ☐ sirloin steak, 2 pounds
- ☐ tomato paste, 2 ounces
- ☐ tomato puree, 4 cups (32 ounces)
- ☐ turnips, 1 pound
- ☐ Vidalia onions, 2 small
- ☐ yellow squash, 2 pounds
- ☐ zucchini or yellow squash, 3 large (about 1½ pounds)

\* If not using homemade.

## additional items you might need

**If making Pesto Sauce**

- ☐ basil, fresh, 2½ ounces
- ☐ garlic, 3 cloves
- ☐ lemon, ½
- ☐ olive oil, extra-virgin, ⅓ cup (5 ounces)
- ☐ pine nuts, ⅓ cup (1⅔ ounces)

**If making Chicken Stock**

- ☐ apple cider vinegar, 1 tablespoon
- ☐ bay leaves, 2
- ☐ carrots, 3 large (about ¾ pound)
- ☐ celery with leaves, 2 stalks
- ☐ chicken bones and gizzards, 1 to 2 pounds
- ☐ garlic, 4 cloves
- ☐ onion, yellow, 1
- ☐ parsley, fresh, 1 bunch

# week 7 meal plan shopping list

- ☐ asparagus, ¾ pound
- ☐ avocados, 2 (plus 2 more for optional garnish)
- ☐ basil, fresh, 1 sprig
- ☐ beef, ground, 3 pounds
- ☐ Brussels sprouts, 1 pound
- ☐ butternut squash, 1 (2 to 3 pounds), or 4 cups cubed
- ☐ carrots, 8 large (2 pounds)
- ☐ cayenne pepper, ½ teaspoon
- ☐ celery, 2 stalks
- ☐ chili powder, ¼ cup
- ☐ cilantro, fresh, ½ to ¾ ounce
- ☐ coconut crystals, ⅓ cup (2¼ ounces)
- ☐ crushed red pepper, ¼ teaspoon
- ☐ cucumber, 1
- ☐ cumin, ground, 2 teaspoons
- ☐ dill, fresh, 1 sprig
- ☐ dry mustard, 1 tablespoon
- ☐ garlic, 3 heads
- ☐ garlic powder, 1 tablespoon
- ☐ ghee, generous ½ cup (sub bacon fat, extra-virgin olive oil, or coconut oil, depending on recipe)
- ☐ lamb, ground, 3 pounds
- ☐ lemons, 2 large or 3 medium
- ☐ lettuce leaves, romaine, butter, or iceberg, several large
- ☐ limes, 3
- ☐ olive oil, extra-virgin, ⅓ cup (2¾ ounces)
- ☐ onions, red, 2 small and 1 medium plus 2 tablespoons diced
- ☐ onions, yellow, 4 medium
- ☐ oregano, fresh, 1 to 2 sprigs
- ☐ oregano leaves, dried, 2 teaspoons
- ☐ paprika, ¼ cup
- ☐ peaches, 2 large ripe
- ☐ poblano peppers, 2 small
- ☐ pork chops, bone-in, thin-cut, 6 (about 6 ounces each)
- ☐ red wine vinegar, 2 teaspoons
- ☐ roasting chickens, 2 (4 pounds each)
- ☐ Roma tomatoes, 6
- ☐ romaine lettuce, 1 head
- ☐ rosemary, fresh, 5 sprigs
- ☐ salmon, wild, skin-on, 2 pounds fillets
- ☐ sea salt, coarse, 2 tablespoons plus ½ teaspoon
- ☐ thyme leaves, fresh, 8 sprigs
- ☐ tomato juice, 1½ cups (12 ounces)
- ☐ tomato puree, 16 ounces
- ☐ tomatoes, 2
- ☐ yellow squash, 2 medium (about ⅔ pound)
- ☐ yogurt, plain, dairy-free, 1½ cups (13½ ounces)
- ☐ zucchini, 2 medium (about ⅔ pound)

## additional items you might need

### If making Chicken Stock

- ☐ apple cider vinegar, 1 tablespoon
- ☐ bay leaves, 2
- ☐ carrots, 3 large (about ¾ pound)
- ☐ celery with leaves, 2 stalks
- ☐ chicken bones and gizzards, 1 to 2 pounds
- ☐ garlic, 4 cloves
- ☐ onion, yellow, 1
- ☐ parsley, fresh, 1 bunch

### If making Greek Dressing

- ☐ Dijon mustard, ½ teaspoon
- ☐ garlic, 2 cloves
- ☐ lemons, 2 large
- ☐ olive oil, extra-virgin, ½ cup (4 ounces)
- ☐ oregano, fresh, 1 or 2 sprigs
- ☐ red wine vinegar, 2 teaspoons

### If making Taco Seasoning

- ☐ cayenne pepper, 1 to 3 teaspoons
- ☐ chili powder, 2½ tablespoons
- ☐ coriander, ground, 2 teaspoons
- ☐ cumin, ground, 1½ tablespoons
- ☐ onion powder, 2 teaspoons
- ☐ oregano, dried, ground, 1 tablespoon
- ☐ paprika, 2 teaspoons

### If making Guacamole

- ☐ avocados, ripe, 4
- ☐ cilantro, fresh, 2 sprigs
- ☐ garlic, 2 cloves
- ☐ jalapeño pepper, ½
- ☐ lime, 1
- ☐ onion, red, ½ small
- ☐ tomato, ½ small

# week 8 meal plan shopping list

- ☐ apple cider vinegar, ¼ cup (2 ounces)
- ☐ arrowroot powder, 1½ cups (7 ounces)
- ☐ arugula, 7 cups (about 7 ounces)
- ☐ asparagus, 1 pound
- ☐ baby bok choy, 1 pound
- ☐ baby greens, 6 cups (about 6 ounces)
- ☐ balsamic vinegar, 1 cup (8 ounces)
- ☐ basil, fresh, ¼ ounce
- ☐ bell peppers, yellow, 2
- ☐ broccolini, 1 pound
- ☐ chicken, ground, dark or white meat, 2 pounds
- ☐ cilantro, fresh, several sprigs
- ☐ coconut aminos, ¼ cup plus 2 teaspoons
- ☐ coconut flour, ½ cup
- ☐ coconut oil, 1 teaspoon
- ☐ cremini mushrooms, 3½ ounces
- ☐ crushed red pepper, ¼ teaspoon
- ☐ cumin, ground, 1 tablespoon

- ☐ Dijon mustard, 3 tablespoons
- ☐ eggs, 3 large
- ☐ garlic, 2 heads
- ☐ ghee, ½ cup plus 2 tablespoons (sub coconut oil or extra-virgin olive oil, depending on the recipe)
- ☐ ginger, fresh, ½ ounce
- ☐ honey, 1 tablespoon plus 2 teaspoons
- ☐ hot sauce, dash of
- ☐ lemons, 2
- ☐ lettuce leaves, romaine or butter lettuce several for serving
- ☐ lime, 1
- ☐ maple syrup, grade B, or honey, ⅓ cup (5 ounces)
- ☐ olive oil, extra-virgin, ½ cup plus 3 tablespoons
- ☐ onion, red, 1
- ☐ onions, sweet, 3 small
- ☐ oregano leaves, dried, ½ teaspoon
- ☐ paprika, 1½ tablespoons
- ☐ pears, 2
- ☐ pineapple rings, fresh, 6

- ☐ pork tenderloins, 2 (1½ to 2 pounds each)
- ☐ prosciutto, 4 ounces
- ☐ pumpkin seeds, roasted and salted, 2 tablespoons
- ☐ radish, 1
- ☐ roasting chicken, 1 (4 pounds) cut into 10 parts
- ☐ scallions, 1 bunch plus 2
- ☐ sesame oil, cold-pressed, 2 tablespoons
- ☐ sesame oil, toasted, 1 tablespoon
- ☐ sesame seeds, ¾ teaspoon
- ☐ snow peas, ½ pound
- ☐ sweet potatoes, 1½ pounds
- ☐ tarragon, fresh, ½ ounce
- ☐ tomato, 1
- ☐ tri-tip roast, 1 (about 2½ to 3 pounds)
- ☐ watermelon, seedless, 2 pounds
- ☐ white vinegar, 2 tablespoons

## additional items you might need

### If making Barbecue Dry Rub

- ☐ cayenne pepper, ½ teaspoon
- ☐ chili powder, ¼ cup (1¼ ounces)
- ☐ coconut crystals, ⅓ cup (2¼ ounces)
- ☐ cumin, ground, 2 teaspoons
- ☐ dry mustard, 1 tablespoon
- ☐ garlic powder, 1 tablespoon
- ☐ oregano leaves, dried, 2 teaspoons
- ☐ paprika, ¼ cup (1 ounce)

### If making Mayonnaise

- ☐ Dijon mustard, ¼ teaspoon
- ☐ egg, 1 large
- ☐ lemon, ½ small
- ☐ macadamia nut oil, ¾ cup (6 ounces)
- ☐ white vinegar, 1 teaspoon

# recipe index

## breakfast

50
southwestern frittata

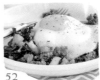
52
autumn breakfast skillet

54
breakfast burritos

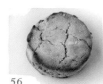
56
biscuits

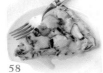
58
quiche with bacon, zucchini, and chard

60
nut-free granola

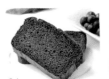
62
overnight breakfast casserole

64
pumpkin bread

66
freezer waffles

68
fluffy pancakes

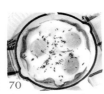
70
shirred eggs with ham

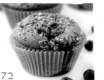
72
blueberry muffins

74
sausage breakfast sandwiches

76
quick smoothies

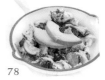
78
simple scrambles

## soups and hearty salads

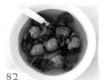
82
italian wedding soup

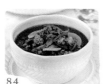
84
minestrone soup

86
roasted chicken and vegetable soup

88
mexican chicken soup

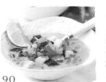
90
white pork chili

92
roasted beet and bacon salad

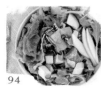
94
spa salad

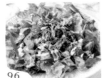
96
buffalo chicken salad

98
roasted chicken, butternut, and apple salad

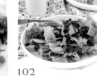
100
chicken waldorf salad

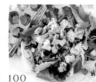
102
warm taco salad with creamy avocado-cilantro vinaigrette

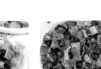

104
BLT salad

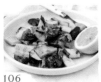
106
grilled greek summer squash salad

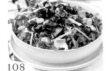
108
barbecue chicken chopped salad

110
greek salad with garlic-oregano lamb

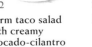
112
tuna salad

# poultry

116 peruvian-style chicken

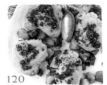
118 roasted chickens with thyme gravy

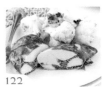
120 garlic-herb chicken thighs

122 pesto-stuffed prosciutto chicken

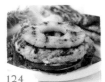
124 hawaiian chicken burgers

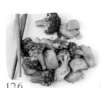
126 ginger chicken and broccoli

128 california chicken wraps

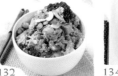
130 chicken tikka masala

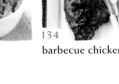
132 chicken curry

134 barbecue chicken

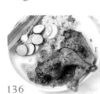
136 chicken verde

138 lemon-oregano chicken kabobs

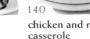
140 chicken and rice casserole

# beef, pork, and lamb

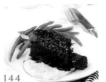
144 barbecue beef short ribs

146 beef tacos

148 meatloaf meatballs

150 beef stroganoff

152 enchilada stuffed peppers

154 chipotle barbacoa

156 sausage and peppers arrabbiata

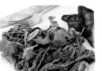
158 ropa vieja

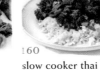
160 slow cooker thai beef stew

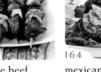
162 pineapple beef kabobs

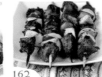
164 mexican burgers

166 pepperoni pizza pasta

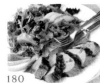
168 shortcut spaghetti with meat sauce

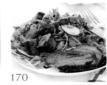
170 barbecue tri-tip with grilled watermelon salad

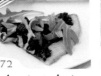
172 balsamic steak pizza

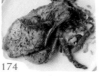
174 rosemary-lemon pork chops

176 mediterranean braised lamb

178 greek lamb burgers with tzatziki sauce

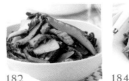
180 maple-dijon pork tenderloin

182 pork stir-fry

184 slow cooker braised pork shoulder

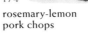
186 pork ragu

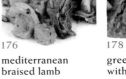
188 cuban pork panini

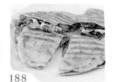

# seafood

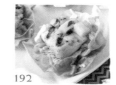
192
fish tacos

194
pesto pasta with scallops

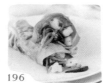
196
summer shrimp rolls

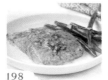
198
creamy dill salmon

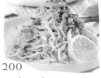
200
crab and asparagus linguine

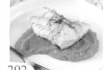
202
poached cod with butternut squash and carrot puree

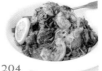
204
roasted tomato and shrimp pasta

206
pesto orange roughy

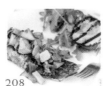
208
barbecue salmon with grilled peach salsa

# sides

212
green beans almondine

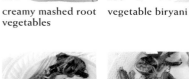
214
creamy mashed root vegetables

216
vegetable biryani

218
cauliflower rice three ways

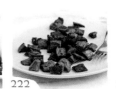
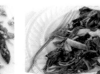
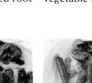

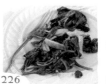

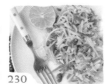

220
grilled sesame asparagus and scallions

222
smoky roasted sweet potatoes

224
lemon-roasted asparagus and brussels sprouts

226
catalan-style spinach

228
thyme-roasted fennel and carrots

230
jicama apple bacon slaw

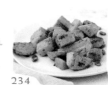
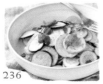

232
roasted basil eggplant

234
roasted squash and beets in tahini sauce

236
cumin-garlic summer squash

# basics

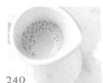

240

almond milk

242

chicken stock

244

barbecue dry rub

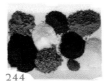

244

taco seasoning

247

champagne
vinaigrette

247

herb ranch dressing

247

greek dressing

248

mayonnaise

250

barbecue sauce

252

hollandaise sauce

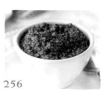

254

ketchup

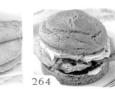

256

pesto sauce

258

mango-pineapple
salsa

258

roasted tomatillo
salsa

258

guacamole

260

pancake mix

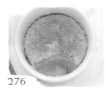

262

wraps

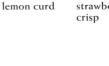

264

sandwich rolls

# simply sweets

268

no-cook chocolate
pudding

270

mint chocolate
milkshake

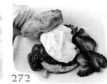

272

strawberry
shortcake

274

tarragon-vanilla
stone fruits

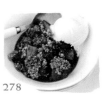

276

meyer lemon curd
cakes

278

strawberry-rhubarb
crisp

280

real deal chocolate
chip cookies 2.0

282

fudgy brownies

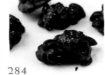

284

dark chocolate
almond clusters

286

carrot cake
cupcakes

danielle walker | 311

# index

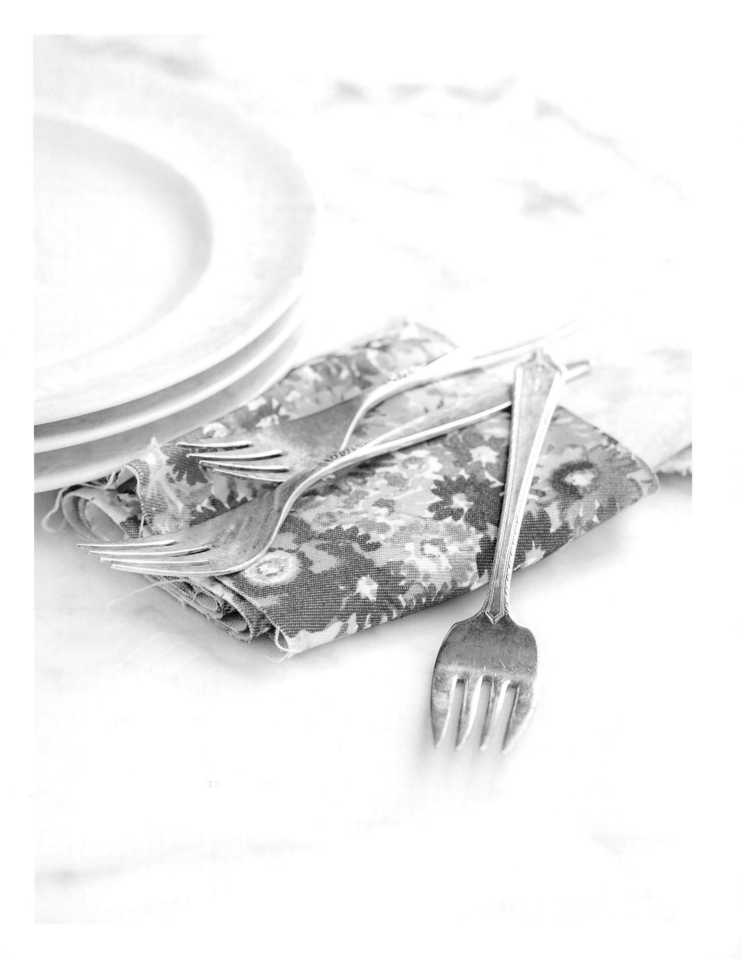

# danielle walker's
## AGAINST all GRAIN

# paleo cheat sheet

## eat

**FISH**
- *low-mercury*
- *wild-caught*

**GRASS-FED, PASTURE-RAISED MEATS**
- *beef*
- *bison*
- *lamb*
- *pork*

**POULTRY**
- *chicken*
- *duck*
- *turkey*
- *eggs*

**VEGETABLES,** including root vegetables

**FRUIT**

**FERMENTED FOODS**

**NUTS and SEEDS**

**HEALTHY OILS and FATS**
- *avocado oil*
- *bacon fat*
- *coconut oil*
- *ghee*
- *grass-fed butter*
- *olive oil*

## avoid

**GRAINS**
- *barley*
- *wheat*
- *rice*
- *corn*
- *rye*
- *cereals*
- *quinoa\**
- *breads*
- *oats*
- *pastas*

*\* While quinoa is not technically a grain, most people find that their bodies process it as such and are not able to tolerate it.*

**LEGUMES**
- *beans*
- *peanuts*
- *lentils*

**WHITE POTATOES**

**REFINED SUGAR**

**DAIRY**

**SOY**

**REFINED, HYDROGENATED VEGETABLE OILS**

**PROCESSED FOODS**

## key words to look for

grass-fed

organic

pasture-raised

wild-caught

natural

local

sustainable

hormone-free

pesticide-free

GMO-free

## words to avoid

agave nectar

cane sugar or juice

carrageenan

corn
*(syrup, starch, dextrose, dextrin)*

xanthan & guar gum

hydrogenated oils

monosodium glutamate (MSG)

potato starch

sucrose, galactose, & maltose

## swap this for that

| PASTA | RICE | WHITE POTATOES | MASHED POTATOES | MILK |
|---|---|---|---|---|
| spiral-sliced sweet potato or squash, spaghetti squash (pages 156, 166, & 204) | Cauliflower Rice (page 218) | white sweet potatoes, celeriac, parsnips | mashed parsnips (page 214) or cauliflower | coconut milk or Almond Milk (page 240) |
| **SUGAR** | **CANOLA OIL** | **FLOURS** | **SOY SAUCE** | **TABLE SALT** |
| raw honey, grade B maple syrup, coconut crystals | coconut oil, ghee | nut flours, coconut flour | coconut aminos | sea salt |

# danielle walker's
## AGAINST all GRAIN

1. apples
2. strawberries
3. grapes
4. celery
5. peaches
6. spinach
7. bell peppers
8. nectarines (imported)
9. cucumbers
10. cherry tomatoes
11. hot peppers
12. kale/collard greens

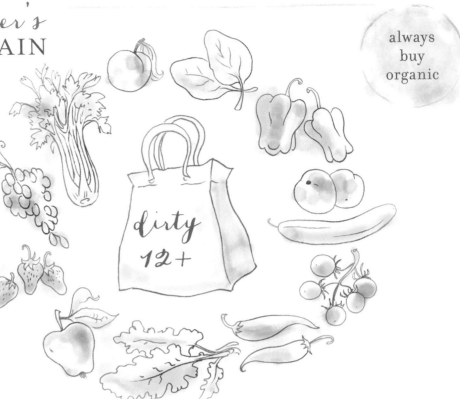

dirty 12+

---

1. avocados
2. pineapple
3. cabbage
4. sweet peas
5. onions
6. asparagus
7. mangoes
8. papaya
9. kiwi
10. eggplant
11. grapefruit
12. cantaloupe
13. cauliflower
14. sweet potatoes
15. mushrooms

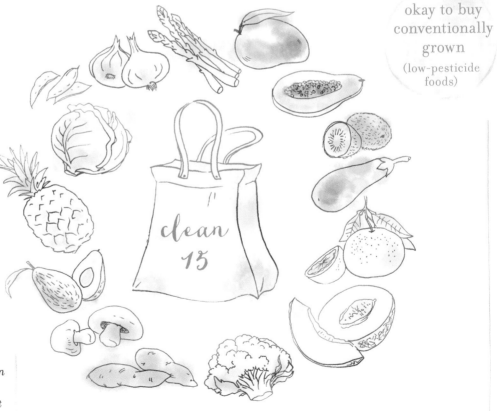

clean 15

*The "Dirty Dozen" and "Clean Fifteen" lists are updated yearly. To check out the latest versions, visit www.ewg.org.*

# grocery list for beginners

For those just starting out on a grain-free diet, the task of identifying hidden ingredients that are often snuck into food and deciphering marketing jargon can be slightly overwhelming. Use this basic grocery list to help guide you through the store when you are looking to buy basics and stock your fridge and pantry. For more specific grocery lists pertaining to the recipes in this book, see the meal plans on pages 44–47 and the meal plan grocery shopping lists on pages 300–307. (Note that this grocery list for beginners is also offered as a tear-out in the back of the book.)

## key words to look for

grass-fed

organic

pasture-raised

wild-caught

natural

local

sustainable

hormone-free

pesticide-free

GMO-free

## hidden ingredients and terms to avoid

agave nectar

cane sugar or juice

carrageenan

corn (*syrup, starch, dextrose, dextrin*)

xanthan & guar gum

hydrogenated oils

monosodium glutamate (MSG)

potato starch

sucrose, galactose, & maltose

## protein

*(100% grass-fed, organic, pasture-raised when possible)*

beef, bison, lamb, elk, etc.

poultry (*turkey, chicken, duck, etc.*)

pork

sausages, bacon, deli meat*

fish and shellfish (*wild-caught and fresh when possible*)

eggs

* *Avoid added sugars, carrageenan, nitrates, sulfates, and MSG.*

## vegetables and fruits

Pick fruits and vegetables that are in season and local if possible. If you cannot afford to purchase all organic produce, consult the Dirty Dozen cheat sheet (page 25) for a guide on which to buy organic. Refer to the Paleo Cheat Sheet (page 35) for which vegetables are off-limits, such as white potatoes and corn.

| | | | |
|---|---|---|---|
| acorn squash | carrots | leeks | spaghetti squash |
| artichoke | cauliflower | lettuce | spinach |
| asparagus | celery | mushrooms | sweet potato |
| beets | cucumbers | parsley | Swiss chard |
| bell peppers | eggplant | parsnips | watercress |
| broccoli and broccoli rabe | fennel | pumpkin | yam |
| Brussels sprouts | herbs | radishes | yellow onion |
| butternut squash | jicama | red onion | zucchini |
| cabbage | kabocha squash | scallions | |
| | kale | shallots | |

apples
apricots
avocados
bananas
berries
cantaloupe
cherries
dates

figs
grapefruit
grapes
lemons
limes
mangoes
nectarines
oranges

papaya
peaches
pears
pineapple
plums
pomegranates
raspberries
strawberries

tangerines
tomatoes
watermelon
dried fruits *(without added sugar or preservatives)*

## fats

avocado oil

butter *(grass-fed and pastured)*

coconut oil *(virgin or expeller-pressed for mild flavor)*

duck fat

bacon fat

extra-virgin olive oil

ghee

lard *(pastured)*

macadamia oil

palm shortening *(sustainable and organic)*

sesame oil *(toasted or cold pressed)*

## baking

almond flour *(blanched)*

arrowroot flour

baking powder *(grain-free)*

baking soda

coconut crystals or palm sugar

coconut flour

cream of tartar

dark chocolate *(85% cacao)*

grade B maple syrup

honey

pure vanilla extract

raw cacao powder or cocoa powder

## nuts, seeds, and nut or seed butters *(purchase raw and organic when possible)*

almonds

cashews

flaxseeds

hazelnuts

macadamia nuts

pecans

pepitas (pumpkin seeds)

pine nuts

pistachios

sesame seeds

sunflower seeds

walnuts

almond butter

cashew butter

sunflower seed butter

tahini

## seasonings

fresh herbs

sea salt *(fine-grained)*

organic spices

## jarred and canned goods

organic tomato products *(no citric acid or sugars added)*
- *diced tomatoes in juices*
- *strained tomatoes or tomato puree*
- *tomato paste*

olives

curry paste

unsweetened applesauce

full-fat coconut milk

capers

pickles

vinegars *(apple cider, pure balsamic, champagne, red wine)*

fish sauce *(Red Boat brand)*

coconut aminos

# 8-week meal plans

I have designed eight weeks' worth of dinners to offer variety at mealtime and minimize waste. I left one day open each week to utilize leftovers or for special occasions and dining out.

Saturdays or Sundays should be used for shopping and prepping. The meals are designed to use the most perishable items first. Freeze fresh fish and poultry the day it is purchased and defrost it in the refrigerator the night before to avoid having to shop twice in a week. I've listed a few desserts if there are items to be used up, such as coconut milk, but of course you are welcome to enjoy dessert whenever you choose!

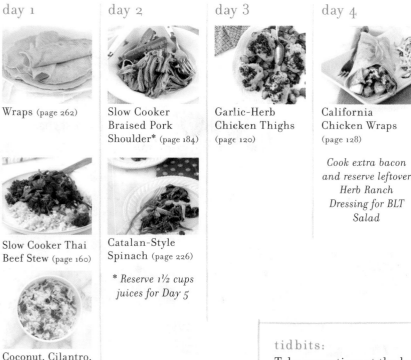

| day 1 | day 2 | day 3 | day 4 | day 5 | day 6 |
|---|---|---|---|---|---|
| Wraps (page 262) | Slow Cooker Braised Pork Shoulder* (page 184) | Garlic-Herb Chicken Thighs (page 120) | California Chicken Wraps (page 128) | Pork Ragu (page 186) | BLT Salad (page 104) |
| Slow Cooker Thai Beef Stew (page 160) | Catalan-Style Spinach (page 226) | | *Cook extra bacon and reserve leftover Herb Ranch Dressing for BLT Salad* | | *Use leftover Herb Ranch Dressing* |
| Coconut, Cilantro, & Lime Cauli-Rice (page 218) | * Reserve 1½ cups juices for Day 5 | | | | |

tidbits:
Take some time at the beginning of each week to prepare the basics you will use throughout the week. Stock your refrigerator with things like Mayonnaise (page 248), Chicken Stock (page 242), Wraps (page 262), and salad dressings (page 247) to make meal preparation quicker during the week.

*danielle walker's*
AGAINST all GRAIN

*week*
1

## week 2

### day 1

Roasted Chickens with Thyme Gravy (page 118)

*Make Chicken Stock (page 242) with leftover bones*

### day 2

Roasted Chicken, Butternut, and Apple Salad (page 98)

### day 3
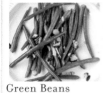

Creamy Dill Salmon (page 198)

Green Beans Almondine (page 212)

Meyer Lemon Curd Cakes (page 276)

*Save remaining coconut milk for Day 6*

### day 4

Roasted Chicken and Vegetable Soup (page 86)

*Add a simple green salad of your choice to complete this meal*

### day 5

Beef Tacos (page 146)

### day 6

Ropa Vieja (page 158)

Coconut, Cilantro, & Lime Cauli-Rice* (page 218)

*\* Double and save half for Week 3*

---

### day 1
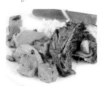

Mediterranean Braised Lamb* (page 176)

Roasted Squash and Beets in Tahini Sauce (page 234)

Roasted Tomatillo Salsa** (page 258)

*\* Save 2 cups braised lamb for Greek Salad*
*\*\* Prepare salsa to use on Days 2 and 6, or buy store-bought*

### day 2

Chicken Verde (page 136)

Coconut, Cilantro, & Lime Cauli-Rice* (page 218)

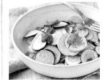

Cumin-Garlic Summer Squash (page 236)

*\* Use leftover from Day 6 of Week 2*

### day 3

Maple-Dijon Pork Tenderloin* (page 180)

Tarragon-Vanilla Stone Fruits (page 274)

*\* Save 2 cups cooked pork tenderloin for White Pork Chili*

### day 4
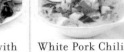

Greek Salad with Garlic-Oregano Lamb (page 110)

### day 5

White Pork Chili (page 90)

*Add a simple green salad of your choice to complete this meal*

### day 6
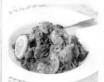

Roasted Tomato and Shrimp Pasta (page 204)

*danielle walker's*
AGAINST *all* GRAIN

## week 3

## week 4

### day 1

Crab and
Asparagus
Linguine
(page 200)

### day 2

Lemon-Oregano
Chicken Kabobs
(page 138)

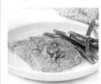
Grilled Greek
Summer Squash
Salad (page 106)

### day 3

Ginger Chicken
and Broccoli
(page 126)

Basic Cauli-Rice*
(page 218)

*Double and use
leftover for Day 5*

### day 4
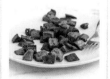
Mexican Burgers
(page 164)

Smoky Roasted
Sweet Potatoes
(page 222)

### day 5

Chicken Curry
(page 132)

Basic Cauli-Rice*
(page 218)

*Use leftover
from Day 3*

### day 6

Sausage and
Peppers
Arrabbiata
(page 156)

---

## week 5

### day 1

Barbecue Chicken
(page 134)

Jicama Apple
Bacon Slaw
(page 230)

Barbecue Sauce
(page 250)

### day 2
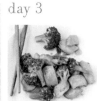
Creamy Dill
Salmon (page 198)

Green Beans
Almondine
(page 212)

### day 3

Barbecue Chicken
Chopped Salad
(page 108)

### day 4

Slow Cooker Thai
Beef Stew
(page 160)

Coconut, Cilantro,
& Lime Cauli-Rice
(page 218)

### day 5
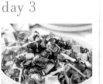
Pesto Orange
Roughy (page 206)

Roasted Basil
Eggplant (page 232)

### day 6

Garlic-Herb
Chicken Thighs
(page 120)

*danielle walker's*
AGAINST all GRAIN

## week 6

**day 1**

Pesto-Stuffed Prosciutto Chicken (page 122)

**day 2**

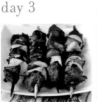

Beef Stroganoff (page 150)

**day 3**

Pineapple Beef Kabobs (page 162)

**day 4**

Poached Cod with Butternut Squash and Carrot Puree (page 202)

**day 5**

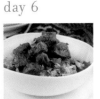

Meatloaf Meatballs (page 148)

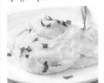

Creamy Mashed Root Vegetables (page 214)

**day 6**

Chicken Tikka Masala (page 130)

Saffron Cauli-Rice (page 219)

---

## week 7

**day 1**

Roasted Chickens with Thyme Gravy (page 118)

*Make Chicken Stock (page 242) with leftover bones*

*Reserve 3 cups of shredded roasted chicken for Mexican Chicken Soup*

**day 2**

Rosemary-Lemon Pork Chops (page 174)

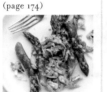

Lemon-Roasted Asparagus and Brussels Sprouts (page 224)

**day 3**

Greek Lamb Burgers (page 178)

Grilled Greek Summer Squash Salad (page 106)

**day 4**

Mexican Chicken Soup (page 88)

*Add a simple green salad of your choice to complete this meal*

**day 5**

Barbecue Salmon with Grilled Peach Salsa (page 208)

**day 6**

Beef Tacos (page 146)

---

## week 8

**day 1**

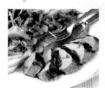

Maple-Dijon Pork Tenderloin (page 180)

*Save 2½ cups cooked pork tenderloin for Pork Stir-Fry on Day 4*

**day 2**

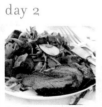

Barbecue Tri-Tip with Grilled Watermelon Salad (page 170)

*Save ¾ cups cooked Tri-Tip for Balsamic Steak Pizza on Day 5*

**day 3**

Peruvian-Style Chicken (page 116)

**day 4**

Pork Stir-Fry (page 182)

**day 5**

Balsamic Steak Pizza (page 172)

**day 6**

Hawaiian Chicken Burgers (page 124)

Grilled Sesame Asparagus and Scallions (page 220)

*danielle walker's*
AGAINST all GRAIN

# week 1 meal plan shopping list

- [ ] apple, 1 small
- [ ] arrowroot powder, ½ cup
- [ ] avocados, 2
- [ ] baby spinach, 2 pounds
- [ ] bacon, 1½ pounds
- [ ] beef stew meat, 3 pounds
- [ ] broccoli, 1 pound
- [ ] Brussels sprouts, 1 pound
- [ ] butternut squash, 1 (4 pounds)
- [ ] carrots, 2 pounds
- [ ] cauliflower, 1 small head
- [ ] cherry tomatoes, ¾ pound
- [ ] chicken breasts, boneless, skinless, 2 pounds
- [ ] chicken thighs, bone-in, skin-on, 4 pounds
- [ ] cilantro, fresh, ½ small bunch
- [ ] coconut flour, 6 tablespoons
- [ ] coconut milk, full-fat, 2 (13½-ounce) cans
- [ ] coconut oil, 3 tablespoons
- [ ] Dijon mustard, 3 tablespoons
- [ ] dry red wine, ¾ cup
- [ ] eggs, 6 large
- [ ] extra-virgin olive oil, 2 tablespoons (sub ghee)
- [ ] fennel bulb, 1 small
- [ ] fennel seeds, 1½ teaspoons
- [ ] fish sauce, 2 tablespoons
- [ ] garlic, 1 large head
- [ ] ghee, about ½ cup (sub bacon fat or palm shortening)
- [ ] ginger, fresh, ½ ounce
- [ ] honey, 2 tablespoons
- [ ] jicama, ¼ pound
- [ ] lime, 1 medium
- [ ] onions, yellow, 1 medium plus 2 small
- [ ] pancetta, 6 ounces
- [ ] parsley, fresh, ½ ounce
- [ ] pork shoulder roast, boneless, 1 (5 pounds)
- [ ] raisins, 3 tablespoons
- [ ] red wine vinegar, 2 teaspoons
- [ ] romaine lettuce, 3 heads
- [ ] sage, fresh, 2 or 3 sprigs
- [ ] sea salt
- [ ] Thai red curry paste, 4 ounces
- [ ] tomato paste, 4 ounces
- [ ] tomato puree, 8 ounces
- [ ] sea salt and cracked black pepper

## additional items you might need

**If making Almond Milk**
- [ ] almonds, raw, 5 ounces
- [ ] date, 1 small

**If making Mayonnaise**
- [ ] Dijon mustard, ¼ teaspoon
- [ ] egg, 1 large
- [ ] lemon, ¼ small
- [ ] macadamia nut oil, ¾ cup
- [ ] white vinegar, 1 teaspoon

**If making Herb Ranch Dressing**
- [ ] chives, fresh, ½ small bunch
- [ ] coconut milk, full-fat, ½ cup
- [ ] dill, fresh, 2 or 3 sprigs
- [ ] garlic, 2 cloves
- [ ] lemon, ½ small
- [ ] onion powder, ½ teaspoon
- [ ] parsley, fresh, 6 sprigs

**If making Chicken Stock**
- [ ] apple cider vinegar, 1 tablespoon
- [ ] bay leaves, 2
- [ ] carrots, 3 large (about ¾ pound)
- [ ] celery, with leaves, 2 stalks
- [ ] chicken bones and gizzards, 1 to 2 pounds
- [ ] garlic, 4 cloves
- [ ] onion, yellow, 1
- [ ] parsley, fresh, 1 bunch

*danielle walker's*
AGAINST *all* GRAIN

# week 2 meal plan shopping list

- [ ] almonds, sliced, ¼ cup (about 1 ounce)
- [ ] apple cider vinegar, 1 tablespoon
- [ ] apples, Fuji, 2
- [ ] baby spinach, 8 ounces
- [ ] bay leaf, 1
- [ ] bell pepper, red, 1
- [ ] bell pepper, yellow, 1
- [ ] butter lettuce, 1 head
- [ ] butternut squash, 1 (2½ to 3 pounds)
- [ ] carrots, 2 pounds
- [ ] cauliflower, 2 small heads or 1 large head
- [ ] celery, 2 stalks
- [ ] chicken, boneless breasts or thighs, 2½ pounds
- [ ] cilantro, ½ bunch (about 1 ounce)
- [ ] coconut flour, 1½ tablespoons
- [ ] coconut milk, full-fat, 8 ounces
- [ ] coconut oil, 2 tablespoons
- [ ] cumin, ground, 2 teaspoons
- [ ] Dijon mustard, 2 teaspoons
- [ ] dill, fresh, ½ ounce
- [ ] dry white wine, ½ cup (sub Chicken Stock)
- [ ] eggs, 3 large
- [ ] escarole, 1 head
- [ ] flank steak, 2 pounds
- [ ] garlic, 2 large heads
- [ ] ghee, scant 1 cup (sub coconut oil or extra-virgin olive oil)
- [ ] green beans, 1½ pounds
- [ ] ground beef, 3 pounds
- [ ] honey, ⅔ cup (8 ounces)
- [ ] jalapeños, 2
- [ ] lemon, 1
- [ ] lime, 1 large
- [ ] Meyer lemons, 2
- [ ] onions, yellow, 6 medium (about 1¼ pounds)
- [ ] oregano leaves, dried, 2 teaspoons
- [ ] parsley, dried, 2½ teaspoons
- [ ] pimento-stuffed green olives, ¼ cup (about 2 ounces)
- [ ] prosciutto or bacon, 4 ounces
- [ ] roasting chickens, 2 (4 pounds each)

- [ ] rosemary, dried, 1½ teaspoons
- [ ] salmon, wild, skin-on, 6 (6-ounce) fillets
- [ ] sea salt, coarse, 1 tablespoon plus 1½ teaspoons
- [ ] sweet potato, 1 small
- [ ] thyme, fresh, 8 sprigs
- [ ] thyme leaves, dried, 1½ teaspoons
- [ ] tomatoes, diced, 1 (18-ounce) jar
- [ ] tomato puree, 16 ounces
- [ ] vanilla bean, 1

## additional items you might need

For Chicken Stock. If making stock for all recipes in Week 2, you'll need a double batch.

- [ ] apple cider vinegar, 1 tablespoon
- [ ] bay leaves, 2
- [ ] carrots, 3 large (about ¾ pound)
- [ ] celery with leaves, 2 stalks
- [ ] chicken bones and gizzards, 1 to 2 pounds
- [ ] garlic, 4 cloves
- [ ] onion, yellow, 1
- [ ] parsley, fresh, 1 bunch

If making Champagne Vinaigrette

- [ ] champagne vinegar, 2 teaspoons
- [ ] Dijon mustard, 1 teaspoon
- [ ] lemon, 1 small
- [ ] olive oil, extra-virgin, ¼ cup

If making Taco Seasoning

- [ ] cayenne pepper, 1 to 3 teaspoons
- [ ] chili powder, 2½ tablespoons
- [ ] coriander, ground, 2 teaspoons
- [ ] cumin, ground, 1 tablespoon plus 1½ teaspoons
- [ ] onion powder, 2 teaspoons
- [ ] oregano, dried ground, 1 tablespoon
- [ ] paprika, 2 teaspoons

Serving suggestions for Beef Tacos

- [ ] avocado
- [ ] cilantro, fresh
- [ ] Guacamole
- [ ] lime quarters
- [ ] onion, red
- [ ] lettuce leaves, romaine, butter, or iceberg, large
- [ ] tomatoes

If making Guacamole for Beef Tacos

- [ ] avocados, 4 ripe
- [ ] black pepper, cracked, pinch of
- [ ] cilantro, fresh, 2 sprigs
- [ ] garlic, 2 cloves
- [ ] jalapeño pepper, ½
- [ ] lime, 1
- [ ] onion, red, ½ small
- [ ] tomato, ½ small

If making Pan-Fried Plantains

- [ ] coconut oil
- [ ] lime juice, fresh
- [ ] plantains, 2 very ripe

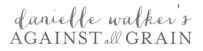

# week 3 meal plan shopping list

- ☐ apple cider vinegar, ¼ cup (2 ounces)
- ☐ apricots, 2
- ☐ arrowroot powder, 2 teaspoons
- ☐ baby greens, 6 ounces
- ☐ bell pepper, red, 1
- ☐ butternut squash, 1 pound
- ☐ cashew butter, raw, ½ cup (4½ ounces)
- ☐ chard, 1 small bunch (¾ to 1 pound) (sub spinach or baby kale)
- ☐ chicken legs, bone-in, skin-on, 6 (about 1½ pounds)
- ☐ coconut crystals or honey, 1 tablespoon
- ☐ coconut oil, 2 tablespoons
- ☐ coriander, ground, 1 teaspoon
- ☐ cumin, ground, 1 tablespoon plus 1 teaspoon
- ☐ Dijon mustard, 3 tablespoons
- ☐ English cucumber, 1
- ☐ garlic, 2 large heads
- ☐ ghee, ⅓ cup (sub bacon fat, coconut oil, cold-pressed

- ☐ sesame oil, or olive oil, depending on recipe)
- ☐ golden beets, 1 pound
- ☐ green olives, pitted, ¼ cup (about 2 ounces)
- ☐ hard cider or dry white wine, 1 cup (8 ounces)
- ☐ Kalamata olives, pitted, ¼ cup (about 2 ounces)
- ☐ lamb shoulder roast, trimmed and tied, 1 (5 pounds)
- ☐ lemons, 3
- ☐ lime, 1
- ☐ maple syrup, grade B, ⅓ cup (2¾ ounces) (sub honey)
- ☐ nectarines, 2
- ☐ olive oil, extra-virgin, ¾ cup (6 ounces)
- ☐ onion, red, ½
- ☐ onion, yellow, ½ medium
- ☐ oregano leaves, dried, 2 teaspoons
- ☐ oregano leaves, fresh, ¾ ounce (sub 3 tablespoons dried)
- ☐ parsley, fresh, ½ ounce
- ☐ peaches, 2

- ☐ pears, 2
- ☐ pepperoncini
- ☐ pistachios, raw, shelled, 2 tablespoons (½ ounce)
- ☐ plums, 2
- ☐ poblano peppers, 2
- ☐ pork tenderloins, 2 (1½ to 2 pounds each)
- ☐ prosciutto, 4 ounces
- ☐ Roma tomatoes, 2¾ pounds
- ☐ romaine lettuce, 2 heads
- ☐ rosemary, fresh, 1 sprig
- ☐ spaghetti squash, 1 (3 pounds)
- ☐ tahini, 2 tablespoons
- ☐ tarragon, fresh, 8 sprigs
- ☐ vanilla bean, 1
- ☐ white sweet potatoes, 2 medium (about ¾ pound)
- ☐ shrimp, wild-caught, medium, 2 pounds
- ☐ zucchini, 2 medium (about ¾ pound)

## additional items you might need

If making Roasted Tomatillo Salsa

- ☐ garlic, 4 cloves
- ☐ onion, yellow, ½
- ☐ serrano peppers, 2, or 1 medium jalapeño
- ☐ tomatillos, 2 pounds

If using toppings for Tarragon-Vanilla Stone Fruit

- ☐ dairy-free vanilla ice cream
- ☐ sliced almonds

If making Greek Dressing

- ☐ Dijon mustard, ½ teaspoon
- ☐ garlic, 2 cloves
- ☐ lemons, 2
- ☐ olive oil, extra-virgin, ½ cup (4 ounces)
- ☐ oregano, fresh, 2 sprigs
- ☐ red wine vinegar, 2 teaspoons

If making Chicken Broth

- ☐ apple cider vinegar, 1 tablespoon
- ☐ bay leaves, 2
- ☐ carrots, 3 large (about ¾ pound)
- ☐ celery with leaves, 2 stalks
- ☐ chicken bones and gizzards, 1 to 2 pounds
- ☐ garlic, 4 cloves
- ☐ onion, yellow, 1
- ☐ parsley, fresh, 1 bunch

# week 4 meal plan shopping list

- ☐ allspice, ground, ¼ teaspoon
- ☐ asparagus, ¾ pound
- ☐ bacon, ½ pound
- ☐ basil, fresh, ¼ ounce
- ☐ beef, ground, 3 pounds
- ☐ bell pepper, red, 1
- ☐ bell pepper, yellow, 1
- ☐ broccoli, 3 heads
- ☐ carrots, 5 large (about 1¼ pounds)
- ☐ cashew pieces, raw, ½ cup (about 3 ounces)
- ☐ cauliflower, 2 small heads
- ☐ cayenne pepper, ¼ teaspoon
- ☐ chicken breasts or thighs, boneless, skinless, 3 pounds
- ☐ chicken breasts, boneless, skinless, 2 pounds
- ☐ chicken thighs, boneless, skinless, 3 pounds
- ☐ chili powder, 1½ teaspoons
- ☐ cilantro, fresh, ¼ ounce plus more for optional garnish
- ☐ cinnamon, ground, ½ teaspoon
- ☐ coconut aminos, 8½ ounces
- ☐ coconut milk, full-fat, 2 cups (about 1¼ [13½-ounce] cans)
- ☐ coconut oil, expeller-pressed, 3 tablespoons (sub ghee)
- ☐ coriander, ground, 1¾ teaspoons
- ☐ crab meat, fresh, lump and claw, 1½ pounds
- ☐ cremini mushrooms, 8 ounces
- ☐ crushed red pepper, 1¼ teaspoons
- ☐ cumin, ground, 1 tablespoon plus 1 teaspoon
- ☐ dry white wine, such as Sauvignon Blanc, 8 ounces
- ☐ eggs, 2 large
- ☐ fish sauce, 1½ teaspoons
- ☐ garlic, 3 heads
- ☐ ghee, ⅓ cup (sub extra-virgin olive oil or bacon fat, depending on recipe)
- ☐ ginger, fresh, 1½ to 2 ounces
- ☐ Italian seasoning, 1½ teaspoons
- ☐ leek, 1 small
- ☐ lemon, 1
- ☐ nutmeg, ground, ¾ teaspoon
- ☐ onion, red, ½
- ☐ onions, yellow, 3 medium
- ☐ parsley, fresh, 1 bunch
- ☐ parsnips, 2 pounds
- ☐ peas, frozen, ½ cup (about 2½ ounces)
- ☐ Roma tomatoes, 2
- ☐ romaine lettuce, 1 head
- ☐ salsa of choice, ½ cup (4 ounces)
- ☐ scallions, 6
- ☐ sesame oil, cold-pressed, 2 teaspoons
- ☐ sesame oil, toasted (or dark), 2 tablespoons
- ☐ spicy Italian sausage, 2 pounds
- ☐ sweet potatoes, 5 pounds
- ☐ tomatoes, diced, 1 (18-ounce) jar
- ☐ turmeric, ground, 2½ teaspoons
- ☐ yellow squash, 2 medium (about ¾ pound)
- ☐ zucchini, 2 medium (about ¾ pound)

## additional items you might need

### If making Greek Dressing

- ☐ Dijon mustard, ½ teaspoon
- ☐ garlic, 2 cloves
- ☐ lemons, 2 large
- ☐ olive oil, extra-virgin, ½ cup (4 ounces)
- ☐ oregano leaves, fresh, 1 to 2 sprigs
- ☐ red wine vinegar, 2 teaspoons

### If making Guacamole

- ☐ avocados, 4 ripe
- ☐ cilantro, fresh, 2 sprigs
- ☐ garlic, 2 cloves
- ☐ jalapeño pepper, ½
- ☐ lime, 1
- ☐ onion, red, ½ small
- ☐ tomatoes, ½ small

*danielle walker's*
AGAINST all GRAIN

# week 5 meal plan shopping list

- ☐ allspice, ground, ½ teaspoon
- ☐ almonds, sliced, ¼ cup (about 1 ounce)
- ☐ apple cider vinegar, 2 tablespoons
- ☐ apples, 2 small
- ☐ avocados, 2 ripe
- ☐ bacon, 3 ounces
- ☐ basil, fresh, 1½ ounces
- ☐ beef stew meat, 3 pounds
- ☐ broccoli, 1 head
- ☐ Brussels sprouts, 1 pound
- ☐ carrots, 2 pounds
- ☐ cauliflower, 1 small head
- ☐ cayenne pepper, 1 teaspoon
- ☐ chicken breasts, boneless, skinless, ¾ pound*
- ☐ chicken parts, bone-in, skin-on, 5 pounds
- ☐ chicken thighs, bone-in, skin-on, 4 pounds
- ☐ chili powder, ¼ cup plus 1 teaspoon
- ☐ cilantro, fresh, scant 1 ounce
- ☐ coconut aminos, 2 tablespoons
- ☐ coconut crystals, ½ cup (3½ ounces)
- ☐ coconut milk, full-fat, 2 (13½-ounce) cans

- ☐ coconut oil, 3 tablespoons
- ☐ cumin, ground, 2 teaspoons
- ☐ Dijon mustard, 1 tablespoon
- ☐ dill, fresh, ¼ ounce
- ☐ dry mustard, 1 tablespoon
- ☐ eggplant, 1½ pounds
- ☐ fish sauce, 2 tablespoons plus 2 teaspoons
- ☐ garlic, 1 head plus 1 clove
- ☐ garlic powder, 1 tablespoon
- ☐ ghee, scant 1 cup (sub bacon fat or extra-virgin olive oil, depending on the recipe)
- ☐ ginger, fresh, ½ ounce
- ☐ green beans, 1½ pounds
- ☐ honey, ¾ cup plus 1 tablespoon (6½ ounces)
- ☐ jicama, 1 pound
- ☐ lemon, 1
- ☐ limes, 2
- ☐ liquid smoke, natural, 1½ teaspoons
- ☐ olive oil, extra-virgin, ⅓ cup (2¾ ounces)
- ☐ onion powder, ½ teaspoon
- ☐ onion, yellow, 1 medium
- ☐ orange roughy fillets or other mild white fish, 1½ pounds

- ☐ oregano leaves, dried, 2 teaspoons
- ☐ paprika, ¼ cup plus 1 teaspoon
- ☐ parsley, fresh, 3 sprigs
- ☐ pine nuts, ½ cup (2½ ounces)
- ☐ romaine lettuce, 2 heads
- ☐ sage, fresh, 1 sprig
- ☐ scallion, 1
- ☐ sea salt, coarse, 1 tablespoon
- ☐ Thai red curry paste, 4 ounces
- ☐ tomato paste, 5 ounces
- ☐ tomato puree, 16 ounces
- ☐ tomatoes, 2 medium
- ☐ white vinegar, ½ cup plus 1 teaspoon
- ☐ salmon, wild, skin-on, 6 (6-ounce) fillets

\* Needed only if you do not have the equivalent of 2 cups leftover diced cooked chicken on hand.

## additional items you might need

### If making Herb Ranch Dressing
- ☐ chives, fresh, ¼ bunch
- ☐ coconut milk, full-fat, ½ cup (4 ounces)
- ☐ dill, fresh, 1 or 2 sprigs
- ☐ garlic, 2 cloves
- ☐ lemon, ½
- ☐ onion powder, ½ teaspoon
- ☐ parsley, fresh, ¼ ounce

### If making Chicken Stock
- ☐ apple cider vinegar, 1 tablespoon
- ☐ bay leaves, 2
- ☐ carrots, 3 large (about ¾ pound)
- ☐ celery with leaves, 2 stalks
- ☐ chicken bones and gizzards, 1 to 2 pounds
- ☐ garlic, 4 cloves
- ☐ onion, yellow, 1
- ☐ parsley, fresh, 1 bunch

### If making Mayonnaise
- ☐ Dijon mustard, ¼ teaspoon
- ☐ egg, 1 large
- ☐ lemon, ¼
- ☐ macadamia nut oil, ¾ cup (12 ounces)
- ☐ white vinegar, 1 teaspoon

# week 6 meal plan shopping list

- ☐ apple cider vinegar, 2 tablespoons plus ¼ teaspoon
- ☐ beef stock, low-sodium, 8 ounces*
- ☐ beef, ground, 1½ pounds
- ☐ bell peppers, red, 2
- ☐ butternut squash, 1 small (about 2 pounds)
- ☐ carrots, 5 large (about 1¼ pounds)
- ☐ cashew pieces, raw, scant ¾ cup (3 ounces)
- ☐ cashews, raw, ½ cup (about 2½ ounces)
- ☐ cauliflower, 2 small heads
- ☐ cayenne pepper, ¼ teaspoon
- ☐ chicken breast halves, boneless, skinless, 6 (about 3 pounds)
- ☐ chicken thighs, boneless, skinless, 2½ pounds
- ☐ chuck, ground, 2 pounds
- ☐ cilantro, fresh, ¼ ounce
- ☐ coconut aminos, ½ cup (4 ounces)
- ☐ coconut flour, 2 tablespoons (sub almond meal, ½ cup)
- ☐ cod, skinless, 6 (6-ounce) fillets

- ☐ cremini mushrooms, 8 ounces
- ☐ crushed red pepper, ¼ teaspoon
- ☐ Dijon mustard, 1 tablespoon plus 1 teaspoon
- ☐ dry sherry, ½ cup (4 ounces)
- ☐ eggs, 2 large
- ☐ garam masala, 2 tablespoons plus 2½ teaspoons
- ☐ garlic, 1 large head
- ☐ ghee, up to ⅔ cup (sub extra-virgin olive oil)
- ☐ ginger, fresh, ½ to ¾ ounce
- ☐ ginger, ground, 1 teaspoon
- ☐ honey, ¼ cup (3¼ ounces)
- ☐ leek, 1
- ☐ lemon, 1 large
- ☐ olive oil, extra-virgin, 1 teaspoon (sub ghee or coconut oil)
- ☐ onion, red, 1 large
- ☐ onion, yellow, 2 medium
- ☐ oregano, dried, ground, 1 teaspoon
- ☐ paprika, ½ teaspoon
- ☐ parsley, fresh, ½ ounce
- ☐ parsnips, 1½ pounds
- ☐ peas, ¼ cup (about 1¼ ounces)

- ☐ pineapple juice, unsweetened, ⅓ cup (2⅔ ounces)
- ☐ pineapple, 1 small (about 1½ pounds)
- ☐ pork, ground, lean, ½ pound
- ☐ prosciutto, thinly sliced, 12 slices
- ☐ saffron threads, ½ teaspoon
- ☐ sage, fresh, 1 sprig
- ☐ scallion, 1
- ☐ sesame oil, cold-pressed, 1 tablespoon
- ☐ shallot, 1
- ☐ sirloin steak, 2 pounds
- ☐ tomato paste, 2 ounces
- ☐ tomato puree, 4 cups (32 ounces)
- ☐ turnips, 1 pound
- ☐ Vidalia onions, 2 small
- ☐ yellow squash, 2 pounds
- ☐ zucchini or yellow squash, 3 large (about 1½ pounds)

* If not using homemade.

## additional items you might need

**If making Pesto Sauce**

- ☐ basil, fresh, 2½ ounces
- ☐ garlic, 3 cloves
- ☐ lemon, ½
- ☐ olive oil, extra-virgin, ⅓ cup (5 ounces)
- ☐ pine nuts, ⅓ cup (1⅔ ounces)

**If making Chicken Stock**

- ☐ apple cider vinegar, 1 tablespoon
- ☐ bay leaves, 2
- ☐ carrots, 3 large (about ¾ pound)
- ☐ celery with leaves, 2 stalks
- ☐ chicken bones and gizzards, 1 to 2 pounds
- ☐ garlic, 4 cloves
- ☐ onion, yellow, 1
- ☐ parsley, fresh, 1 bunch

danielle walker's
AGAINST all GRAIN

# week 7 meal plan shopping list

- ☐ asparagus, ¾ pound
- ☐ avocados, 2 (plus 2 more for optional garnish)
- ☐ basil, fresh, 1 sprig
- ☐ beef, ground, 3 pounds
- ☐ Brussels sprouts, 1 pound
- ☐ butternut squash, 1 (2 to 3 pounds), or 4 cups cubed
- ☐ carrots, 8 large (2 pounds)
- ☐ cayenne pepper, ½ teaspoon
- ☐ celery, 2 stalks
- ☐ chili powder, ¼ cup
- ☐ cilantro, fresh, ½ to ¾ ounce
- ☐ coconut crystals, ⅓ cup (2¼ ounces)
- ☐ crushed red pepper, ¼ teaspoon
- ☐ cucumber, 1
- ☐ cumin, ground, 2 teaspoons
- ☐ dill, fresh, 1 sprig
- ☐ dry mustard, 1 tablespoon
- ☐ garlic, 3 heads
- ☐ garlic powder, 1 tablespoon
- ☐ ghee, generous ½ cup (sub bacon fat, extra-virgin olive oil, or coconut oil, depending on recipe)
- ☐ lamb, ground, 3 pounds
- ☐ lemons, 2 large or 3 medium
- ☐ lettuce leaves, romaine, butter, or iceberg, several large
- ☐ limes, 3
- ☐ olive oil, extra-virgin, ⅓ cup (2¾ ounces)
- ☐ onions, red, 2 small and 1 medium plus 2 tablespoons diced
- ☐ onions, yellow, 4 medium
- ☐ oregano, fresh, 1 to 2 sprigs
- ☐ oregano leaves, dried, 2 teaspoons
- ☐ paprika, ¼ cup
- ☐ peaches, 2 large ripe
- ☐ poblano peppers, 2 small
- ☐ pork chops, bone-in, thin-cut, 6 (about 6 ounces each)
- ☐ red wine vinegar, 2 teaspoons
- ☐ roasting chickens, 2 (4 pounds each)
- ☐ Roma tomatoes, 6
- ☐ romaine lettuce, 1 head
- ☐ rosemary, fresh, 5 sprigs
- ☐ salmon, wild, skin-on, 2 pounds fillets
- ☐ sea salt, coarse, 2 tablespoons plus ½ teaspoon
- ☐ thyme leaves, fresh, 8 sprigs
- ☐ tomato juice, 1½ cups (12 ounces)
- ☐ tomato puree, 16 ounces
- ☐ tomatoes, 2
- ☐ yellow squash, 2 medium (about ⅔ pound)
- ☐ yogurt, plain, dairy-free, 1½ cups (13½ ounces)
- ☐ zucchini, 2 medium (about ⅔ pound)

## additional items you might need

### If making Chicken Stock

- ☐ apple cider vinegar, 1 tablespoon
- ☐ bay leaves, 2
- ☐ carrots, 3 large (about ¾ pound)
- ☐ celery with leaves, 2 stalks
- ☐ chicken bones and gizzards, 1 to 2 pounds
- ☐ garlic, 4 cloves
- ☐ onion, yellow, 1
- ☐ parsley, fresh, 1 bunch

### If making Greek Dressing

- ☐ Dijon mustard, ½ teaspoon
- ☐ garlic, 2 cloves
- ☐ lemons, 2 large
- ☐ olive oil, extra-virgin, ½ cup (4 ounces)
- ☐ oregano, fresh, 1 or 2 sprigs
- ☐ red wine vinegar, 2 teaspoons

### If making Taco Seasoning

- ☐ cayenne pepper, 1 to 3 teaspoons
- ☐ chili powder, 2½ tablespoons
- ☐ coriander, ground, 2 teaspoons
- ☐ cumin, ground, 1½ tablespoons
- ☐ onion powder, 2 teaspoons
- ☐ oregano, dried, ground, 1 tablespoon
- ☐ paprika, 2 teaspoons

### If making Guacamole

- ☐ avocados, ripe, 4
- ☐ cilantro, fresh, 2 sprigs
- ☐ garlic, 2 cloves
- ☐ jalapeño pepper, ½
- ☐ lime, 1
- ☐ onion, red, ½ small
- ☐ tomato, ½ small

*danielle walker's*
AGAINST *all* GRAIN

# week 8 meal plan shopping list

- ☐ apple cider vinegar, ¼ cup (2 ounces)
- ☐ arrowroot powder, 1½ cups (7 ounces)
- ☐ arugula, 7 cups (about 7 ounces)
- ☐ asparagus, 1 pound
- ☐ baby bok choy, 1 pound
- ☐ baby greens, 6 cups (about 6 ounces)
- ☐ balsamic vinegar, 1 cup (8 ounces)
- ☐ basil, fresh, ¼ ounce
- ☐ bell peppers, yellow, 2
- ☐ broccolini, 1 pound
- ☐ chicken, ground, dark or white meat, 2 pounds
- ☐ cilantro, fresh, several sprigs
- ☐ coconut aminos, ¼ cup plus 2 teaspoons
- ☐ coconut flour, ½ cup
- ☐ coconut oil, 1 teaspoon
- ☐ cremini mushrooms, 3½ ounces
- ☐ crushed red pepper, ¼ teaspoon
- ☐ cumin, ground, 1 tablespoon

- ☐ Dijon mustard, 3 tablespoons
- ☐ eggs, 3 large
- ☐ garlic, 2 heads
- ☐ ghee, ½ cup plus 2 tablespoons (sub coconut oil or extra-virgin olive oil, depending on the recipe)
- ☐ ginger, fresh, ½ ounce
- ☐ honey, 1 tablespoon plus 2 teaspoons
- ☐ hot sauce, dash of
- ☐ lemons, 2
- ☐ lettuce leaves, romaine or butter lettuce several for serving
- ☐ lime, 1
- ☐ maple syrup, grade B, or honey, ⅓ cup (5 ounces)
- ☐ olive oil, extra-virgin, ½ cup plus 3 tablespoons
- ☐ onion, red, 1
- ☐ onions, sweet, 3 small
- ☐ oregano leaves, dried, ½ teaspoon
- ☐ paprika, 1½ tablespoons
- ☐ pears, 2
- ☐ pineapple rings, fresh, 6

- ☐ pork tenderloins, 2 (1½ to 2 pounds each)
- ☐ prosciutto, 4 ounces
- ☐ pumpkin seeds, roasted and salted, 2 tablespoons
- ☐ radish, 1
- ☐ roasting chicken, 1 (4 pounds) cut into 10 parts
- ☐ scallions, 1 bunch plus 2
- ☐ sesame oil, cold-pressed, 2 tablespoons
- ☐ sesame oil, toasted, 1 tablespoon
- ☐ sesame seeds, ¾ teaspoon
- ☐ snow peas, ½ pound
- ☐ sweet potatoes, 1½ pounds
- ☐ tarragon, fresh, ½ ounce
- ☐ tomato, 1
- ☐ tri-tip roast, 1 (about 2½ to 3 pounds)
- ☐ watermelon, seedless, 2 pounds
- ☐ white vinegar, 2 tablespoons

## additional items you might need

### If making Barbecue Dry Rub

- ☐ cayenne pepper, ½ teaspoon
- ☐ chili powder, ¼ cup (1¼ ounces)
- ☐ coconut crystals, ⅓ cup (2¼ ounces)
- ☐ cumin, ground, 2 teaspoons
- ☐ dry mustard, 1 tablespoon
- ☐ garlic powder, 1 tablespoon
- ☐ oregano leaves, dried, 2 teaspoons
- ☐ paprika, ¼ cup (1 ounce)

### If making Mayonnaise

- ☐ Dijon mustard, ¼ teaspoon
- ☐ egg, 1 large
- ☐ lemon, ½ small
- ☐ macadamia nut oil, ¾ cup (6 ounces)
- ☐ white vinegar, 1 teaspoon